Molecular Mechanisms in Spermatogenesis

ADVANCES IN EXPERIMENTAL MEDICINE AND BIOLOGY

Recent Volumes in this Series

Volume 628
BRAIN DEVELOPMENT IN DROSOPHILA MELANOGASTER
Edited by Gerhard M. Technau

Volume 629
PROGRESS IN MOTOR CONTROL
Edited by Dagmar Sternad

Volume 630
INNOVATIVE ENDOCRINOLOGY OF CANCER
Edited by Lev M. Berstein and Richard J. Santen

Volume 631
BACTERIAL SIGNAL TRANSDUCTION
Edited by Ryutaro Utsumi

Volume 632
CURRENT TOPICS IN COMPLEMENT II
Edited by John. D. Lambris

Volume 633
CROSSROADS BETWEEN INNATE AND ADAPTIVE IMMUNITY II
Edited by Stephen P. Schoenberger, Peter D. Katsikis, and Bali Pulendran

Volume 634
HOT TOPICS IN INFECTION AND IMMUNITY IN CHILDREN V
Edited by Adam Finn, Nigel Curtis, and Andrew J. Pollard

Volume 635
GI MICROBIOTA AND REGULATION OF THE IMMUNE SYSTEM
Edited by Gary B. Huffnagle and Mairi Noverr

Volume 636
MOLECULAR MECHANISMS IN SPERMATOGENESIS
Edited by C. Yan Cheng

A Continuation Order Plan is available for this series. A continuation order will bring delivery of each new volume immediately upon publication. Volumes are billed only upon actual shipment. For further information please contact the publisher.

Molecular Mechanisms in Spermatogenesis

Edited by
C. Yan Cheng, PhD
Center for Biomedical Research, The Population Council, New York, New York, USA

Springer Science+Business Media, LLC
Landes Bioscience

Springer Science+Business Media, LLC
Landes Bioscience

SoftCover re-print of the Hardcover 1st edition 2008

Please address all inquiries to the Publishers:
Landes Bioscience, 1002 West Avenue, Austin, Texas 78701, USA
Phone: 512/ 637 6050; FAX: 512/ 637 6079
http://www.landesbioscience.com

Molecular Mechanisms in Spermatogenesis, edited by C. Yan Cheng, Landes Bioscience / Springer Science+Business Media, LLC dual imprint / Springer series: Advances in Experimental Medicine and Biology.

ISBN: 978-1-4899-8145-5

Molecular mechanisms in spermatogenesis / edited by C. Yan Cheng.
p. ; cm. -- (Advances in experimental medicine and biology ; v. 638)
Includes bibliographical references and index.
ISBN 978-0-387-79990-2
1. Spermatogenesis. 2. Testis--Molelcular aspects. I. Cheng, C. Yan. II. Series.
[DNLM: 1. Spermatogenesis--physiology. 2. Testis--physiology. 3. Tight Junctions--physiology. W1 AD559 v.638 2008 / WJ 834 M718 2008]

QP255.M638 2008
612.6'1--dc22

2008023382

ABOUT THE EDITOR...

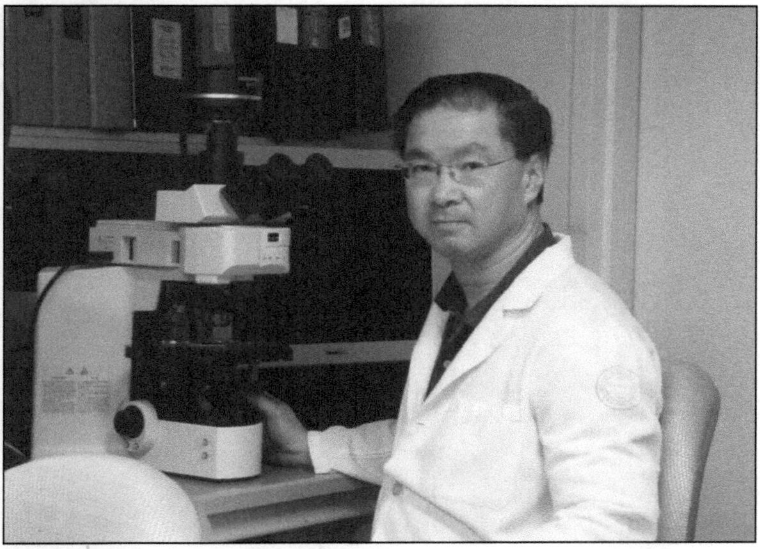

C. YAN CHENG, PhD, is a Senior Scientist at the Population Council's Center for Biomedical Research, inside the campus of the Rockefeller University in New York City. Dr. Cheng is a native of Hong Kong, graduated from the Chinese University of Hong Kong, and received his PhD in biochemistry and cell biology in the Laboratory of Professor Barry Boettcher at the University of Newcastle. He then received postdoctoral training in the laboratory of Drs. Wayne Bardin, Neal Musto and Glen Gunsalus at the Population Council in New York City. He has since stayed there, becoming a Senior Scientist in 1990. His studies in recent decades are focused mostly on the biology of the apical ectoplasmic specialization and the blood-testis barrier in the seminiferous epithelium. Working with a team of young scientists and collaborating with Professor Will M. Lee at the School of Biological Sciences, The University of Hong Kong, Dr. Cheng and his colleagues, Drs. Dolores Mruk, Helen Yan and Elissa Wong and Professor Will Lee have recently identified a novel autocrine regulatory loop in the seminiferous epithelium. This new autocrine-based loop utilizes laminin chains, polarity complex proteins and integrins to functionally link the apical ectoplasmic specialization, the blood-testis barrier and the hemidesmosome together to coordinate the events of spermiation and BTB restructuring to facilitate spermatid and preleptotene spermatocyte movement, respectively, that occur at stage VIII of the seminiferous epithelial cycle. These findings have now provided a framework for investigators in the field to design functional studies to understand the biology of spermatogenesis. Dr. Cheng is the recipient of several NIH grants and the CONRAD Program, and he serves as ad hoc reviewer for a number of leading journals in the field, such as *Journal of Cell Biology*, *Nature Cell Biology*, *PNAS*, *Molecular Endocrinology*, and *Endocrinology*.

PREFACE

In the past thirty years, significant advances have been made in the field of reproductive biology in "unlocking" the molecular and biochemical events that regulate spermatogenesis in the mammalian testis. It was possible because of the unprecedented breakthroughs in molecular biology, cell biology, immunology and biochemistry. I am fortunate to have personally witnessed such rapid changes in the field since I was a graduate student and a postdoctoral fellow in the late '70s through the early '80s. In this book, entitled *Molecular Mechanisms in Spermatogenesis*, I have included a collection of chapters written by colleagues on the latest developments in the field using genomic and proteomic approaches to study spermatogenesis, as well as different mechanisms and/or molecules including environmental toxicants and transcription factors that regulate and/or affect spermatogenesis.

The book begins with a chapter that provides the basic concept of cellular regulation of spermatogenesis. A few chapters are also dedicated to some of the latest findings on the Sertoli cell cytoskeleton and other molecules (e.g., proteases, adhesion proteins) that regulate spermatogenesis. These chapters contain thought-provoking discussions and concepts which shall be welcomed by investigators in the field. It is obvious that many of these "concepts" will be updated and some may be amended in the years to come. However, they will serve as a guide and the basis for investigation by scientists in the field. Due to the page limit, I could not cover all areas of interest in this monograph; instead, I tried to present this subject area with a balanced approach.

I hope this book will be helpful to young investigators who consider entering reproductive biology to get a balanced view of the latest developments in the field. For established investigators, these chapters will be helpful for their studies in the laboratory.

I am indebted to members of my laboratory who have provided insightful and critical discussion in the course of preparing this book. I am also grateful to all the staff at Landes Bioscience, in particular Cynthia Conomos, Celeste Carlton, Kristen Shumaker, and Megan Klein, who have helped me to work on this book from its inception through publication. Furthermore, I am grateful to my colleagues who have taken their time and worked with me these past two years on their chapters amidst the intensive day-to-day routines in their laboratories: teaching, administration, research and writing manuscripts and grant applications. Finally, I also want to thank my former mentors and friends Drs. Wayne Bardin, Barry Boettcher, Neal Musto,

Glen Gunsalus and Bruno Silvestrini for their critiques, help, encouragement and discussion during my graduate student and postdoctoral years in their laboratories in different parts of the world, who have introduced me to the fascinating areas of research in reproductive biology and animal/pharmaceutical models, set up a high standard of quality research, and unknowingly shaped my scientific personality and my approach to science.

C. Yan Cheng, PhD

PARTICIPANTS

R. John Aitken
ARC Centre of Excellence
in Biotechnology and Development
Discipline of Biological Sciences
University of Newcastle
Callaghan
Australia

Carla Boitani
Department of Histology
and Medical Embryology
"Sapienza" University of Rome
Rome
Italy

Guorong Chen
The Population Council
and
The Rockefeller University
New York, New York
USA

C. Yan Cheng
Center for Biomedical Research
The Population Council
New York, New York
USA

Luiz Renato de Franca
Department of Morphology
Universidade Federal de Minas Gerais
Belo Horizonte
Brazil

Renshan Ge
The Population Council
and
The Rockefeller University
New York, New York
USA

Julian A. Guttman
Michael Smith Laboratories
The University of British Columbia
Vancouver, British Columbia
Canada

Matthew P. Hardy
The Population Council
and
The Rockefeller University
New York, New York
USA

Mark P. Hedger
Monash Institute of Medical Research
Monash University
Melbourne
Australia

Rex A. Hess
Reproductive Biology and Toxicology
Department of Veterinary Biosciences
University of Illinois
Urbana, Illinois
USA

Bernard Jégou
Inserm U625
IFR 140
University of Rennes I
Campus de Beaulieu
Rennes
France

Nikki P.Y. Lee
Departments of Surgery and Medicine
Queen Mary Hospital
University of Hong Kong
Hong Kong
China

Will M. Lee
School of Biological Sciences
The University of Hong Kong
Hong Kong
China

Brigitte Le Magueresse-Battistoni
Inserm U418
INRA UMR 1245
Université Lyon 1
Hospital Debrousse
Lyon
France

Wing-Yee Lui
School of Biological Sciences
The University of Hong Kong
Hong Kong
China

Dolores D. Mruk
Center for Biomedical Research
The Population Council
New York, New York
USA

Moira K. O'Bryan
Monash Institute of Medical Research
and
The ARC Centre of Excellence
in Biotechnology and Development
Monash University
Melbourne
Australia

Charles Pineau
Inserm U625
IFR 140
University of Rennes I
Campus de Beaulieu
Rennes
France

Rossella Puglisi
Department of Histology
and Medical Embryology
"Sapienza" University of Rome
Rome
Italy

Antoine D. Rolland
Inserm U625
IFR 140
University of Rennes I
Campus de Beaulieu
Rennes
France

Shaun D. Roman
ARC Centre of Excellence
in Biotechnology and Development
Discipline of Biological Sciences
University of Newcastle
Callaghan
Australia

Brian P. Setchell
Department of Anatomical Sciences
University of Adelaide
Adelaide
Australia

Chandrima Shaha
Cell Death and Differentiation
Laboratory
National Institute of Immunology
Aruna Asaf Ali Marg
New Delhi
India

Michelle K.Y. Siu
Department of Pathology
Queen Mary Hospital
University of Hong Kong
Hong Kong
China

Kuljeet S. Vaid
Department of Cellular and
Physiological Sciences
Division of Anatomy and Cell Biology
The University of British Columbia
Vancouver, British Columbia
Canada

A. Wayne Vogl
Department of Cellular and Physiological Sciences
Division of Anatomy and Cell Biology
The University of British Columbia
Vancouver, British Columbia
Canada

Helen H.N. Yan
Center for Biomedical Research
The Population Council
New York, New York
USA

CONTENTS

CHAPTER 1

Spermatogenesis and Cycle of the Seminiferous Epithelium

Rex A. Hess* and Luiz Renato de Franca

Abstract

Spermatogenesis is a complex biological process of cellular transformation that produces male haploid germ cells from diploid spermatogonial stem cells. This process has been simplified morphologically by recognizing cellular associations or 'stages' and 'phases' of spermatogenesis, which progress through precisely timed and highly organized cycles. These cycles of spermatogenesis are essential for continuous sperm production, which is dependent upon numerous factors, both intrinsic (Sertoli and germ cells) and extrinsic (androgens, retinoic acids), as well as being species-specific.

Introduction

Spermatogenesis is the transformation of spermatogonial cells into spermatozoa over an extended period of time within seminiferous tubule boundaries of the testis. The seminiferous epithelium (Fig. 1) consists of germ cells that form numerous concentric layers penetrated by a single type of somatic cell first identified by Enrico Sertoli in 1865.[1] The cytoplasm of Sertoli cells extends as thin arms around all the germ cells to nurture and maintain their cellular associations throughout the process of spermatogenesis. Germ cells multiply first by repeated mitotic divisions and then by meiosis, which involves the duplication of chromosomes, genetic recombination, and then reduction of chromosomes through two cell divisions to produce spherical haploid spermatids that differentiate into highly compacted spermatozoa for release into the tubule lumen. To study this complex and lengthy process, spermatogenesis has been organized by several different approaches, including the more popular method of 'Staging' or the recognition of germ cell association in time and the 'phases' of spermatogenesis (mitosis, meiosis and spermiogenesis). This review will examine the stages and their cycle in the production of sperm in several species, but the mouse will receive special emphasis, as it is currently the most commonly used species in research.

Cellular Components—Stages of Spermatogenesis

The seminiferous epithelium consists of only one somatic cell type, the Sertoli cell,[2,3] but many different germinal cell types.[4] The complexity of this epithelium was simplified when Leblond and Clermont[5] were able to divide the epithelium into separate stages, according to the cellular associations observed in each tubular cross section. Stages of spermatogenesis are artificial definitions that are based upon rules established by the investigator. The original

*Corresponding Author: Rex A. Hess—Reproductive Biology and Toxicology, Department of Veterinary Biosciences, University of Illinois, 2001 S. Lincoln Ave., Urbana, IL 61802-6199, USA. Email: rexhess@uiuc.edu

Molecular Mechanisms in Spermatogenesis, edited by C. Yan Cheng. ©2008 Landes Bioscience and Springer Science+Business Media.

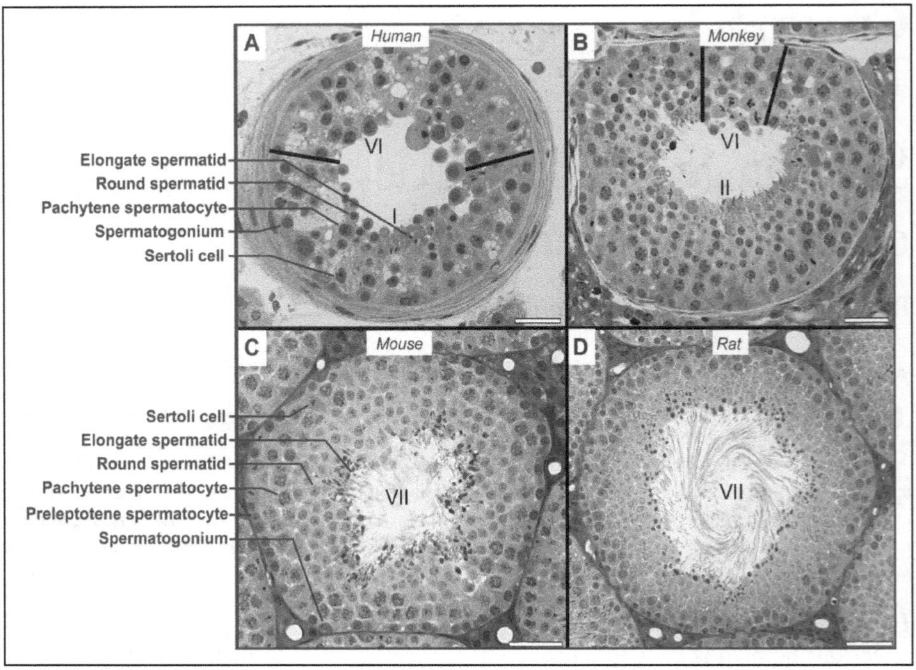

Figure 1. Seminiferous tubule cross-sections in different mammalian species. In the human (A) and marmoset *Callithrix penicillata* (B), two stages of the cycle or germ cells association (delimited by a black line) are observed, whereas in mouse (C) and rat (D) only one stage is found. Bars = 40 μm in A, B, and C; and 60 μm in D.

stages were defined according to changes observed in the Golgi region of spermatids, an area where the forming acrosomic system can be visualized by the periodic acid-Schiff's reaction (PAS). In the mouse, XII stages are well defined by this method (Fig. 2). However, spermatogenesis is a continuum, which results in transitional areas being observed between two stages.[6] In such cases, a preponderance of cell types can be used for stage identification. PAS staining and higher microscopic resolution is required to identify specific stages. However, for most research purposes, grouping stages into three categories is adequate and much easier for evaluation. For example, it is possible to group Stages I-V as 'early'; Stages VI-VIII as 'middle'; and Stages IX-XII as 'late' (Fig. 2).

Phases of Spermatogenesis

Mitosis

Spermatogonia are diploid germ cells (2n) that divide by mitosis and reside on the basement membrane (Figs. 1, 2). Currently, it is not possible to identify spermatogonial stem cells by routine microscopy, but different types of spermatogonia are recognized as type-A, intermediate, and type-B. In well-studied laboratory rodents, such as rats and mice, four classes of spermatogonia are present: undifferentiated type A spermatogonia [A single (A_s), A paired (A_{pr}), A aligned (A_{al})]; differentiated type A spermatogonia (A_1, A_2, A_3, A_4); intermediate spermatogonia (In); and type B spermatogonia (B).[4,7] In these species, the different spermatogonial classes can be characterized by light and transmission electron microscopy according to the presence and distribution of heterochromatin.[8,9] It has also been suggested that undifferentiated spermatogonia, including A_s or stem cell, are located in niches of the seminiferous epithelium, which are regulated by the Sertoli cell.[8-18]

Meiosis

B-spermatogonia divide by mitosis forming two preleptotene spermatocytes, cells representing the beginning of meiotic prophase (Fig. 2). These small cells rest on the basement membrane, but leptotene and zygotene spermatocytes become transit and move through the blood-testis-barrier (or Sertoli-Sertoli barrier).[19,20] Preleptotene, leptotene and zygotene spermatocytes are located in specific stages and are identifiable by routine microscopy, although fixation artifact results in the leptotene and zygotene cells appearing to be attached to the basement membrane. Spermatocytes are found in all stages, because meiosis is a prolonged period of spermatogenesis that extends over approximately 14 days in the mouse. Thus, any attempt to isolate specific stages of spermatogenesis for molecular analysis, will include cells of this phase. Spermatocytes are the cells of meiosis and their regulation requires a special focus. Of special note, meiotic cell division occurs in and defines a single stage (XII). In the mouse, stage XII is found in approximately 10% of the seminiferous tubular cross sections and meiotic division is completed in approximately 1 day.[21] This cellular division goes through three categories, all occurring in stage XII: (a) meiosis I, the division of 4n cells; (b) formation of secondary spermatocytes (2n), which are larger than step 1 spermatids, but rarely are found as the only spermatocyte in a tubular cross section; and (c) meiosis II, the division of 2n secondary spermatocytes to form haploid (1n) round spermatids. Studies in rats, buffalos, rams, and pigs revealed a striking increase in size for primary spermatocytes, from preleptotene to diplotene.[22,23] This increase is followed by a dramatic decrease of cell size during spermiogenesis in such a way that, due to changes in chromatin and nuclear condensation, in rats, for instance, before spermiation spermatid nuclear volume reaches only 1/50th (~500 to 10μm^3) of its initial volume.

Spermiogenesis

The transformation of spherical, haploid spermatids (1n) into elongate, highly condensed and mature spermatozoa that are released into the seminiferous tubule lumen is called spermiogenesis (Fig. 2). The differentiation of spermatids proceeds through at least 4 prolonged steps (or phases): Golgi, capping, acrosomal, and maturation. These steps are useful for the identification of specific stages in the cycle of the seminiferous epithelium.

Golgi

Golgi apparatus is very important during the early steps of spermiogenesis,[4,6,24] as the formation of the acrosome is dependent upon this organelle's ability to produce vesicles and granules containing the enzymatic components of the acrosomic system that will cover the developing sperm nucleus. Differentiation of the first three steps of round spermatid formation involves a prominent Golgi apparatus that is identified by PAS staining. Step 1 spermatids have a small, perinuclear Golgi region without an acrosomic vesicle or granule. Subsequent steps 2-3 show proacrosomal vesicles and granules within the Golgi apparatus, with the formation of a single, large acrosomal granule within a larger vesicle that will indent the nucleus (Fig. 2).

Capping

Capping involves steps 4-5 round spermatids, where the acrosomic granule touches the nuclear envelope and the vesicle begins to flatten into a small cap over the nuclear surface. In steps 6-7, the acrosomic vesicle becomes very thin and the granule flattens. Step 8 is the last round spermatid, and the acrosome flattens over approximately 1/3 of the nuclear surface. In late stage VIII, step 8 nuclei begin to change shape.

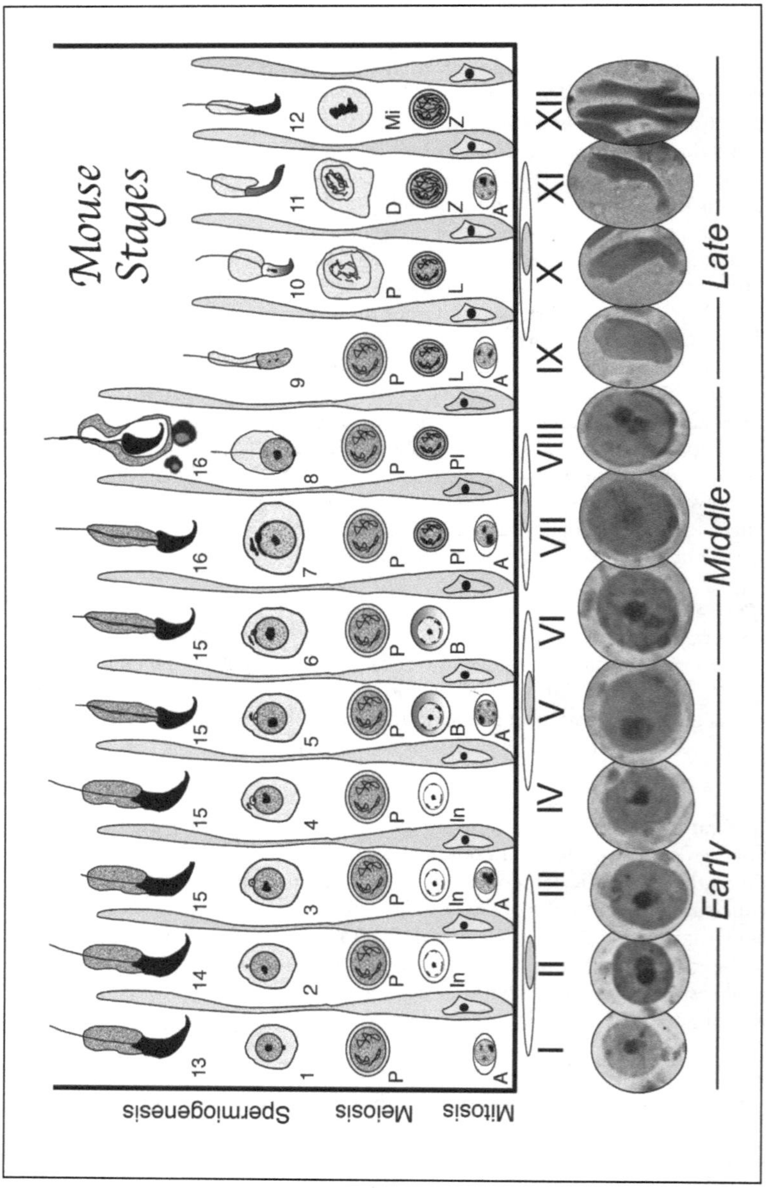

Figure 2. Legend viewed on following page.

Figure 2, viewed on previous page. Mouse Stages in the cycle of the seminiferous epithelium (I-XII). Layers depicting the cellular associations are drawn with Sertoli cells separating each stage. Along the base are photos of early, middle and late spermatid nuclei, stained with the PAS reaction and hematoxylin. Spermatogonia (A, In, B); spermatocytes (Pl: preleptotene, L: leptotene, Z: zygotene, P: pachytene, D: diakinesis, Mi: meiotic division); round spermatids (1-8); elongate spermatids (9-16). Adapted with permission from Dr. Robert E. Braun.

Stage I. Two generations of spermatids are found in Stages I-VIII, round and elongate spermatids. In this stage, the round spermatid nucleus is smaller than in subsequent stages and contains a typical large central nucleolus. The Golgi is also small and lacks PAS+ granular material.

Stage II. Small PAS+ proacrosomal granules are seen in the center of the Golgi apparatus, which is attached to the nucleus of round spermatids.

Stage III. An acrosomic granule is well formed within the larger round Golgi vesicle, which forms an indentation of the round spermatid nucleus.

Stage IV. The acrosomic granule begins to flatten in this stage.

Stage V. The acrosomic system is clearly defined now and there is a straight line formed by the acrosomic granule lying on the PAS+ dark line that caps the round spermatid nucleus, surrounded by the vesicle. Along the basement membrane, B-type spermatogonia are prominent.

Stage VI. The acrosomic system begins to spread, but remains thick and the granules are distinct. In this stage, B-type spermatogonia undergo mitosis to form preleptotene spermatocytes. Elongate spermatids begin to migrate toward the lumen.

Stage VII. The acrosomic system spreads across the nucleus and becomes thinner, allowing the central acrosomic granule to bulge slightly above the acrosomic vesicle. Elongate spermatids are located at the luminal edge of the tubule, but the cytoplasm covers the sperm head and about 1/2 of the tail.

Early VII. There is more cytoplasm covering the mid region of elongate spermatids and no cytoplasmic lobe has formed. Numerous small preleptotene cell nuclei are found on the basement membrane.

Middle VII. The cytoplasmic lobe begins to form and elongate spermatid cytoplasm no longer covers the midpiece of tail. Large dark granules in cytoplasmic lobes are still absent.

Late VII. The cytoplasmic lobe is well formed and much of it is now between the sperm head and the basement membrane. Dark granules are beginning to appear distinct near the sperm head and sometimes below it. Preleptotene cell nuclei are enlarging as these cells transform into leptotene and chromatin begins to disperse into smaller, finer clumps.

Stage VIII. The acrosome is flattened and forms a cap that covers nearly half of the round spermatid nucleus. Many of the nuclei have migrated to the cytoplasmic plasmalemma and the acrosomic system may be oriented toward the basement membrane. Elongate spermatids are being released into the lumen through a process called spermiation, while excess spermatid cytoplasm forms large cytoplasmic lobes with large dark bodies beneath the head of step 16 spermatids.

Stage IX. Only one generation of spermatids is found in Stages IX-XII, the transition from round into elongate. Cross sections of step 9 spermatid nuclei are oblong, as they begin the elongation process, with the thin PAS+ acrosomic system off center and extending from the apex toward the caudal region of the nucleus. Cytoplasmic lobes fuse into very large residual bodies that are phagocytized by the Sertoli cell and disappear by Stages X-XI.

Stage X. The spermatid head forms a distinct protrusion with a sharp angle. Only the protrusion is covered by the PAS+ acrosome on the ventral side, while the dorsal side is covered to the caudal surface of the nucleus. Pachytene spermatocyte nuclei reach their maximum diameter prior to diplotene phase.

Stage XI. Step 11 spermatid nuclei become thinner, more elongated and begin to stain more intensely, indicating chromatin condensation. Diplotene spermatocyte nuclei become excessively large and begin to lose nuclear envelope as the cells enter diakinesis of meiosis I.

Stage XII. In this stage the most important identifying feature is the presence of meiotic and secondary spermatocytes. Step 12 spermatid nuclei are thinner and nuclear staining is intensely dark throughout except for the most caudal region. PAS+ acrosomic system forms a ventral and dorsal fin over the apical protrusion.

Acrosomal

Acrosomal steps 9-14 involve migration of the acrosomal system over the ventral surface of the elongating spermatid nucleus (Fig. 2). This migration of the acrosome is completed approximately by step 14 spermatid and is difficult to identify in typical histological sections, due to its presence in different planes of sections and angles or orientation. Thus, recognition of specific stages of spermatogenesis will typically rely on the acrosomal system observed in the round spermatids, rather than in the elongate cells. These spermatid steps also involve condensation of the chromatin, as the chromosomes are packed more tightly and stain more intensely with hematoxylin.

Maturation

Maturation steps 15-16 appear across Stages III-VIII and show fewer changes in nuclear shape and acrosomal migration. The nucleus continues to condense and the acrosome matures into a thin PAS+ structure that protrudes at the apex but covers nearly all the nucleus, except for that portion connected to the tail.[4] Excess cytoplasm is removed in Stages VII-VIII, resulting in the formation of prominent cytoplasmic lobes and residual bodies, which contain unused mitochondria, ribosomes, lipids, vesicles and other cytoplasmic components.[4,25,26]

The Cycle and Wave of Spermatogenesis

Germ cells within each layer of the seminiferous epithelium change in synchrony with the other layers over time, producing the sequence of Stages described above (Fig. 2). The cells do not migrate laterally along the length of the seminiferous tubule; however, an unusual successive order of the Stages is observed, whereby sequential Stages occur with repetition along the length of the tubules, in a 'wave' of the seminiferous epithelium.[27] That is, at least in the rodent, Stage I is followed by II, followed by III, etc. through Stage XIV, which is then repeated by Stage I. The Stages are found in ascending order from the rete testis to the center of the seminiferous tubule, where the Stages are reversed.[4] The wave is produced by synchronous development of clonal units of germ cells through a mechanism of biochemical signaling that remains a subject of inquiry.

Sperm Production

The precise mechanisms by which spermatogonial stem cells (A_s) and other early proliferative spermatogonia (A_{pr}-A_{al}) transform into differentiating spermatogonia (type A, In, and type B) and simultaneously renew their own population is now a major focus of reproductive biology.[10-12,16-18,28-46] In addition to c-kit and vitamin A, which are important for differentiation of A_{al} into A_1, other important factors are emerging as being involved in the regulation of spermatogonial stem cells. These proteins include the following: GFRα1, PLZF, OCT4, NGN3, NOTCH-1, SOX3, c-RET, RBM, EP-CAM, STRA8, and EE2.[7,10,17,31,47,48]

Spermatogonia give rise to spermatocytes after a fixed number of mitotic divisions that are characteristic of each species,[49] as two to six differentiated spermatogonial generations have been observed in mammals (Table 1). Besides being useful for comparative studies among different species,[49] the precise knowledge of the number of spermatogonial generations is essential for better understanding of regulatory mechanisms of spermatogenesis.[7] Compared to many other well-known self-renewing cell systems in the body, spermatogenesis is thought to have the greatest number of cell divisions during its expansion. For instance, in mice, rats, and pigs, about ten generations of spermatogonia are necessary to form preleptotene spermatocytes from one spermatogonia stem cell ($A_s \rightarrow A_{pr} \rightarrow A_{al4} \rightarrow A_{al8\text{-}16} \rightarrow A_1 \rightarrow A_2 \rightarrow A_3 \rightarrow A_4 \rightarrow$ In $\rightarrow$ B); whereas in humans this figure is much lower and estimated to be only 4 mitotic divisions. As will be shown later, both the kinetics and rate of germ cell loss have an impact on the number of sperm produced.

Knowledge of the spermatogenic cycle length is fundamental for determining the spermatogenic efficiency and performing comparative studies among species. The total duration of

Table 1. Number of differentiated spermatogonial generations and germ cell ratios[1]

Species	Spermatogonial Generations	Meiotic Index (%)[2]	Overall Rate of Spermatogenesis[3]
Bull	6 (A_{1-3}, In, B_{1-2})[4]	3.6 (10)[5]	65 (75)
Buffalo	6 (A_{1-3}, In, B_{1-2})	3.4 (15)	74 (71)
Ram	6 (A_{1-3}, In, B_{1-2})	3.1 (23)	37 (85)
Goat	6 (A_{1-3}, In, B_{1-2})	2.8 (30)	91 (65)
Boar	6 (A_{1-4}, In, B)	3.2 (20)	68 (73)
Peccary	6 (A_{1-4}, In, B)	3.2 (20)	74 (71)
Wild boar	6 (A_{1-4}, In, B)	2.7 (33)	29 (89)
Dog	6 (A_{1-4}, In, B)	3.4 (15)	51 (80)
Rat	6 (A_{1-4}, In, B)	3.4 (15)	97 (62)
Mouse	6 (A_{1-4}, In, B)	2.3-3.1 (23-43)	44-84 (67-83)
Gerbil	5 (A_{1-3}, In, B)	2.8 (30)	34 (73)
Capybara	5 (A_{1-3}, In, B)	2.1 (48)	21 (84)
Agouti paca	5 (A_{1-3}, In, B)	3.2 (20)	31 (76)
Dasyprocta sp	5 (A_{1-3}, In, B)	3.0 (25)	28 (78)
Chinchilla	5 (A_{1-3}, In, B)	3.0 (25)	49 (62)
Jaguar	5 (A_{1-3}, In, B)	2.8 (30)	45 (65)
Cat	5 (A_{1-3}, In, B)	2.8 (30)	19 (85)
Rabbit	5 (A_{1-2}, In_{1-2}, B)	3.3 (18)	39 (69)
Marmoset	4 (A_{1-2}, B_{1-2})	3.4 (15)	25 (60)
Man	2 (A_{pale}, B)	1.3 (68)	3.2 (80)

[1] Data from our laboratory and compiled from the literature (see reviews in França and Russell, 1998; França et al, 2002; França et al, 2005).[2] Number of spermatids per each primary spermatocyte.[3] Number of spermatids formed per each differentiated type A_1 spermatogonia. [4] Type A spermatogonia (A); intermediate spermatogonia (In); and type B spermatogonia (B).[5] Numbers in parentheses show the percentage of germ cell loss based on the theoretical yield.

spermatogenesis based on 4.5 spermatogenic cycles ranges from approximately 30 to 78 days in mammals (8.6-8.9 for each cycle and 39-40 days for total duration in mice) (see reviews by refs. 4,23,50-51), and is under the control of the germ cell genotype, according to a study using xenogenic (rats to mice) spermatogonial transplantation.[52] Also, similar results were found utilizing porcine and ovine testis xenografts.[53] Although strain or breed differences can be found among members of the same species, the length of the spermatogenic cycle has been generally considered to be constant for a given species and is not phylogenetically determined. However, it is suggested in the literature that the temperature and some drugs may influence the duration of spermatogenesis,[54-56] probably altering the cell cycle.[57,58] In most mammals, each spermatogenic cycle lasts around 9 to 12 days, whereas the total duration of spermatogenesis lasts nearly 40 to 54 days. Particularly in humans, the entire spermatogenic process is very long and lasts more than 70 days. As a general pattern for mammals, and probably related to the synchronized development of different germ cell types per seminiferous tubule cross-sections (Stages), each phase of spermatogenesis (spermatogonial, spermatocyte, and spermatid) lasts approximately one third of the duration of the entire process.

Germ cell loss (apoptosis) occurs normally during spermatogenesis in all mammals investigated,[59] playing a critical role in determining total sperm output. However, the greatest influence on germ cell production is the capacity for mitosis, and the number of generations of spermatogonial divisions, which will dictate, at least in part, the number of cells that enter meiosis. Taking into account the number of generations of differentiated spermatogonia and the two meiotic divisions prior to the formation of haploid spermatids, only 2-3 spermatozoa out of 10 are produced from each differentiated type A_1 spermatogonia in most mammalian species (see overall rate of spermatogenesis in Table 1).[23,60] Thus, significant germ cell loss occurs during the spermatogonial phase, called 'density-dependent regulation', primarily during mitotic divisions of type A_2 to A_4 spermatogonia, possibly mediated by the p53 tumor suppressor protein, as well as Bcl-2, Bax and Fas. One possibility, as yet untested, is that the degeneration is a homeostatic mechanism to limit germ cells to the number that can be supported by available Sertoli cells. Apoptosis is also frequent during meiosis (Table 1), especially in humans, and is probably related to chromosomal damage. Also, it should be mentioned that missing generations of spermatocytes and spermatids in the seminiferous epithelium, plus apoptosis, contribute to the low efficiency of human spermatogenesis.[60,61]

The Sertoli cell has several important roles in spermatogenesis, including the following: support and nutrition of the developing germ cells; compartmentalization of the seminiferous tubule by tight junctions, which provides a protected and specialized environment for the developing germ cells; controlled release of mature spermatids into the tubular lumen (spermiation); secretion of fluid, proteins and several growth factors; and phagocytosis of the degenerating germ cells and phagocytosis of the excess cytoplasm (residual body) that remains from released sperm.[2] The Sertoli cell also mediates the actions of FSH and luteinizing hormone (LH)-stimulated testosterone production in the testis, apparently in a stage-dependent manner.[62] Although it is strongly suggested that FSH plays a major role in the initiation, maintenance and restoration of spermatogenesis in primates, it appears that in most mammalian species testosterone has this important role in maintaining *'quantitatively'* normal spermatogenesis, whereas FSH plays a qualitative role and is not strictly necessary for fertility.[62] Recent investigations of the Sertoli cell specific knockout of androgen receptor (SCARKO) mouse found that spermatogenesis rarely advanced beyond diplotene spermatocytes.[63] Thus, at least in this species, androgens are crucial for late meiosis and spermiogenesis.

The relative mass of seminiferous tissue determines how much space is devoted to sperm production. In general, species whose testes have a high proportion of seminiferous tubular tissue produce more sperm per unit mass (Fig. 3).[23,50,60] Regardless of other factors, the number of Sertoli cells is now well established as being one of the most important determining factors that defines maximum sperm production.[64-73] In all mammalian species investigated, no Sertoli cell proliferation has been observed after puberty. Thus, the perinatal and prepubertal period, when the size of the Sertoli cell population is established, ultimately dictates the magnitude of testis size and sperm production. This occurs because Sertoli cells have differing capacities to support germ cell development and each Sertoli cell is able to support only a relatively fixed number of germ cells in a species-specific manner (Fig. 3).[23,50,60] Thus, animals with more Sertoli cells have more germ cells per testis, and the number of Sertoli cells per gram of tissue combined with the number of spermatids per Sertoli cell is positively correlated with sperm production per gram of testis.

There also appears to be species-specific regulation of the total Sertoli cell population.[66,71,74-84] Volume density of Sertoli cells in the seminiferous epithelium changes considerably in mammals (from ~15% in mice to ~40% in humans) and is inversely related to the efficiency of sperm production. Thus, in contrast to humans, species with a lower proportion of Sertoli cells in the seminiferous epithelium, such as mice, rabbits, rats, hamsters, and pigs are among those with the highest Sertoli cell and spermatogenic efficiencies (Fig. 3).[23]

Daily sperm production per gram of testicular parenchyma is a measure of spermatogenic efficiency in sexually mature animals and is useful for species comparisons. In mammalian species, four to sixty million spermatozoa are produced daily per gram of testis tissue (Fig. 3), and in humans for instance approximately 1,500 spermatozoa are produced with each heartbeat. Usually, species that have shorter spermatogenic cycle lengths have higher spermatogenic efficiency (Table 1; Fig. 3). However, the higher efficiency of spermatogenesis observed in some mammalian species results from the combination of higher Sertoli cell support capacity

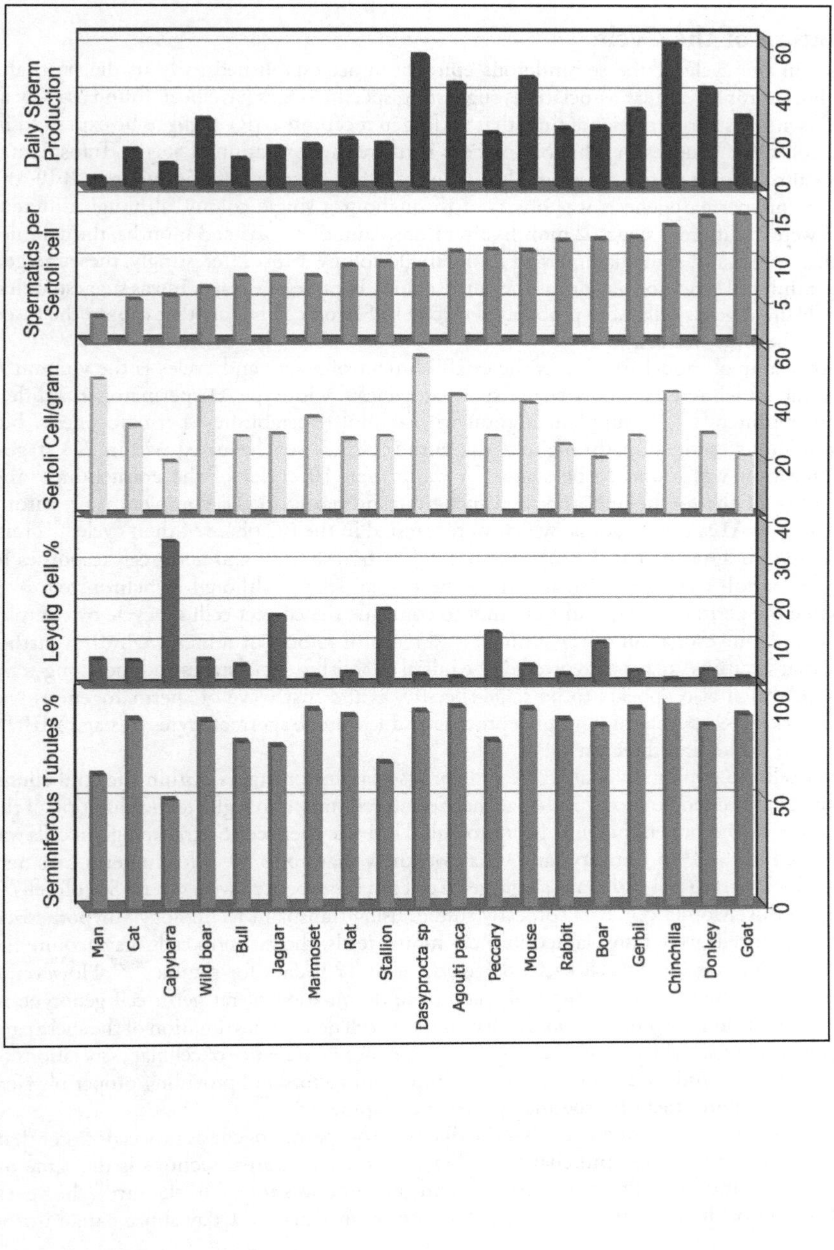

Figure 3. Comparative species testicular data for percentage of seminiferous tubules (%), Leydig cell or interstitial space (%), Sertoli cells (millions)/gram of testis parenchyma, spermatids per Sertoli cell, and daily sperm production per gram of testis (millions).

for germ cells and greater number of Sertoli cells per gram of testis. Data shown in Figure 3 for the domestic boar and wild boar illustrate this assumption, because the lower Sertoli efficiency observed for the wild boar is compensated for by the higher Sertoli cell number per gram of testis, resulting in similar daily sperm production per gram of testis in both species. Higher seminiferous tubule volume density (%) in the testis, lower Sertoli cell volume density (%) in the seminiferous epithelium, greater number of spermatogonia generations, and lower germ cell loss during spermatogenesis, also correlate significantly with spermatogenic efficiency.

Regulation of the Cycle

Stages in the cycle of the seminiferous epithelium are established early in the postnatal period. For example, cellular associations suggesting specific stages have been found as early as day 10,[85] which is about the same time that androgen receptors (AR) begin to be expressed in early Sertoli cells,[86] suggesting that Sertoli cells regulate the formation of stages. Transplantation data also support this conclusion. Using the green fluorescence protein mouse (GFP), the same stage of spermatogenesis was observed throughout a single colony, although different colonies were in different stages, 2 months after transplantation.[87] After 3 months, the colonies were much larger and some had merged into a single colony. Most interestingly, these merged colonies exhibited synchronization, as the entire colony became one stage. It was suggested that the transplanted germ cells were probably sensitive to Sertoli cell factors that caused the fused colonies to become one stage.[87]

Another animal model to address the establishment of stages and cycles is the vitamin A deficient rat, which results in an arrest of spermatogenesis, with type A1 spermatogonia differentiation inhibited.[88-91] Resupplementation with retinol re-establishes spermatogenesis, but the seminiferous epithelium throughout the entire testis is synchronized within 2-3 stages. Synchronization was found to be stable for more than 10 cycles of the epithelium[92] and repopulation of the epithelium appeared to be due primarily to the completion of mitotic activity by type A1 spermatogonia, which were arrested in the G2 phase of their cycle.[88] Thus, in this model, it appears that the regulation involves both Sertoli and germ cell responses to vitamin A. Sertoli cells appear to maintain the correct stages, although synchronized, over time, while the germ cells respond to retinol to continue the correct cellular cycle by completion of G2. An investigation of the retinoic acid receptor knockout mouse (*RARα-/-*) further revealed that vitamin A may be involved in the initial establishment of stages and their long-term regulation, which also appears to be stage-specific, as the first wave of spermatogenesis was arrested at step 8-9 spermatids and preleptotene and leptotene spermatocytes in stage VIII-IX were delayed in the first three waves.[93]

Sertoli cells do appear to regulate the cellular associations or 'stages' within the epithelium; therefore, it has been logical to hypothesize that Sertoli cells may also regulate the 'duration of the cycle of the seminiferous epithelium'. Morphological intimacy between Sertoli and germ cells was first observed in the 19th Century[1] and today we know that up to 50 different germ cells may contact a single Sertoli cell and that a single germ cell can be associated with several Sertoli cells.[94] Based upon this 'Mother cell' concept, early studies using transplant technology[95] hypothesized that if rat germ cells were transplanted into the mouse testis, the rat germ cells may acquire the mouse testis duration of the cell cycle, 8.6 days versus 12.9 days for the rat.[96,97] However, a subsequent experiment demonstrated "the complete domination of rat germ cell genotype in differentiation timing."[52] Thus, it appears that the germ cell determines duration of the spermatogenic cycle, while the resident Sertoli cell is responsible for maintenance of cellular associations or stages through the production and secretion of important factors and providing proper physical and functional environment for spermatogenesis development.[3,98,99]

It has been known for many years that the first wave of spermatogenesis proceeds faster than does the adult seminiferous epithelial cycle. Stage frequency in cross sections is the same on days 13, 23, 30 and in adult mouse testes[100] and the same was found in the rat;[101] however, mean duration of the cycle from 10 to 30 days was approximately 1 day shorter than in the adult rodents.[85,102,103] When germ cells from the GFP mouse were transplanted into the adult testis, the rate of growth was 2x faster during the first 2 months compared to the third month post transplant.[87] It is often pointed out that this reduction in the rate of the spermatogenetic cycle during development is correlated with testicular descent; therefore, it is possible that a higher intra-abdominal temperature may result in acceleration of the cell cycle and mitotic events, as observed in fish (tilapias) maintained at elevated temperatures.[58] Although this explanation may have some credibility, other data suggest that the first wave may be different simply because the spermatogonia are filling clonal niches and establishing an epithelial wave. For example, the first wave has a unique regulation that is dependent on a subpopulation of neurogenin 3 (Ngn3) negative spermatogonia that differentiate into the first wave germ cells, while Ngn3+ cells are reserved for stem cells and subsequent waves of spermatogenesis.[28]

Finally, there are numerous studies showing stage and Sertoli cell specific expressions of proteins and it appears that different stages have different dependences upon androgens and FSH, with these factors having a greater influence just before spermiation in stage VII-VIII.[62,104-109] However, understanding the individual contribution of factors to the maintenance of the cycle and stages of spermatogenesis will require careful analysis and interpretation, because disruption of individual factors will often lead to an initial stage-specific and/or cell-specific effect, but the long term consequence is secondary degeneration of the entire process of spermatogenesis.[110,111] This very important aspect of mammalian spermatogenesis is still poorly understood and should be a focus of intensive research in the coming years, mainly because appropriate animal models are now available for dissecting molecular regulation of the cycle of the seminiferous epithelium.

References

1. Hess R, França LR. History of the sertoli cell discovery. In: Griswold M, Skinner M, eds. Sertoli Cell Biology. New York: Academic Press, 2005.
2. Russell LD, Griswold MD, eds. The Sertoli Cell. Clearwater: Cache River Press, 1993.
3. Hess R, França LR. Structure of the Sertoli cell. In: Griswold M, Skinner M, eds. Sertoli Cell Biology. New York: Academic Press, 2005.
4. Russell LD, Ettlin RA, Sinha Hikim AP et al. Histological and Histopathological Evaluation of the Testis. Clearwater: Cache River Press, 1990.
5. Leblond CP, Clermont Y. Definition of the stages of the cycle of the seminiferous epithelium in the rat. Ann NY Acad Sci 1952; 55:548-573.
6. Hess RA. Quantitative and qualitative characteristics of the stages and transitions in the cycle of the rat seminiferous epithelium: Light microscopic observations of perfusion-fixed and plastic-embedded testes. Biol Reprod 1990; 43(3):525-542.
7. de Rooij DG, Russell LD. All you wanted to know about spermatogonia but were afraid to ask. J Androl 2000; 21(6):776-798.
8. Chiarini-Garcia H, Hornick JR, Griswold MD et al. Distribution of type A spermatogonia in the mouse is not random. Biol Reprod 2001; 65(4):1179-1185.
9. Chiarini-Garcia H, Russell LD. High-resolution light microscopic characterization of mouse spermatogonia. Biol Reprod 2001; 65(4):1170-1178.
10. Hess RA, Cooke PS, Hofmann MC et al. Mechanistic insights into the regulation of the spermatogonial stem cell niche. Cell Cycle 2006; 5(11):1164-1170.
11. Cooke PS, Hess RA, Simon L et al. The transcription factor Ets-related molecule (ERM) is essential for spermatogonial stem cell maintenance and self-renewal. Anim Reprod 2006; 3(2):98-107.
12. Chen C, Ouyang W, Grigura V et al. ERM is required for transcriptional control of the spermatogonial stem cell niche. Nature 2005; 436(7053):1030-1034.
13. Ryu BY, Orwig KE, Avarbock MR et al. Stem cell and niche development in the postnatal rat testis. Dev Biol 2003; 263(2):253-263.
14. Brinster RL. Germline stem cell transplantation and transgenesis. Science 2002; 296(5576):2174-2176.
15. Dobrinski I. Germ cell transplantation and testis tissue xenografting in domestic animals. Anim Reprod Sci 2005; 89(1-4):137-145.
16. Ogawa T, Ohmura M, Ohbo K. The niche for spermatogonial stem cells in the mammalian testis. Int J Hematol 2005; 82(5):381-388.
17. Oatley JM, Brinster RL. Spermatogonial stem cells. Methods Enzymol 2006; 419:259-282.

18. Ryu BY, Orwig KE, Oatley JM et al. Effects of aging and niche microenvironment on spermatogonial stem cell self-renewal. Stem Cells 2006; 24(6):1505-1511.
19. Russell L. Movement of spermatocytes from the basal to the adluminal compartment of the rat testis. Am J Anat 1977; 148(3):313-328.
20. Russell LD. Sertoli-germ cell interactions: A review. Gamete Res 1980; 3:179-202.
21. Hess RA. STAGES: Interactive Software on Spermatogenesis. 2.2 ed. Champaign: Vanguard Productions and Cache River Press, 1998.
22. Franca LR, Cardoso FM. Duration of spermatogenesis and sperm transit time through the epididymis in the Piau boar. Tissue Cell 1998; 30(5):573-582.
23. Franca LR, Avelar GF, Almeida FF. Spermatogenesis and sperm transit through the epididymis in mammals with emphasis on pigs. Theriogenology 2005; 63(2):300-318.
24. Leblond CP, Clermont Y. Spermiogenesis of rat, mouse, hamster and guinea pig as revealed by the "periodic acid-fuchsin sulfurous acid" technique. Am J Anat 1952; 90:167-215.
25. Hess RA, Miller LA, Kirby JD et al. Immunoelectron microscopic localization of testicular and somatic cytochromes c in the seminiferous epithelium of the rat [published erratum appears in Biol Reprod 1993; 49(2):439]. Biol Reprod 1993; 48(6):1299-1308.
26. Franca LR, Ye SJ, Ying L et al. Morphometry of rat germ cells during spermatogenesis. Anat Rec 1995; 241(2):181-204.
27. Perey B, Clermont Y, Leblond C. The wave of the seminiferous epithelium in the rat. Am J Anat 1961; 108:47-77.
28. Yoshida S, Takakura A, Ohbo K et al. Neurogenin3 delineates the earliest stages of spermatogenesis in the mouse testis. Dev Biol 2004; 269(2):447-458.
29. Braydich-Stolle L, Nolan C, Dym M et al. Role of glial cell line-derived neurotrophic factor in germ-line stem cell fate. Ann NY Acad Sci 2005; 1061:94-99.
30. Hofmann MC, Braydich-Stolle L, Dettin L et al. Immortalization of mouse germ line stem cells. Stem Cells 2005; 23(2):200-210.
31. Hofmann MC, Braydich-Stolle L, Dym M. Isolation of male germ-line stem cells; influence of GDNF. Dev Biol 2005; 279(1):114-124.
32. Kanatsu-Shinohara M, Miki H, Inoue K et al. Long-term culture of mouse male germline stem cells under serum-or feeder-free conditions. Biol Reprod 2005; 72(4):985-991.
33. Kanatsu-Shinohara M, Toyokuni S, Shinohara T. Genetic selection of mouse male germline stem cells in vitro: Offspring from single stem cells. Biol Reprod 2005; 72(1):236-240.
34. Ballow D, Meistrich ML, Matzuk M et al. Sohlh1 is essential for spermatogonial differentiation. Dev Biol 2006; 294(1):161-167.
35. Braydich-Stolle L, Kostereva N, Dym M et al. Role of Src family kinases and N-Myc in spermatogonial stem cell proliferation. Dev Biol 2007; 304(1):34-45.
36. de Rooij DG. Rapid expansion of the spermatogonial stem cell tool box. Proc Natl Acad Sci USA 2006; 103(21):7939-7940.
37. Kanatsu-Shinohara M, Inoue K, Miki H et al. Clonal origin of germ cell colonies after spermatogonial transplantation in mice. Biol Reprod 2006; 75(1):68-74.
38. Kanatsu-Shinohara M, Inoue K, Ogonuki N et al. Leukemia inhibitory factor enhances formation of germ cell colonies in neonatal mouse testis culture. Biol Reprod 2007; 76(1):55-62.
39. Kierszenbaum AL. Cell-cycle regulation and mammalian gametogenesis: A lesson from the unexpected. Mol Reprod Dev 2006; 73(8):939-942.
40. Naughton CK, Jain S, Strickland AM et al. Glial cell-line derived neurotrophic factor-mediated RET signaling regulates spermatogonial stem cell fate. Biol Reprod 2006; 74(2):314-321.
41. Oatley JM, Avarbock MR, Telaranta AI et al. Identifying genes important for spermatogonial stem cell self-renewal and survival. Proc Natl Acad Sci USA 2006; 103(25):9524-9529.
42. Payne C, Braun RE. Glial cell line-derived neurotrophic factor maintains a POZ-itive influence on stem cells. Proc Natl Acad Sci USA 2006; 103(26):9751-9752.
43. Yoshida S, Sukeno M, Nakagawa T et al. The first round of mouse spermatogenesis is a distinctive program that lacks the self-renewing spermatogonia stage. Development 2006; 133(8):1495-1505.
44. Ebisuno S, Kohjimoto Y, Tamura M et al. Histological observations of the adhesion and endocytosis of calcium oxalate crystals in MDCK cells and in rat and human kidney. Urol Int 1997; 58(4):227-231.
45. Ehmcke J, Joshi B, Hergenrother SD et al. Aging does not affect spermatogenic recovery after experimentally induced injury in mice. Reproduction 2007; 133(1):75-83.
46. Nakagawa T, Nabeshima Y, Yoshida S. Functional identification of the actual and potential stem cell compartments in mouse spermatogenesis. Dev Cell 2007; 12(2):195-206.
47. Aponte PM, van Bragt MP, de Rooij DG et al. Spermatogonial stem cells: Characteristics and experimental possibilities. Apmis 2005; 113(11-12):727-742.

48. Brinster RL. Male germline stem cells: From mice to men. Science 2007; 316(5823):404-405.
49. Clermont Y. Kinetics of spermatogenesis in mammals: Seminiferous epithelium cycle and spermatogonial renewal. Physiol Rev 1972; 52(1):198-236.
50. Franca LR, Russell LD. The testis of domestic mammals. In: Martinez-Garcia F, Regadera J, eds. Male Reproduction: A Multidisciplinary Overview. Madrid: Churchill Communications Europe España, 1998:197-219.
51. Hess RA, Schaeffer DJ, Eroschenko VP et al. Frequency of the stages in the cycle of the seminiferous epithelium in the rat. Biol Reprod 1990; 43(3):517-524.
52. Franca LR, Ogawa T, Avarbock MR et al. Germ cell genotype controls cell cycle during spermatogenesis in the rat. Biol Reprod 1998; 59(6):1371-1377.
53. Zeng W, Avelar GF, Rathi R et al. The length of the spermatogenic cycle is conserved in porcine and ovine testis xenografts. J Androl 2006; 27(4):527-533.
54. Hess RA, Chen P. Computer tracking of germ cells in the cycle of the seminiferous epithelium and prediction of changes in cycle duration in animals commonly used in reproductive biology and toxicology. J Androl 1992; 13(3):185-190.
55. Creasy DM. Evaluation of testicular toxicity in safety evaluation studies: The appropriate use of spermatogenic staging. Toxicol Pathol 1997; 25(2):119-131.
56. Creasy DM. Evaluation of testicular toxicology: A synopsis and discussion of the recommendations proposed by the Society of Toxicologic Pathology. Birth Defects Res Part B Dev Reprod Toxicol 2003; 68(5):408-415.
57. Liu Y, Nusrat A, Schnell FJ et al. Human junction adhesion molecule regulates tight junction resealing in epithelia. J Cell Sci 2000; 113(Pt 13):2363-2374.
58. Vilela DAR, Silva SGB, Peixoto MTD et al. Spermatogenesis in teleost; Insights from the Nile tilapia (Oreochromis niloticus) model. Fish Physiol Biochem 2003; 28:187-190.
59. Russell LD, Chiarini-Garcia H, Korsmeyer SJ et al. Bax-dependent spermatogonia apoptosis is required for testicular development and spermatogenesis. Biol Reprod 2002; 66(4):950-958.
60. Franca LR, Russell LD, Cummins JM. Is human spermatogenesis uniquely poor? ARBS 2002; 4:19-42.
61. Johnson L, Chaturvedi PK, Williams JD. Missing generations of spermatocytes and spermatids in seminiferous epithelium contribute to low efficiency of spermatogenesis in humans. Biol Reprod 1992; 47(6):1091-1098.
62. Sharpe R. Regulation of spermatogenesis. In: Knobil E, Neill J, eds. The Physiology of Reproduction. 2nd ed. New York: Raven Press, 1994:1363-1434.
63. De Gendt K, Atanassova N, Tan KA et al. Development and function of the adult generation of Leydig cells in mice with Sertoli cell-selective or total ablation of the androgen receptor. Endocrinology 2005; 146(9):4117-4126.
64. Sharpe RM, McKinnell C, Kivlin C et al. Proliferation and functional maturation of Sertoli cells, and their relevance to disorders of testis function in adulthood. Reproduction 2003; 125(6):769-784.
65. van Haaster LH, De Jong FH, Docter R et al. The effect of hypothyroidism on Sertoli cell proliferation and differentiation and hormone levels during testicular development in the rat. Endocrinology 1992; 131(3):1574-1576.
66. van Haaster LH, de Jong FH, Docter R et al. High neonatal triiodothyronine levels reduce the period of Sertoli cell proliferation and accelerate tubular lumen formation in the rat testis, and increase serum inhibin levels. Endocrinology 1993; 133(2):755-760.
67. Holsberger DR, Cooke PS. Understanding the role of thyroid hormone in Sertoli cell development: A mechanistic hypothesis. Cell Tissue Res 2005; 322(1):133-140.
68. Holsberger DR, Kiesewetter SE, Cooke PS. Regulation of neonatal Sertoli cell development by thyroid hormone receptor alpha1. Biol Reprod 2005; 73(3):396-403.
69. Cooke PS, Arambepola NK, Kirby JD et al. Thyroid hormone regulation of the development of the testis and its constituent cell types. Polish J Endocrinol 1997; 48(Suppl. 3):43-58.
70. Cooke PS, Hess RA, Kirby JD et al. Neonatal propylthiouracil (PTU) treatment as a model system for studying factors controlling testis growth and sperm production. In: Bartke A, ed. Function of Somatic Cells in the Testis. New York: Springer-Verlag, 1994:400-407.
71. Hess RA, Cooke PS, Bunick D et al. Adult testicular enlargement induced by neonatal hypothyroidism is accompanied by increased Sertoli and germ cell numbers. Endocrinol 1993; 132(6):2607-2613.
72. Cooke PS, Porcelli J, Hess RA. Induction of increased testis growth and sperm production in adult rats by neonatal administration of the goitrogen propylthiouracil (PTU): The critical period. Biol Reprod 1992; 46(1):146-154.
73. Cooke PS, Hess RA, Porcelli J et al. Increased sperm production in adult rats after transient neonatal hypothyroidism. Endocrinol 1991; 129(1):244-248.

74. Holsberger DR, Buchold GM, Leal MC et al. Cell-cycle inhibitors p27Kip1 and p21Cip1 regulate murine Sertoli cell proliferation. Biol Reprod 2005; 72(6):1429-1436.
75. Franca LR, Hess RA, Cooke PS et al. Neonatal hypothyroidism causes delayed Sertoli cell maturation in rats treated with propylthiouracil: Evidence that the Sertoli cell controls testis growth. Anat Rec 1995; 242(1):57-69.
76. Sharpe RM, Turner KJ, McKinnell C et al. Inhibin B levels in plasma of the male rat from birth to adulthood: Effect of experimental manipulation of Sertoli cell number. J Androl 1999; 20(1):94-101.
77. Petersen C, Soder O. The sertoli cell—A hormonal target and 'super' nurse for germ cells that determines testicular size. Horm Res 2006; 66(4):153-161.
78. Tan KA, De Gendt K, Atanassova N et al. The role of androgens in sertoli cell proliferation and functional maturation: Studies in mice with total or Sertoli cell-selective ablation of the androgen receptor. Endocrinology 2005; 146(6):2674-2683.
79. Schulz RW, Menting S, Bogerd J et al. Sertoli cell proliferation in the adult testis—Evidence from two fish species belonging to different orders. Biol Reprod 2005; 73(5):891-898.
80. McCoard SA, Wise TH, Lunstra DD et al. Stereological evaluation of Sertoli cell ontogeny during fetal and neonatal life in two diverse breeds of swine. J Endocrinol 2003; 178(3):395-403.
81. Neves ES, Chiarini-Garcia H, Franca LR. Comparative testis morphometry and seminiferous epithelium cycle length in donkeys and mules. Biol Reprod 2002; 67(1):247-255.
82. Franca LR, Silva Jr VA, Chiarini-Garcia H et al. Cell proliferation and hormonal changes during postnatal development of the testis in the pig. Biol Reprod 2000; 63(6):1629-1636.
83. Leal MC, Franca LR. The seminiferous epithelium cycle length in the black tufted-ear marmoset (Callithrix penicillata) is similar to humans. Biol Reprod 2006; 74(4):616-624.
84. Almeida FF, Leal MC, Franca LR. Testis morphometry, duration of spermatogenesis, and spermatogenic efficiency in the wild boar (Sus scrofa scrofa). Biol Reprod 2006; 75(5):792-799.
85. Kluin PM, Kramer MF, de Rooij DG. Spermatogenesis in the immature mouse proceeds faster than in the adult. Int J Androl 1982; 5(3):282-294.
86. Sharpe RM. Sertoli cell endocrinology and signal transduction: Androgen regulation. In: Griswold M, Skinner M, eds. Sertoli Cell Biology. New York: Academic Press, 2005:199-216.
87. Ventela S, Ohta H, Parvinen M et al. Development of the stages of the cycle in mouse seminiferous epithelium after transplantation of green fluorescent protein-labeled spermatogonial stem cells. Biol Reprod 2002; 66(5):1422-1429.
88. Ismail N, Morales C, Clermont Y. Role of spermatogonia in the stage-synchronization of the seminiferous epithelium in vitamin-A-deficient rats. Am J Anat 1990; 188(1):57-63.
89. Morales CR, Griswold MD. Variations in the level of transferrin and SGP-2 mRNAs in Sertoli cells of vitamin A-deficient rats. Cell Tissue Res 1991; 263(1):125-130.
90. Ismail N, Morales CR. Effects of vitamin A deficiency on the inter-Sertoli cell tight junctions and on the germ cell population. Microsc Res Tech 1992; 20(1):43-49.
91. van Pelt AM, van Dissel-Emiliani FM, Gaemers IC et al. Characteristics of A spermatogonia and preleptotene spermatocytes in the vitamin A-deficient rat testis. Biol Reprod 1995; 53(3):570-578.
92. Bartlett JM, Weinbauer GF, Nieschlag E. Stability of spermatogenic synchronization achieved by depletion and restoration of vitamin A in rats. Biol Reprod 1990; 42(4):603-612.
93. Chung SS, Sung W, Wang X et al. Retinoic acid receptor alpha is required for synchronization of spermatogenic cycles and its absence results in progressive breakdown of the spermatogenic process. Dev Dyn 2004; 230(4):754-766.
94. Weber JE, Russell LD, Wong V et al. Three-dimensional reconstruction of a rat stage V Sertoli cell: II. Morphometry of Sertoli-Sertoli and Sertoli-germ-cell relationships. Am J Anat 1983; 167(2):163-179.
95. Brinster RL, Avarbock MR. Germline transmission of donor haplotype following spermatogonial transplantation. Proc Natl Acad Sci USA 1994; 91(24):11303-11307.
96. Russell LD, Franca LR, Brinster RL. Ultrastructural observations of spermatogenesis in mice resulting from transplantation of mouse spermatogonia. J Androl 1996; 17(6):603-614.
97. Russell LD, Brinster RL. Ultrastructural observations of spermatogenesis following transplantation of rat testis cells into mouse seminiferous tubules. J Androl 1996; 17(6):615-627.
98. Ye SJ, Ying L, Ghosh S et al. Sertoli cell cycle: A re-examination of the structural changes during the cycle of the seminiferous epithelium of the rat. Anat Rec 1993; 237(2):187-198.
99. Franca LR, Ghosh S, Ye SJ et al. Surface and surface-to-volume relationships of the Sertoli cell during the cycle of the seminiferous epithelium in the rat. Biol Reprod 1993; 49(6):1215-1228.
100. McKinney TD, Desjardins C. Postnatal development of the testis, fighting behavior, and fertility in house mice. Biol Reprod 1973; 9(3):279-294.

101. Clermont Y, Perey B. Quantitative study of the cell population of the seminiferous tubules in immature rats. Am J Anat 1957; 100(2):241-267.
102. Oakberg EF. Duration of spermatogenesis in the mouse and timing of stages of the cycle of the seminiferous epithelium. Am J Anat 1956; 99(3):507-516.
103. van Haaster LH, de Rooij DG. Spermatogenesis is accelerated in the immature Djungarian and Chinese hamster and rat. Biol Reprod 1993; 49(6):1229-1235.
104. Tan KA, Turner KJ, Saunders PT et al. Androgen regulation of stage-dependent cyclin D2 expression in Sertoli cells suggests a role in modulating androgen action on spermatogenesis. Biol Reprod 2005; 72(5):1151-1160.
105. Zhang YQ, He XZ, Zhang JS et al. Stage-specific localization of transforming growth factor beta1 and beta3 and their receptors during spermatogenesis in men. Asian J Androl 2004; 6(2):105-109.
106. Xu J, Beyer AR, Walker WH et al. Developmental and stage-specific expression of Smad2 and Smad3 in rat testis. J Androl 2003; 24(2):192-200.
107. O'Donnell L, McLachlan RI, Wreford NG et al. Testosterone withdrawal promotes stage-specific detachment of round spermatids from the rat seminiferous epithelium. Biol Reprod 1996; 55(4):895-901.
108. Sharpe RM, Maddocks S, Millar M et al. Testosterone and spermatogenesis: Identification of stage-specific, androgen-regulated proteins secreted by adult rat seminiferous tubules. J Androl 1992; 13(2):172-184.
109. Vihko KK, Toppari J, Parvinen M. Stage-specific regulation of plasminogen activator secretion in the rat seminiferous epithelium. Endocrinology 1987; 120(1):142-145.
110. Liu D, Matzuk MM, Sung WK et al. Cyclin A1 is required for meiosis in the male mouse. Nat Genet 1998; 20(4):377-380.
111. Shang E, Salazar G, Crowley TE et al. Identification of unique, differentiation stage-specific patterns of expression of the bromodomain-containing genes Brd2, Brd3, Brd4, and Brdt in the mouse testis. Gene Expr Patterns 2004; 4(5):513-519.

Chapter 2

Testicular Development and Spermatogenesis: Harvesting the Postgenomics Bounty

Antoine D. Rolland, Bernard Jégou and Charles Pineau*

Introduction

Spermatogenesis is a sophisticated process facilitating transmission of the genetic patrimony and, thus, perpetuation of the species. Mammalian spermatogenesis is classically divided into three 3 phases. In the first—the proliferative or mitotic phase—primitive germ cells or spermatogonia undergo a series of mitotic divisions. In the second—the meiotic phase—the spermatocytes undergo two consecutive divisions to produce the haploid spermatids. In the third—spermiogenesis—spermatids differentiate into spermatozoa. The entire process is regulated by paracrine, autocrine and endocrine pathways, an array of structural elements and chemical factors modulating somatic and germ cell activity (for reviews, see refs. 1-4). The communication network linking the various cellular activities during spermatogenesis is highly complex and sophisticated.[5,6]

Determination of the function and regulation of genes and their products is one of the key objectives of human biology. The advances in molecular biology and genomics of the last 20 years have greatly improved our global knowledge of spermatogenesis, by identifying numerous genes essential for the development of functional male gametes (for reviews, see refs. 7,8). Significant progress has recently been made in the large-scale analysis of testicular function, deepening our insight into normal and pathological spermatogenesis. Several laboratories have built on rapid progress in genome sequencing and microarray development, by carrying out genome-wide expression studies, leading to the identification of hundreds of genes differentially expressed within the testis (for review see ref. 9). The development of tools for high-throughput protein identification has allowed a few laboratories to undertake differential protein profiling expression studies and/or the systematic analysis of testicular proteomes from various species, based either on the entire organ[10] or on isolated cells.[11-13]

This chapter reviews the current state of large-scale gene expression analyses of spermatogenesis, from gonad development during sex determination to hormonal regulation. It also deals with the advantages and limitations of transcriptomics and proteomics for studies of the expression program of testicular germ cells. Finally, the concept of systems biology—which involves integrative 'omics' (i.e., combining genomics, transcriptomics and proteomics) together with bioinformatics and modeling—is discussed.

Gene Expression Profiling Technologies: The Underlying Differences

Several different technologies are now available for studying gene expression by assessing mRNA and protein levels. However, there are fundamental differences between these technologies.

*Corresponding Author: Charles Pineau—Inserm, U625, IFR 140, University of Rennes I, Campus de Beaulieu, Rennes, F-35042, France. Email: charles.pineau@rennes.inserm.fr

Molecular Mechanisms in Spermatogenesis, edited by C. Yan Cheng. ©2008 Landes Bioscience and Springer Science+Business Media.

Transcriptome and Transcriptomics

The complete set of ribonucleic acid (RNA) transcripts produced by the genome in any given organism is called the transcriptome. Transcriptomics—the global analysis of gene expression, also called genome-wide expression profiling—is now widely used to investigate the genes and pathways involved in various biological processes. This approach is based on the principle that genes with similar patterns of expression may have related functions and may be regulated by the same genetic control mechanism. Common technologies for the genome-wide or high-throughput analysis of gene expression include spotted and oligonucleotide microarrays and tag-based approaches, such as serial analysis of gene expression (SAGE), cap-analysis gene expression (CAGE) and gene identification signature (GIS) methods. Microarray methods are dependent on the choice of sequences to be screened at the outset, whereas sequencing-based approaches require no such prior sequence selection. The various transcriptomic technologies used in these two approaches allow scientists to study tens of thousands of genes simultaneously, rather than considering one gene at a time.

Proteome and Proteomics

The word "proteome"—a contraction of "protein" and "genome"—was first coined by Marc Wilkins at the 4th 2D Gel Electrophoresis Meeting in Sienna in 1994.[14] This term encapsulates the complex and dynamic nature of protein production, at reference points spanning from individual cells to organisms. Genomes are essentially identical in the different cells of an organism, whereas proteomes and transcriptomes vary between cells, over time and as a function of environmental stimuli and stress.

Proteomics research deals with the temporal dynamics of protein production in a given biological compartment at a given time. Until recently, "proteins" were considered solely as the direct products of genes for the purposes of this definition. The definition of proteomics has recently been altered so that this field now covers not only direct gene products, but also proteins undergoing structural alterations due to cell metabolism and turnover (posttranslational modifications).[15] The experimental basis of proteomics, which has become one of the most important areas of research in the postgenomics era, is not new. Nonetheless, proteomics has undoubtedly benefited from unprecedented advances in genome sequencing, bioinformatics and the development of robust, sensitive, reliable and reproducible analytical techniques.

Transcriptomics Versus Proteomics, Finding the Right Balance

The recent completion of the first high-quality drafts of the mouse[16] and human[17,18] genomes has provided scientists with access to a wealth of relevant sequence information essential for the systematic and comprehensive characterization of gene product function. These genome sequencing projects surprisingly revealed that mammalian genomes contain far fewer protein-coding genes than previously thought. The mouse and human genomes have each been found to contain about 22,000 genes (Ensembl[19] release 43), corresponding to 22,000 functional proteins according to the original one gene-one protein dogma of molecular biology. However, alternative splicing can routinely generate 100,000 proteins from 22,000 genes.[20,21] If we include posttranslational modifications (e.g., phosphorylation, glycosylation and proteolysis),[22,23] then the 22,000 genes may give rise to a million proteins,[24,25] each with different functions. This complexity of multilayered gene expression mechanisms is partly responsible for the frequently reported discrepancies between mRNA and protein abundance.[26-28] Thus, although transcriptomics probably still has a greater throughput capacity than proteomics, it is clear that protein diversity cannot be fully characterized by gene expression analyses alone. Great attention must be paid to selecting the most appropriate methods for large-scale experiments, according to whether the biological question addressed relates more to the transcriptional and/or splicing mechanisms underlying a particular process or to role in the process considered of the proteins generated and their subtly different isoforms.

Gonad Development During Sex Determination

The primary event in mammalian sexual development is the differentiation of the bipotential gonad into either a testis or an ovary. The transient expression of a single gene, *Sry* (sex-determining region, chromosome Y), in the supporting cell lineage of mice, from embryonic day (ed) 11.5 onwards, is necessary and sufficient to direct the differentiation of an XY gonad into a testis. This suggests that ovary development may be the "default" pathway of gonad differentiation (Fig. 1). Small et al[29] investigated the molecular mechanisms underlying gonad differentiation, using high-density oligonucleotide microarrays to compare the gene expression profiles of male and female mouse gonads from 11.5 to 18.5 days post-coitum (dpc). They reported the differential expression of thousands of genes during the development of ovaries or testes and between gonads at various time points. The genes identified as differentially expressed included all those previously identified as involved in this process, such as *Sry* itself, *Sox9, Dax1, Sf1* and *Wt1*. Major differences between the sexes were found for genes encoding proteins involved in meiosis, steroidogenesis and apoptosis, consistent with the initiation of meiosis I in the ovary, the differentiation of Leydig and Sertoli cells and the burst of cell apoptosis observed in the testis. Nef et al[30] carried out a similar study on transgenic mice synthesizing green fluorescent protein (GFP) in the somatic compartment of the genital ridge of both male and female embryos. They specifically isolated somatic cells, including both supporting cell (future Sertoli and granulosa cells) and steroidogenic cell (future Leydig and theca cells) precursors, from 10.5 to 13.5 dpc. This made it possible to monitor very early events directly associated with the Sry-signaling pathway, without germ-cell "contamination". This is important because of the potential effects of the expression program of germ cells. At 10.5 dpc, only nine genes on the sexual chromosomes displayed differential expression between XX and XY gonads, indicating that sex determination had not yet occurred. Thereafter, the number of differentially expressed genes increased, eventually reaching more than two thousand by 13.5 dpc. Three genes encoding Cdk inhibitors were found to be more strongly expressed in the ovary than in the testis. This led the authors to suggest that the higher levels of proliferation of testicular somatic cells immediately after *Sry* expression—a crucial event in male sex differentiation—might be a direct or indirect consequence of the inhibitory effect of Sry on Cdk inhibitor production, rather than a reflection of the activation of gene products involved in proliferation. Another identical study investigated gene expression in differentiating mouse gonads at 10.5 and 11.5 dpc.[31] The results obtained were consistent with those of Nef et al,[30] but with a larger number of dimorphic genes identified at 11.5 dpc, probably due to differences in normalization and data processing. Nef's study was remarkable for the identification of several differentially expressed genes for which human orthologs mapped to loci associated with sexual disorders. These three studies demonstrate the existence of strong expression programs in both the developing testis and the ovary, calling into question the notion that ovary differentiation is the "default" pathway of gonad differentiation. One 2D gel-based proteomic study recently investigated gonad development during sex determination.[32] The authors compared whole gonads from mice 13.5 dpc and demonstrated differential expression between male and female gonads for 36 protein spots (6% of the total), three of which they went on to identify. The smaller proportion of proteins than of genes displaying differential expression[30] (10%) may be due to the larger amounts of protein required for visualization on a 2D gel. This would favor the detection of ubiquitous proteins, which are likely to be produced in larger amounts. Although only three proteins displaying differential expression between male and female gonads were identified, none of the corresponding transcripts was demonstrated as differentially expressed in any of the transcriptomic experiments described above. One protein displayed a specific phosphorylation pattern in male extracts. This pattern clearly could not be picked up through a transcriptome-based approach, and indicated the presence of potentially more abundant or active kinases in male gonads.

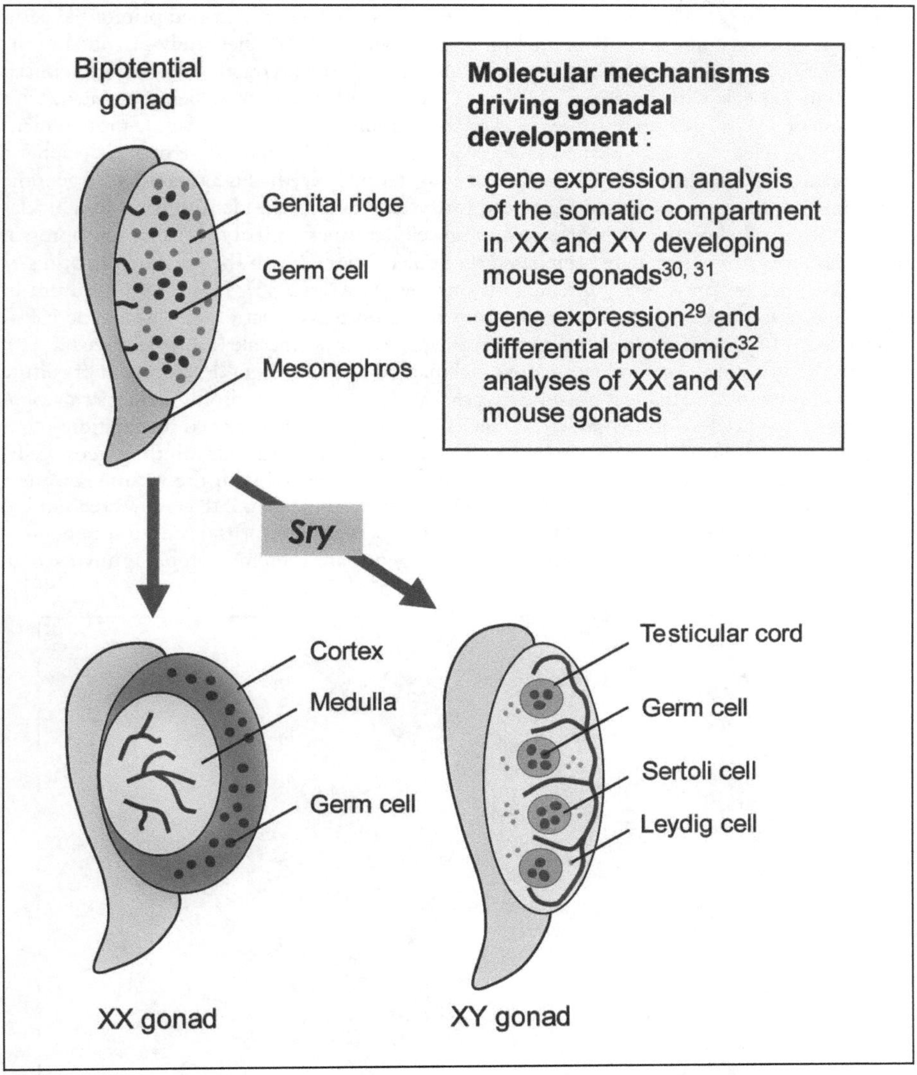

Figure 1. Testis or ovary? During embryological development, a unique anatomical structure present in both males and females, the "bipotential" gonad, is formed before the sexually dimorphic gonads. The differentiation pathways underlying the morphological and functional differences between the testis and ovary are driven principally by the expression of a single gene in the somatic cells of the XY gonad, *SRY*, at about embryonic day 11.5 in the mouse. *SRY*: sex-determining region Y.

Gene Expression Profiling in Spermatogonial Cells

The molecular identity of spermatogonial cells and the signaling events triggering their renewal or entry into spermatogenesis remained largely unknown until recently. Several studies aimed to establish reference proteome maps for these cells, with the aim of gaining insight into their biology (Fig. 2). These studies included proteomic analyses of cultured primordial germ cells from chicken[33] and freshly isolated rat spermatogonia.[34] Another study provided information about discrete low-copy number proteins, through the prefractionation of protein cell extracts on 2D gels with a narrow pH range.[11] This work is currently being pursued, with reverse-phase HPLC used to separate the extracts into subproteome pools before protein identification (Couvet et al, unpublished). Global approaches of this type, designed to decipher a static proteome, should be rewarding in the long term. Indeed, the availability of genome sequence data has generated an urgent need for systematic protein identification for elucidation of the encoded protein networks governing cellular function. Large-scale protein-protein interaction maps have generally been based on results obtained with the yeast two-hybrid system, which detects only binary interactions (for review, see ref. 35). However, the advent of highly sensitive protein identification methods based on mass spectrometry has made it feasible to identify protein complexes directly, at the proteome-wide scale (for review, see ref. 18).

The identification of several spermatogonial markers and the recent development of culture systems in rodents have made it possible to carry out gene expression profiling on spermatogonial cells in various developmental states (Fig. 2). Hamra et al used enriched preparations of rat spermatogonial stem cells (SSC) (type I collagen-non-binding/laminin-binding germ cells) cultured on different feeder cell lines to identify genes associated with the maintenance (on MSC-1 cells) or loss (on STO cells) of stem cell activity.[36] As many as 248 genes were found to be downregulated during the loss of stem cell activity, their level of transcription remaining stable whilst this activity was maintained. These genes are therefore probably involved in

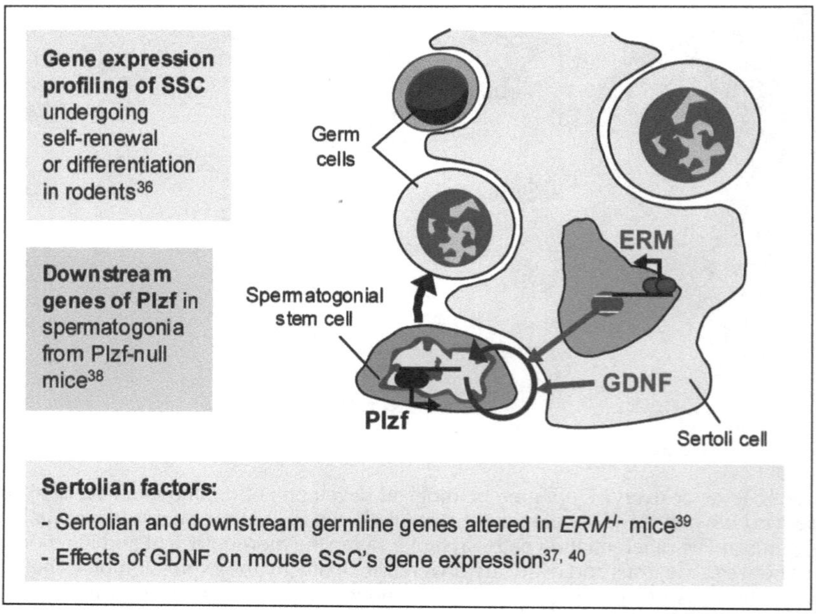

Figure 2. Pathways for the self-renewal and differentiation of spermatogonial stem cells (SSC). The daily production of millions of spermatozoa in mammals is ensured by the presence within the male germ line of stem cells able to maintain their own stock and to differentiate and continuously initiate new waves of spermatogenesis. The balance between proliferation, differentiation and the maintenance of spermatogonial stem cells is governed by intrinsic factors, such as PLZF, and by signals from the testicular stem cell niche, including Sertolian signals, such as GDNF or ERM. GDNF: glial cell line-derived neurotrophic factor; ERM: Ets-related molecule; PLZF: promyelocytic leukemia zinc finger.

self-renewal rather than differentiation. The authors focused on a subset of 115 genes for which mouse homologs also displayed downregulation during germ cell differentiation in vivo, including Bcl6b (see below, ref. 37). Mean expression levels for these genes, referred to as the "stem cell index" (SCI), were strongly correlated with SSC activity, and with the expression of individual genes, such as *Erg3*, expressed only in undifferentiated stem cells. Other studies have investigated specific pathways related to single factors involved in SSC self-renewal and spermatogonial differentiation, as demonstrated by targeted disruption in the mouse. *Zfp145*-null mice lack a transcriptional repressor specifically expressed in spermatogonia in the testis (promyelocytic leukemia zing finger, PLZF) and are unable to maintain their spermatogonia. An analysis of gene expression in isolated spermatogonia (α^6-integrin-positive cells) from one-week-old mutant mice identified more than 230 genes as differentially expressed with respect to the wild type.[38] Analyses of gene expression have also been used to investigate the signaling pathway triggered by the sertolian factor Ets-related molecule (ERM) in mutant mice with impaired spermatogenesis during adulthood.[39] The authors studied total testes from four-week-old mice—no obvious phenotype being visible at this age—and identified specific alterations in the pattern of expression of many spermatogonial genes, thereby demonstrating an effect of ERM on the SSC/spermatogonial expression program. They also showed that a large number of genes were differentially expressed in isolated Sertoli cells. The genes concerned were found to encode secreted factors previously reported to regulate the hematopoietic stem cell niche, and which also seemed to regulate SSC behavior. The SSC self-renewal and differentiation pathways mediated by one such factor, the glial cell line-derived neurotrophic factor (GDNF), have also been analyzed by gene expression profiling experiments.[37,40] Hofmann et al sorted GRFα-1 (the GDNF coreceptor)-positive germ cells from six-day-old mice after isolation by sedimentation under gravity and differential plating. They monitored the gene expression profiles of these cells cultured in the presence or absence of GDNF for 10 hours.[40] They identified more than a thousand genes differentially expressed in the presence and absence of GDNF and focused on one upregulated gene, that encoding fibroblast growth factor-receptor 2 (FGFR2). They found that bFGF amplified the proliferative effects of GDNF on SSC in culture and concluded that GNDF rendered germ-line stem cells more responsive to bFGF. Oatley et al cultured Thy1-positive cells from adult mice on STO feeders (which do not maintain SSC activity), with or without GDNF/GFRα-1.[37] They identified 199 genes that were downregulated 18 hours after the elimination of GNDF/GFRα-1 from the medium ("self-renewal"-associated genes) and 79 genes that were upregulated in these conditions ("differentiation"-associated genes). They found 193 and 63 genes to be upregulated and downregulated, respectively, following the reintroduction of GDNF/GFRα-1 (2, 4 and 8 hours later). They then focused on the transcriptional repressor gene *Bclb6*, one of the six genes both downregulated following the elimination of GDNF/GFRα-1 and upregulated following its reintroduction, regardless of the reintroduction time (these genes also included *Egr3*, see above ref. 36). The pattern of changes in *Bclb6* expression demonstrated that the protein encoded by this gene played a significant role in SSC maintenance. In vitro, cultured SSC treated with Bclb6-siRNA were smaller, fewer in number and had a lower colonization capacity than untreated cells, whereas, in vivo, Bclb6-null mice were found to have a higher proportion of tubules displaying impaired spermatogenesis than wild-type mice. These studies have identified many factors as involved in SSC signaling pathways, but they also highlight the importance of these factors for other stem cell lineages. These findings suggest that the expression of a specific combination of factors, with its own specific regulatory system, rather than the expression of germ line-specific factors may account for the unique ability of SSC to promote spermatogenesis (see below).

Postnatal Testis Development and Spermatogenesis

The development of germ cells through spermatogenesis is probably the aspect of male reproduction most frequently investigated in large-scale experiments. Spermatogenesis—an amazing cellular differentiation process leading to the daily production of millions of spermatozoa—involves the coordinated expression of specific genes and the generation of specific gene products at each step of the process, together with continuous communication between developing germ cells and testicular somatic cells.[1]

Basic strategies have been used to address this issue through the global characterization of genes and proteins expressed in the testis or germ cell-enriched samples of animals, from invertebrates through to humans (Fig. 3). These strategies include the systematic identification of chromatin-associated proteins in *C. elegans* germ cells,[41] insoluble chromatin-associated proteins in mouse elongated spermatids,[42] testicular proteins in pig[10] and mouse[43] and analysis of germline gene expression in *C. elegans*,[44] mouse[45,46] and human[47] testis. Some of these studies used filtering strategies to identify germ line-specific, male germ line-specific or testis-specific genes and proteins, but none was able to provide meaningful results deepening our understanding of spermatogenesis, given the amount of data generated and the various cell types from which they originated.

Several groups have also undertaken more sophisticated analyses, based on different strategies, to identify genes or proteins preferentially or specifically expressed at each stage of spermatogenesis. One of these strategies involved comparisons of different categories of purified germ cells, combined with a SAGE experiment in mice,[48] GeneChip microarray experiments in mice[49-51] and rats,[52,51] or differential proteomic analysis in the rat[13] (Fig. 3). Another involved comparisons of total testis samples from animals of various ages during the first wave of spermatogenesis, in mice, and involved differential display analysis,[53] spotted PCR microarray experiments[54,55] and GeneChip microarray experiments[49,56] (Fig. 3). Both strategies have advantages and disadvantages. The use of isolated cells makes it possible to detect the differential expression of transcripts produced in only small amounts that could not be detected in total testis samples, but the time-consuming isolation procedures required may also alter the expression pattern. Conversely, the use of total testes overcomes the problem of artifacts related to sample preparation and can allow more precise profiling by increasing the number of time points analyzed. However, the observed changes in expression cannot be unambiguously attributed to any particular cell type. Indeed, during the postnatal testis development, the changes in expression observed in such experiments result not only from the different types of germ cell, but also from the various somatic cells, which may display changes in expression pattern during this period.[57,58] This matter was partially resolved by Shima et al, who used both approaches in parallel.[49] They first identified transcripts particularly abundant in each cell type (isolated type A and B spermatogonia, pachytene spermatocytes, round spermatids, Leydig cells, Sertoli cells and peritubular cells) and then monitored levels of these transcripts during the ontological development of the testis. They found that the pattern of gene expression during postnatal development was consistent with the cell type of origin for most transcripts. For example, somatic and premeiotic genes displayed a rapid decrease in expression due to their "dilution" by the genes expressed in maturing germ cells, whereas meiotic and postmeiotic genes displayed a dramatic increase in expression from puberty onwards. This suggests that neither changes in expression during isolation nor the diversity of cell types in total testis samples pose a real problem for the monitoring of spermatogenesis. Correlations have also been reported between expression profiling experiments, not only between purified germ cells and total testis samples, but between species.[9] Indeed, the high reproducibility of commercial GeneChips makes cross-species comparisons and the inclusion of external data possible (see below ref. 51). Furthermore, PCR microarrays can be used to identify new genes or transcripts not yet picked up. This advantage is clearly illustrated by two studies using spotted PCR microarrays consisting of testis-subtracted and germ cell-enriched libraries to investigate the testicular transcriptome of mice carrying Y-chromosome deletions.[59,60] These studies identified several new X- and Y-linked spermatid transcripts as up- or downregulated. These transcripts and the corresponding

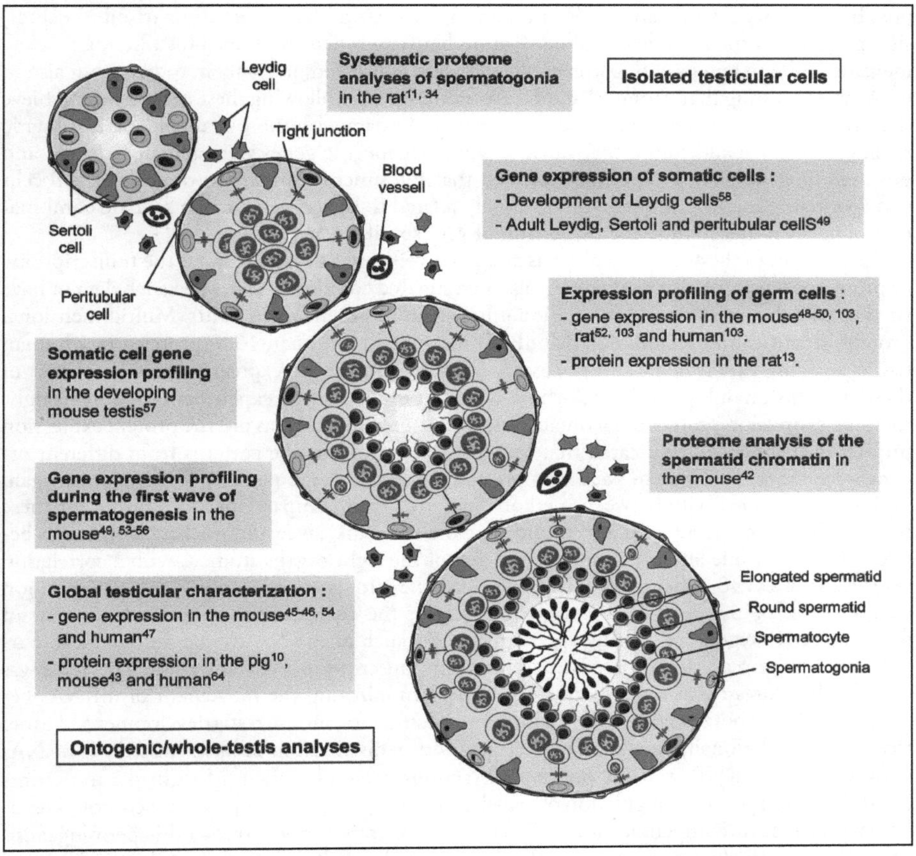

Figure 3. Deciphering spermatogenesis through expression analyses. Spermatogenesis is a complex, coordinated and continuous process by which spermatogonia give rise to mature spermatozoa. In rodents, the first wave of this process starts a few days after birth, when gonocytes (prespermatogonia) resume proliferation and become undifferentiated spermatogonia or spermatogonial stem cells. Once SSC are engaged in differentiation process (i.e., they become differentiated spermatogonia) they undergo six successive mitotic divisions, giving rise to meiotic spermatocytes, which go through two consecutive divisions, with a single round of DNA replication, to give rise to haploid spermatids. The final step in spermatogenesis consists of the transformation of spermatids into spermatozoa and is called spermiogenesis.

genes were difficult to identify as up- or downregulated, because of the many multicopy gene families found on gonosomes.

The use of these different approaches has led to the identification of thousands of genes differentially expressed during germ cell development. This massive body of data is of great interest for an overall understanding of spermatogenesis, but its mining for the identification of key factors remains a huge challenge, as high-throughput in vivo gene inactivation is not yet feasible in rodents. Many other strategies are possible, including identification of the genes operating downstream from relevant transcription factors[61-63] and focusing on testis-specific genes or genes conserved throughout evolution. We recently compared mouse, rat and human spermatogenesis transcriptomes.[51] Several thousands of genes were found to be differentially expressed in the three species, and about one thousand orthologs were identified. It was not possible to prepare some samples for humans, so we instead based our comparison of expression patterns on the high degree of correlation between rodent profiles. This filtering strategy identified 888 orthologs with patterns of expression conserved, not only in rodents, but also in humans, suggesting that strong selection constraints operate, allowing these orthologs to achieve their functions at a given step. We also compared our data with those available for 17 somatic tissues from mice and found that most of the testis-specific genes were actually meiotic and postmeiotic genes. These findings indicated that the functional identity of both Sertoli cells and spermatogonia was probably more closely related to the expression of a specific combination of genes rather than to the expression of very specific genes.

In addition to these analyses of testis and germ cell expression patterns at the transcriptome or proteome levels, several studies have also investigated correlations between such data or have tried to take the regulation of translation into account in their experiments. Multidimensional protein identification technology (MudPIT) identified more than 1600 proteins in a human tissue-profiling experiment, and it was possible to compare the expression profiles of 683 of these proteins unambiguously with those obtained in microarray experiments.[64] Surprisingly, the gene expression profiles of all organs tissues clustered together, as did the protein expression profiles of these organs indicated that transcriptome or proteome patterns from different organs were more similar than were transcriptome and proteome patterns for the same organ. Differences in sensitivity between methods may bias data comparisons, accounting for these results. However, the authors also found that the testis displayed the weakest correlation between transcriptome and proteome data of any of the eight organs studied, with a correlation coefficient of 0.138, whereas the liver displayed the strongest correlation, with a correlation coefficient of 0.432. This weak correlation may be the consequence of particular aspects of gene/transcript regulation during spermatogenesis, such as mRNA storage in free RNP particles with repressed translation or delays between transcription and translation. This issue was specifically addressed in a microarray experiment monitoring the movement of mRNAs between RNPs and polysomes during meiotic and postmeiotic mouse testis development.[65] More than 700 translationally regulated transcripts (with redistribution of at least 20% of mRNAs between the free RNPs and the polysomal fractions) were identified. Most of the transcripts identified displayed an upregulation of translation during late spermiogenesis, a common regulatory mechanism compensating for the cessation of transcription from mid-spermiogenesis onwards. A small cluster of meiotic mRNAs translated only in postmeiotic cells was also identified. The translational regulation of the genes identified in this study may not necessarily lead to a significant difference in RNA and protein expression profiles. For example, an mRNA may be produced in large amounts but inefficiently translated at one stage, whereas it may be produced in small amounts but efficiently translated at another. It is entirely possible for there to be larger amounts of protein present in the first of these cases than in the second, despite the much lower translation efficiency. Several genes identified by Iguchi as displaying translational regulation were found to have similar mRNA and protein expression patterns in our transcriptome[51] and proteome[13] data for male germ cells in the rat (Table 1). Conversely, certain genes with divergent RNA and protein patterns were not found to be translationally regulated.[65] These apparent discrepancies may be accounted for by differences in the species studied. However, some of our rat data profiles were confirmed by in situ analyses in mice. The observed discrepancies may also result from additional mechanisms affecting the ratio of transcript to protein, such as protein stability and turnover.

Focus on Spermatozoa

Transcriptomics usually generates larger datasets than proteomics, but spermatozoa are a special case, for which proteome-based studies have probably generated more relevant data. Most of the studies described in this review were carried out on rodents or non mammalian models. Human samples have been widely studied only in investigations concerning sperm constituents and fecundation. Such studies are therefore the only studies in which human

Table 1. A first set of genes whose mRNA and protein expression levels were compared in transcriptomic and proteomic differential analyses of rat spermatogenesis

Correlated RNA and Protein Expression Patterns				
Spermatogonia				
Aco1	Anxa2	Gstm1	Ltb4dh	Pygb
Actb	Anxa5	Gstm2	Mdh1	Set_predicted
Actg1	Arhgdia	Gstm3	P4hb	Tkt
Ahcy	Crabp1	Hadhsc	Pgk1	Tpm4
Akr1b4	Eef2	Hpcal1	Pkm2	Tpt1
Aldh1a1	Eno1	Hspd1	Prdx1	Txnl1
Aldh2	Fh1	Idh3a	Prdx2	Ube1x
Aldh7a1	Gapdh	Lap3	Psma1	Uchl1
Aldh9a1	Gsn	Ldha	Psme1	Vcl_predicted
Aldoa	Gsta3	Ldhb	Psme2	
Spermatocytes				
Ciapin1	Hyou1	Ptbp2	Ruvbl2	Tra1_predicted
Diablo	Kars	RGD1305235	Sugt1	Tubb2c
Spermatids				
Acrbp	Nudt9	Ranbp5_predicted	Rsd6	Spata20
Asns	Pgam2	Rnpep	Spa17	

Continued on next page

Table 1. Continued

Uncorrelated RNA and Protein Expression Patterns In Spermatogonia versus Spermatocytes				
Adk	Hnrpk	Pcna	Tufm_predicted	
Apoa1bp_predicted	Lrpprc	Rpsa	Uble1a	
Bpnt1	Nudc	Stmn1	Vcp	
In Spermatocytes Versus Spermatids				
Asrgl1	Fkbp4	Hspa4l_predicted	Pcmt1	RGD1311026
Cct5	Ganab_predicted	Hspca	Pebp1	Thop1
Cpt2	Gstm5	Ldhc	Ppp1cc	Tpi1
Fabp9	Hint1_predicted	Lztfl1	Ppp2r4_predicted	
Fbp1	Hspa2	Park7	RGD1307773_predicted	
In Spermatogonia Versus Spermatids				
Fth1	Hnrpa2b1_predicted	LOC360504	Pdia3	
Hbb	Hspa5	Mcm7	Uchl5	

"Correlated" genes displayed similar mRNA and protein expression levels while "uncorrelated" genes displayed discrepancies in mRNA and protein expression levels in between 2 germ cell types. Adapted from references 13 and 51.

physiopathology has been addressed directly. Spermatozoa are transcriptionally inactive and contain only very small amounts of RNA. Nevertheless, several groups have investigated the human sperm transcriptome, through both microarray-based experiments[66,67,68] and SAGE library construction[69] (Fig. 4). These studies highlighted an unexpected diversity of mRNA species and led to two major conclusions: (1) The RNA content of spermatozoa is representative of spermatogenesis and can therefore be used to assess sperm quality and/or to explore certain cases of male sterility and (2) the spermatozoon may deliver more than just its DNA to the oocyte. It may also concern coding and noncoding transcripts playing an important role in early zygote development. However, it remains difficult to discriminate between the thousands of sperm transcripts that will be translated into "true spermatozoon proteins" and residual transcripts used at earlier steps of spermatogenesis.

The possibility of recovering large numbers of spermatozoa in highly pure preparations has led to many groups trying to decipher the proteome of mature male gametes. Various strategies have been used (Fig. 4). Martínez-Heredia et al aimed to map the human sperm proteome, using 2DE combined with MALDI-TOF MS, leading to the resolution of over 1000 protein spots and the unambiguous identification of 98 proteins.[70] More detail of the human sperm proteome emerged from the differential extraction of proteins followed by nano-LC-MS/MS analysis.[71] This approach led to the identification of 1760 proteins (of the 2300 predicted by the authors to be present in human sperm), constituting the largest catalog of proteins potentially involved in or important for fertilization and a myriad of potential contraceptive targets. In an experiment similar to that carried out by Martínez-Heredia, but with greater success, 382 of 600 2DE protein-spots, corresponding to 342 unique proteins, were identified in the *Drosophila melanogaster* sperm proteome. These proteins include several conserved throughout evolution, from invertebrates to mammals, and crucial for sperm function.[72]

In addition to these attempts to characterize the complete sperm proteome, several studies have involved the use of sample prefractionation, making it possible to investigate the protein content of diverse subcellular compartments of spermatozoa, leading to localization of the proteins identified. This, in turn, makes it possible to formulate hypotheses concerning the processes in which these proteins are involved. Protein localization and the formulation of hypotheses relating to protein function are two prerequisites for proteome analysis, as defined by Anderson.[73] Such analyses have focused on the flagellum and/or fibrous sheath, acrosomal content and sperm head membrane (Fig. 4). Sixty proteins from the accessory structures of mouse sperm flagellum—the outer dense fibers, fibrous sheath and mitochondrial sheath, recovered by sucrose density gradient centrifugation of SDS-resistant tail structures—were identified by 2DE combined with MALDI-TOF/TOF-MS/MS.[74] Four of eight proteins identified were also found in the human sperm fibrous sheath.[75] Both the acrosomal content (soluble proteins released after the acrosomal reaction) and membrane constituents (surface-biotinylated proteins of intact sperm and proteins from acrosomal vesicles released after acrosomal reaction) were investigated in mouse by 1DE combined with HPLC-MS/MS identification, so as to focus on proteins likely to be involved in fecundation.[76] Several hundred proteins were identified, 114 of which were predicted to be transmembrane or signal peptide-containing proteins. One third of male mice with the corresponding gene deletions were found to be sterile or subfertile, onfirming the pertinence of this strategy.

Proteomics has also been used for the investigation of posttranslational modifications during sperm maturation and capacitation and for the identification of proteins responsible for some of these modifications (Fig. 4). Thus, 2D-DIGE has been applied to rat spermatozoa from the cauda and caput epididymis, to highlight changes in protein profile during the transit of the sperm through the epididymis.[77] Significant differences were observed for 60 protein spots, and eight proteins were identified by MALDI-TOF MS, including one protein undergoing serine phosphorylation as demonstrated by 2D western blotting. Non capacitated and in vitro capacitated mouse spermatozoa were also compared, to investigate membrane protein redistribution during capacitation.[78] In total, 27 proteins were shown to be dissociated from lipid rafts and,

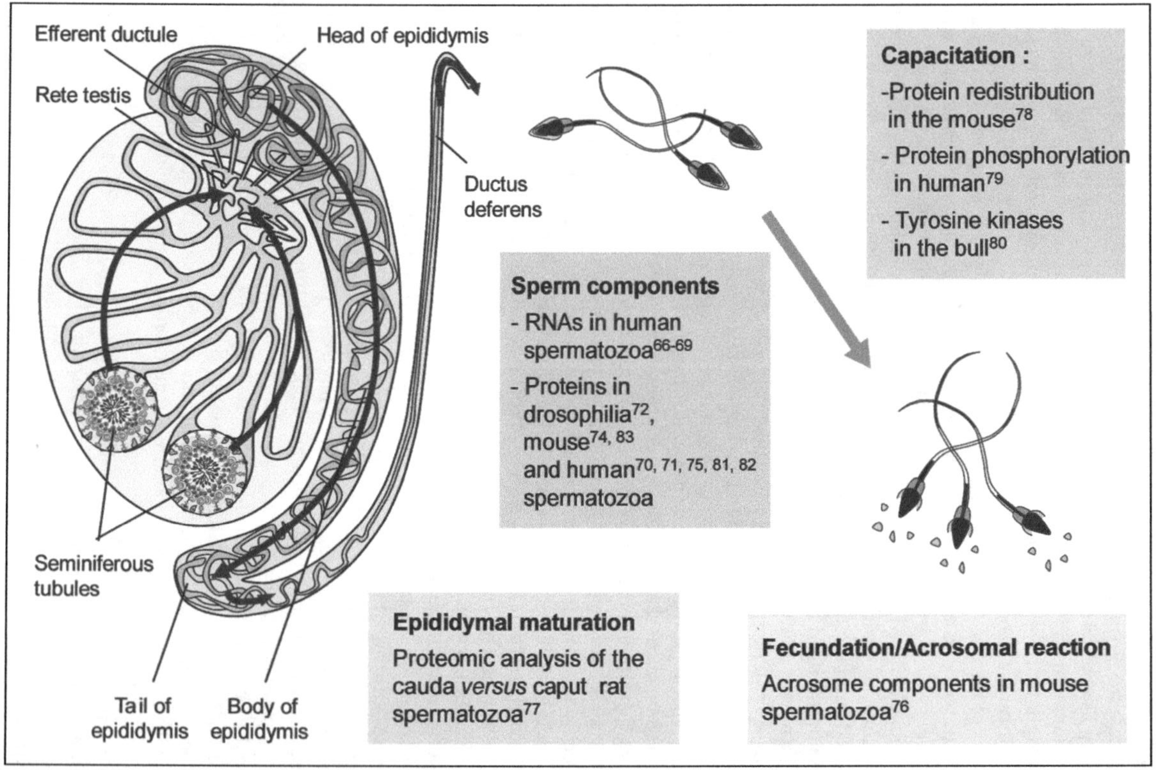

Figure 4. The main components and maturation of spermatozoa. Once released from the seminiferous epithelium, spermatozoa are transferred to the epididymis. During their transit in the epididymis, spermatozoa become motile. However, they are not yet competent for fertilization. Within the female reproductive tract, they finally acquire the ability to fertilize eggs, during a time-dependent process called capacitation, making it possible for them to undergo the acrosomal reaction and to bind to the oocyte membrane.

therefore, potentially involved in the signaling pathways associated with the initiation of capacitation. These signaling pathways included tyrosine phosphorylation, a major process that has also been specifically addressed in proteomic studies. Combining anti-phospho-tyrosine 2D western blots, IMAC, post-IMAC dephosphorylation and LC-MS/MS analysis, Ficarro et al reported the identification of more than 60 phosphorylation sites in 15 proteins from human capacitated sperm and 16 additional proteins undergoing tyrosine phoshorylation during capacitation.[79] Proteins potentially responsible for these tyrosine phosphorlation events were investigated in capacitated bull sperm.[80] A cytosolic fraction enriched in tyrosine kinase activity was generated by poly-Glu-Tyr affinity chromatography, with MALDI-TOF MS, QTOF MS and LC-MS/MS analyses subsequently used to identify 126 proteins.

Finally, several groups have used antisperm antibodies (ASA) from seminal plasma to identify proteins potentially involved in immunological diseases causing infertility. Six and four proteins, from membrane extracts of normal human and mouse sperm, respectively, were identified on 2D western blots with human ASA.[81-83] A similar approach was also used to identify seven testicular proteins recognized by sera from rats subjected to experimental autoimmune orchitis.[84]

Hormonal Regulation of Spermatogenesis

Spermatogenesis is regulated by two gonadotropins released from the anterior pituitary in response to GnRH stimulation: luteinizing hormone (LH) and follicle-stimulating hormone (FSH). LH induces the synthesis of testosterone by Leydig cells, influencing the subsequent development of peritubular and Sertoli cells, and then germ cells, whereas FSH directly induces Sertoli cell division and differentiation, thereby increasing the spermatogenetic capacity of the testis (Fig. 5).

FSH

In vitro cultures of rat Sertoli cells and transcriptomic experiments have led to the identification of several hundreds of genes regulated by FSH treatment.[85] Major effects, essentially involving upregulation, were observed within the first eight hours, with fewer genes shown to be altered 24 hours after treatment. Expression profiles for several genes previously shown to be regulated by FSH were confirmed in the microarray experiment. However, as cultures at time 0 were used as a control (rather than untreated cells at each time point), it remains possible that the changes in expression profile observed for several genes reflects natural changes in gene expression by Sertoli cells during culture. Sadate-Ngatchou et al evaluated the testicular effects of FSH in vivo, using hypogonadal (*hpg*) mice, a model in which circulating LH and FSH are undetectable.[86] As in the in vitro experiment, most of the effects were observed shortly after the FSH treatment (within 4 hours) and corresponded to an overall increase in gene expression. Hundreds of transcripts displayed differential expression profiles, including some encoding proteins with relevant molecular functions, such as DNA and RNA metabolism, particularly after four hours. By contrast, transcripts encoding proteins involved in cell adhesion, cell growth, cell communication and signal transduction displayed differential expression profiles throughout the analysis. Testicular regulation by FSH was also investigated by immune suppression, with 60 genes identified as differentially expressed in 18 dpp rats after four days of anti-FSH antiserum injections.[87] These genes included some already known to be regulated by FSH and/or identified in the other transcriptomic studies, and additional genes involved in the cell cycle. There is a marked correlation between in vitro and in vivo effects, as FSH receptor expression is strongly restricted to Sertoli cells. However, it is impossible, in studies carried out in vivo, to distinguish between genes directly altered in Sertoli cells and genes indirectly altered in other cell types (particularly germ cells) in response to Sertoli cell stimulation. This is particularly true of immunosuppression experiments, in which expression profiling is carried out several days after the reduction/suppression of circulating FSH is observed.

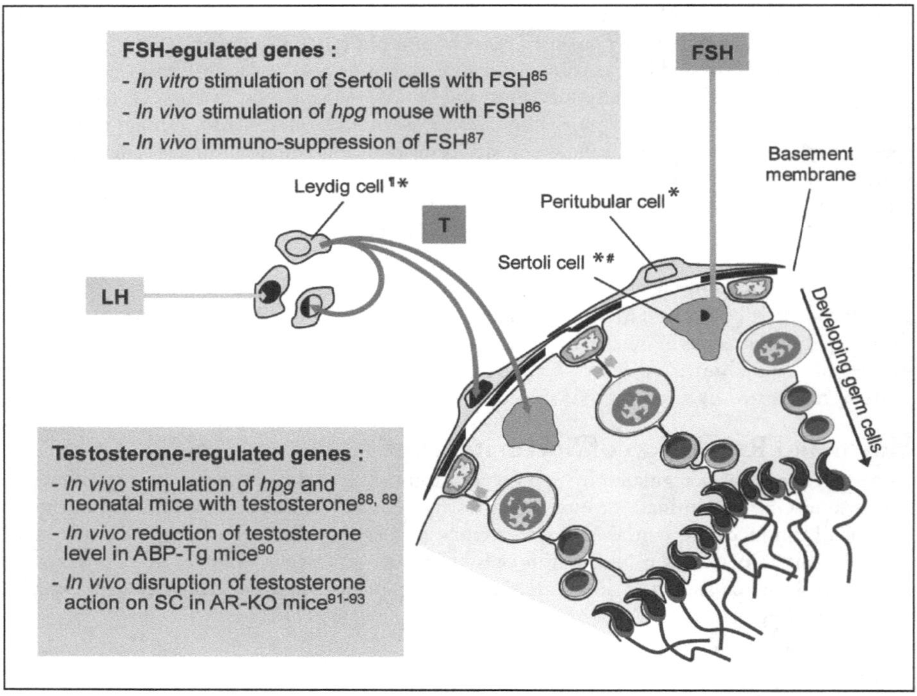

Figure 5. Hormonal regulation of spermatogenesis. Testis development and its capacity to support spermatogenesis depends heavily on endocrine regulation. In the testis, follicle-stimulating hormone exerts its specific effects on Sertoli cells by binding to the FSH receptor. Luteinizing hormone binds to the LH receptor on Leydig cells, thereby promoting testosterone synthesis and secretion. In turn, testosterone acts on Leydig cells themselves and on peritubular and Sertoli cells, via the androgen receptor. Therefore, both follicle-stimulating hormone and testosterone act on Sertoli cell physiology and the ability to drive germ-cell development. FSH: follicle-stimulating hormone; #: FSH receptor; LH: luteinizing hormone; ¶: LH receptor; T: testosterone; ✳: androgen receptor.

Androgens

The *hpg* mouse model has been used to investigate the regulation of spermatogenesis by androgens.[88] As *hpg* mice lack LH, they have little or no detectable testosterone (T). Two experiments were carried out to evaluate the effects of T on immature testes of *hpg* mice not previously exposed to androgens (24-hour time course experiment after a single injection of T) and more mature testes progressing through spermatogenesis (a single experiment 4 hours after an injection of T in *hpg* mice previously treated with T for a period of five days, followed by a 14-day washout period). Unlike the effects of FSH, the early effects of T (within the first 12 hours) on testicular expression profiles were weak, consisting of an overall decrease in expression, whereas later effects (after 24 hours) were more marked and resulted in an increase in gene expression. Interestingly, most of the genes affected by T also showed a decrease in expression, but very few genes were retrieved in both experiments, suggesting that the primary effects of androgens in the testis at the onset of spermatogenesis are different from those in more mature testes in which spermatogenesis is already occurring. Early transcriptome alterations (4-16 hours) following testosterone injections were followed in neonatal mouse (8dpp) testes in another study by the same group.[89] Several hundreds of genes differentially expressed in treated and untreated animals were identified, but only a few correlations with the results of the previous experiment were observed, probably due to the lack of FSH in *hpg* mice and/or of the non physiological amounts of T administered to neonatal mice.

In a different approach, ABP-transgenic mice, a model of chronic androgen depletion, have been used for the identification of genes regulated by testosterone.[90] This study highlighted several hundreds of genes as differentially expressed in 30 dpp WT and ABP-transgenic mice, most of these genes being upregulated in the transgenic mice. Statistical analyses identified several pathways/functions displaying significant alterations, including genes encoding proteins involved in cell adhesion, proteolysis and peptidolysis, the GPCR signaling pathway, cytokine and growth factor activity. Finally, the authors investigated possible interactions between the genes highlighted in a functional network analysis, and identified several proteins (including interleukins 2, 4, 6 and 10, MYC, AGT and MAPK8) likely to be key factors in the effects mediated by androgens, based on the large number of interactions in which they were engaged.

As the androgen receptor (Ar) is expressed in peritubular cells, Leydig cells and Sertoli cells, the changes in gene expression reported in the three studies above cannot be assigned to any particular cell type. Several groups have therefore addressed the issue of spermatogenesis regulation by androgens in mutant mice displaying Sertoli cell-selective knockout of the androgen receptor Ar (*Arinvflox(ex1-neo)/Y*;Tg (*Amh-Cre*) mice,[91,92] SCARKO mice[93]). In one study, the testicular transcriptomes of two-month-old wild-type (WT) and mutant mice were compared and about 60 genes with altered expression patterns (up- or downregulated by a factor of at least two) were highlighted.[91] A downregulated gene, *claudin 3* (*Cln3*), was then studied, as this gene had a putative androgen response element in its promoter and was therefore thought likely to be a direct target of androgens. The Cln3 protein is specifically expressed and located in newly formed tight junctions (TJs) and mutant mice seemed to display greater permeability to small molecules despite the persistence of other TJs components. It was therefore suggested that androgens may regulate the permeability of the blood-testis barrier.

In another study, Denolet et al compared the testicular transcriptome of 10 days post partum (dpp) SCARKO mice and their control littermates.[93] They identified several hundreds of genes differentially expressed in these two groups of mice at this age, about 40 of which displayed a change in expression by a factor of at least two, most of which were underexpressed in SCARKO mice. A significant proportion of the downregulated genes were related to MAPK activity and serine-type endopeptidase activity, whereas a significant proportion of upregulated genes were associated with cell cycle regulation, cell growth, cell adhesion and signal transduction. The expression profiles of genes identified as differentially expressed at 10 dpp during prepubertal development (from 8 to 20 dpp) in WT and SCARKO mice were also monitored. All genes displaying transient upregulation in the WT during this period were found to be downregulated, as early as 8 dpp, in SCARKO mice. This suggests that androgens play an important role in initiating meiosis.

Although these last three studies all addressed the specific question of the role of androgens in Sertoli cells,[91-93] they all highlighted several genes potentially only indirectly regulated by androgens, as the animals used for these experiments were several days to several weeks older than the age at which Ar is first detected in the Sertoli cells (3 to 5 dpp). Screening for potential androgen response elements (AREs) within the genomic sequences of genes found to be differentially expressed in wild-type, *Arinvflox(ex1-neo)/Y* and *Arinvflox(ex1-neo)/Y*;Tg (*Amh-Cre*) mice was carried out to address this problem.[92] This study identified more than 3000 putative AREs within 59 genes, 108 of which were also conserved in 32 human orthologs. Other experiments with neonatal and *hpg* mice focused on very early events more likely to be directly mediated by androgens, but the cell types (i.e., Leydig cells, peritubular cells or Sertoli cells) responsible for these events could not be distinguished.[88,89] Very little overlap was observed between these studies for these issues. Many studies have shown that the effects of androgens during spermatogenesis are probably mediated by gene repression, consecutively modifying junction dynamics and tubular remodeling.

Evolution and Reproduction

The genome sequences available for several species have proved a highly useful resource for phylogenic studies and taxonomic classification, and have made it possible to investigate genome-wide changes in gene expression. Khaitovich et al used probes targeting identical sequences in the human and chimpanzee genomes (94% of probes) to investigate gene expression patterns in five organs within and between these two species.[94] They found that a neutral model with negative selection and divergence time as the major factors was a useful null hypothesis for studies of both genome and transcriptome evolution. The testes—which displayed the most rapid divergence of both transcriptome and expressed gene sequences between the two species, suggesting positive selection in terms of both expression and sequences—and the brain—which displayed the lowest level of divergence—were exceptional in terms of their gene expression patterns. It was also shown that brain genes displayed the lowest diversity of expression within species (i.e., divergence between individuals) of the organs tested, closely followed by testicular genes. It was also found that expression in the testis was associated with the largest number of significant reductions in diversity in organs other than the testis, suggesting that strong selective constraints on genes, rather than a weak influence of the environment, accounted for the low level of diversity of gene expression in the testis. A surprising result was obtained in a similar experiment carried out with different mouse strains.[95] In mice, the testis was again found to be the organ with the highest divergence in gene expression between species and with the lowest diversity within both species and subspecies. However, in this study, the testis also displayed the lowest level of divergence between subspecies. The authors therefore suggested that the early phase of speciation may not be driven by regulatory changes in genes that are potential targets of sexual selection, and that the divergence in these genes is established only during a later phase of the speciation process. In addition to such studies investigating quantitative changes in gene expression, the issue of qualitative changes in gene expression has been addressed by comparing splicing events in mouse and human tissues.[96] By combining the comparison of genomic sequences, the mapping of transcripts to genomic sequences and microarray expression data, the authors identified conserved and divergent alternative splicing events in more than ten thousand mouse and human orthologs. They found a strong correlation between the levels of conserved splice forms in mouse and human genes, suggesting that the functionally important splice forms were established largely before the divergence of humans and rodents and have since been maintained. These results confirm previous results in humans, showing levels of alternative splicing to be highest in the testis and brain,[97,98] but the testis was found to display the largest number of divergent splices, whereas the brain had the highest number of conserved splices. These results suggest that strong evolutionary forces acting on the brain and testis have led to opposite evolutionary profiles but have tended to have similar effects on genomic sequence, gene expression and alternative splicing levels.

The available annotated genome sequences make it possible to map genes expressed in several processes to chromosomal locations. This approach has again generated particularly relevant observations in the field of male reproduction. In their investigations of the correlation between sequence and divergence in the pattern of gene expression in apes, Khaitovich et al observed that only testis-divergent genes were significantly clustered together on a particular chromosome, the X chromosome. They also found that genes expressed in the testis and located on the X chromosome displayed significantly higher levels of sequence divergence than other genes.[94] No such significant enrichment of the X chromosome in testis-divergent genes could be found between mouse species or subspecies, probably due to the small sample size considered.[95] The use of statistical tests is essential in chromosome assignment studies, as gene density varies within and between chromosomes. For example, genes identified during a SAGE analysis of human sperm were considered to be non randomly distributed on chromosomes, with the X chromosome being the third poorest in terms of testicular genes based on the density of expressed genes as a function of the number of expressed genes per million base pairs, but this analysis did not take into account the overall density of genes on each chromosome.[69] By contrast, several studies have analyzed the chromosomal location of testicular genes, using various statistical tests: a proteomic analysis of sperm chromatin in *D. melanogaster*,[72] a microarray experiment of the germ line in *C. elegans*,[44] an analysis of large-scale microarray-based gene expression data and of the distribution of ESTs in various mouse libraries[99] and a SAGE analysis of mouse total testis,[45] all of which also concluded that X-linked genes were underrepresented in the testis or male germ line. However, these results must be interpreted with caution, given the conflicting results published concerning the expression of X-related genes at the different stages of spermatogenesis considered independently. We observed a complete exclusion of X-related gene products from the meiotic clusters of rodents and humans, whereas these genes were preferentially expressed in somatic Sertoli cells, spermatogonia and spermatids, at least in rodents.[51] These results confirm and extend previous gene expression profiling findings for rat testicular cells, developing mouse testis and Spo11 mutant mouse testis.[99] Another experiment, using the same microarrays as Chalmel et al, addressed the specific issue of the expression of genes on the sex chromosomes in mouse germ cells. However, as the authors compared the mean expression of X-related genes between samples rather than comparing the number of genes expressed with that expected by chance, they concluded that the X chromosome underwent persistent inactivation after meiosis.[50] These studies seems to indicate that two main counteracting evolutionary forces affect the distribution of male-biased genes, one force removing these genes from the X chromosome and the other force adding them. Finally, several studies have investigated the location of testicular genes on chromosomes. They have reported, as in many other organs, the existence of a large number of clusters of genes or enriched loci.[30,44,45,50,51,72,100,101] These clusters may be of physiological relevance and are suggestive of potential enhancers or common regulatory elements. However, careful consideration of the results is again required, taking into account whether statistical tests were used, and further promoter analyses and validations are required.

The Complexity of Data Analysis: Towards Holistic Biology of Spermatogenesis

Recent advances in genomics and the results obtained with new technologies for large-scale gene expression analyses have greatly improved our knowledge of male reproduction, by making it possible to investigate the molecular mechanisms underlying this process throughout the genome. The studies reviewed here have led to the identification of factors likely to be of importance for particular steps in testicular development or required for male fertility. However, most of these studies have failed to exploit the large amounts of data generated by such high-throughput approaches to provide useful and meaningful results to enhance our overall understanding of the cellular events involved. Several strategies have been used, focusing on a restricted group of relevant genes or proteins likely to be selected for further investigations. Such strategies include tissue-profiling experiments and cross-species comparisons for the detection of testis-specific genes or genes conserved through evolution, the specific and conserved expression profiles of which may be correlated with essential functions (Fig. 6). These filtering processes have been demonstrated to be efficient for identifying the key factors from very long lists of candidates, but they cannot bridge the gap between the identification of thousands of coexpressed genes or proteins and an understanding of the connections between them, providing the ultimate explanation of the correct progression of a complete biological process.

Elucidation of the complete set of transcriptional regulation mechanisms leading to the coordinated expression of a full set of functional products and identification of the protein network interactions occurring during normal testis and germ cell development are crucial to an understanding of pathological disorders of the human testis and their origins. In the last few years, considerable effort has been made to integrate data from large-scale experiments and to develop tools enabling researchers not only to describe a group of genes or proteins with similar expression profiles, but also to develop new hypotheses from their analyses. One way of analyzing such experiments is to use the gene descriptions (annotations) of the Gene Ontology (GO) Consortium for functional data mining.[102] The GO Consortium provides the scientific community with predictions concerning gene function, the process in which the gene product is involved and subcellular components with which the gene product is associated, using a controlled and structured vocabulary (ontologies). This makes it possible to evaluate whether a particular set of genes or proteins has annotations enriched in GO terms, and thus to demonstrate objectively that specific functions are significantly associated with a given process. This approach is still quite descriptive, but it may facilitate the identification of unexpectedly important pathways and the prediction of functions for uncharacterized genes. Furthermore, it can provide additional insight into observed transcriptional profiles and/or may facilitate the identification of genes or proteins belonging to the same complex from sets of coexpressed genes or proteins. Such multifaceted analysis was recently proposed as a way of deepening analyses of data from a gene expression profiling study of the male germ line.[103] These authors used in silico promoter analysis to evaluate the occurrence of known transcription factor binding sites (TFBSs) within the regulatory sequences of genes coexpressed during mouse spermatogenesis. Combining TFBS predictions, DNA conservation and high-quality expression data, they found that the cAMP response element of the spermiogenesis-related factor *Crem* was indeed significantly more abundant in the genomic regions of loci specifically expressed in the mouse testis- specific post meotic cluster than would be expected by chance (Fig. 6B). The systematic extension of such analyses should make it easier to identify and to discover relevant regulatory elements involved in the establishment of the germline expression program. The authors also investigated the use of data for a large protein network now available for validating the biological significance of clusters of coexpressed genes in terms of protein complexes. They focused on a small group of genes selected by filtering on the basis of testis-specific expression and conserved expression in mammals and for which at least one interacting factor had been identified. This analysis yielded 87 interacting factors for the initial set of 15 genes, corresponding to genes expressed in the testis and other genes not detected on microarrays (Fig. 6C). The large number of interactions detected for genes shown to be important for male reproduction also clearly demonstrates the relevance of this approach for the confirmation and extension of expression data. Finally, transcript and protein expression profiles were compared during male germ cell development, leading to the detection of several genes displaying apparently delayed transcription and translation during spermiogenesis. An analysis similar to that for genomic sequences could be carried out to identify known or new motifs within untranslated regions in such transcripts, making it possible to predict the involvement of specific RNA-binding proteins in these translation regulation mechanisms during spermatogenesis. We are currently initiating such a project in our laboratory. As an example, the discrepancy between mRNA and protein expression levels during germ cell differentiation was confirmed for minichromosome maintenance protein 7 (MCM7) and explained in part by the identification of two additional transcripts in meiotic and post-meiotic germ cells which roles remain to be elucidated (Fig. 7). In this context, a recent study by Liu et al[104] reporting the identification of a number of genes encoding mRNAs specifically subject to alternative 3'-processing during meiosis and postmeiotic development, is of particular interest.

The study by Chalmel et al thus paves the way toward a systems-based analysis of male sexual reproduction, by highlighting the possibility of bridging the gap between DNA sequence, transcriptional activity, and translation regulation, right up to the reconstitution of functional protein complexes, at each step of spermatogenesis. Modeling of the entire process of spermatogenesis will, however, remain a major challenge, as it must include regulation by various hormones and continuous, complex communication between all the cell types present in the testis. The magnitude of this challenge has recently increased, with the arrival of data from the ENCODE project concerning exhaustive analyses of the transcription features of about 1% of the human genome.[105,106] This study has revealed the pattern of gene expression to be much more complex than initially expected, with dispersed regulation and pervasive transcription, together with an abundance of non coding RNAs, dramatically modifying current notions concerning the nature of genes and their expression.

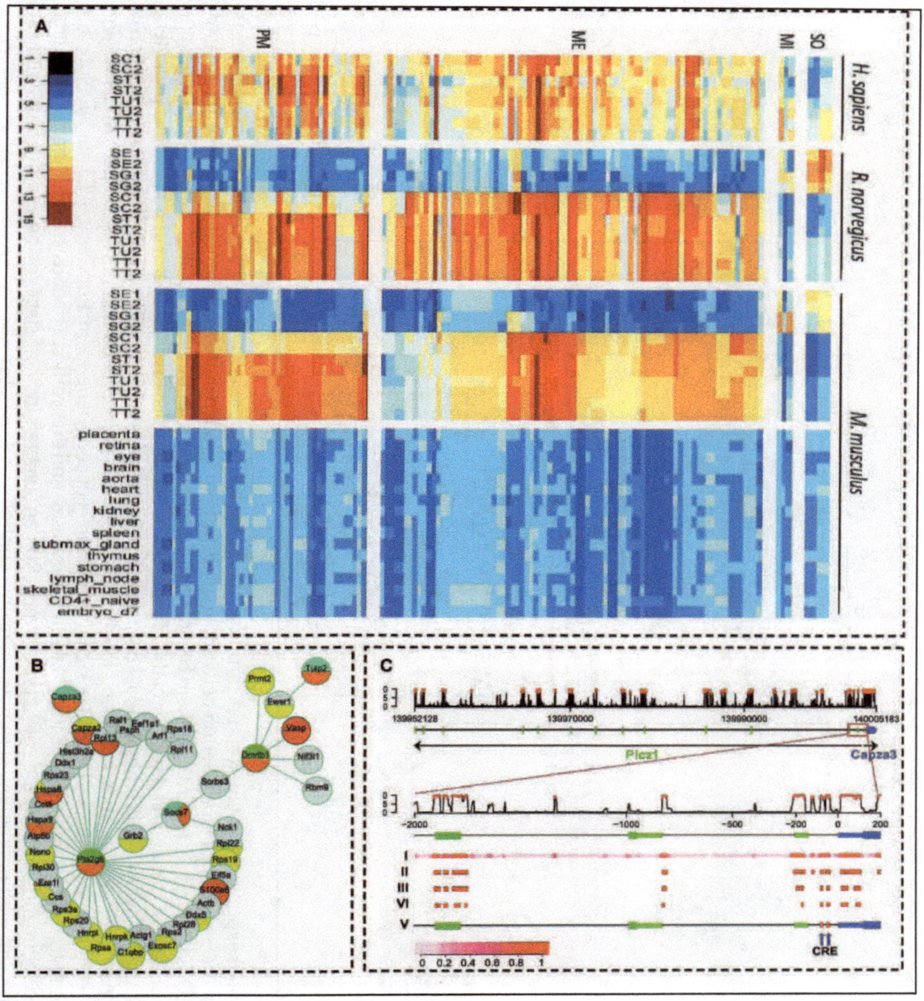

Figure 6. Data mining: Going beyond expression profiles. (Figure adapted from ref. 103). A) Filtering strategy. Cross-species comparison and tissue profiling identified 80 testis-specific orthologs with conserved expression patterns in mouse, rat and human spermatogenesis. Genes differentially expressed during spermatogenesis were identified for each species. Differentially expressed genes corresponding to orthologs represented on microarrays for all 3 species were identified, using the HomoloGene database. Finally, expression data for 17 mouse somatic tissues downloaded from the GEO web server were used to select testis-specific genes. SE, SPG, SC, ST, TU and TT correspond to Sertoli cell, spermatogonia, pachytene spermatocyte, early spermatid, seminiferous tubule and total testis samples, respectively. SO, MI, MEI and PM correspond to the somatic, mitotic, meiotic and postmeiotic expression clusters, respectively. B) Promoter analysis. Automated multi-step promoter analysis showed mouse testis-specific postmeiotic gene promoter regions to be specifically enriched in the CRE motif. We show here the results for Capza3, a gene also identified as present within the interaction node of conserved and testis-specific genes (panel C). C) Interaction network analysis. Data from IntAct, MINT and BioGRID were used to monitor interactions between conserved and testis-specific gene products. Some proteins important for male reproduction were found within these networks and were found to associate with a large number of interacting factors. As not all the interacting factors were detected on microarray analyses, interaction network analysis might help to extend expression data.

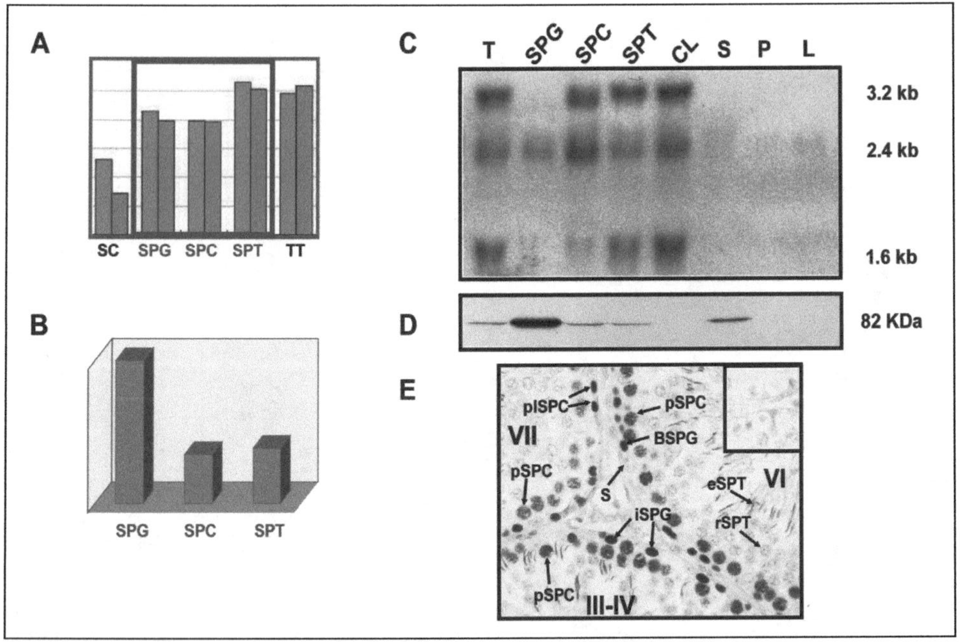

Figure 7. Transcriptomic and proteomic differential expression profiles for minichromosome maintenance protein 7 (MCM7) during rat spermatogenesis. Adapted from reference 111. A) mRNA levels in the 3 germ cell types, Sertoli cells and total testis from 2 independent experiments—Affymetrix data; (B) Relative levels of proteins in the 3 cell types—2D-DIGE data; (C) MCM7 northern blot of rat testis mRNA and for different isolated testicular cell types and total testis; (D) Western blot analysis of MCM7 protein in isolated rat testicular cells. TT: total testis; SC: Sertoli cell; SPG: spermatogonia; SPC: pachytene spermatocyte; SPT: early spermatid; CL: Late spermatid cytoplasmic lobes/residual bodies; PC: peritubular cell; LC: Leydig cell. (E) Immunolocalization of MCM7 protein in the adult rat testis. A transverse testis section showing strong labeling of the nuclei of intermediate and type B spermatogonia and preleptotene spermatocytes (iSPG, BSPG, and plSPC, respectively) and a weaker signal in the nuclei of pachytene spermatocytes (pSPC) nuclei. Note that as spermatocyte differentiation proceeds (stages III to VII), the intensity of MCM7 labeling decreases, and that early spermatids are not labeled. No signal was observed in Sertoli cells, early and elongated spermatids (S, rSPT, and eSPT, respectively). Roman numerals indicate stages of the seminiferous epithelial cycle in rat species [112]. Experiments were carried out with preimmune serum as a negative control.

Conclusions and Future Directions

The large series of "Omics" datasets for the testis collected to date constitute a valuable asset for scientists and doctors working in the field of male reproduction. They may provide us with insight into the molecular events controlling spermatogenesis and a more detailed understanding of human reproductive disorders, making it possible to develop new therapeutic strategies. The contribution made by many groups, through projects carried out on a small scale, as reported here, is vital. The rational compilation of this enormous set of data in a repository system, such as the GermOnline database[107] would itself be a very useful step before the hypothesis-driven mining of the collected data with dedicated bioinformatics tools.

However, as Richard Ivell warned more than a decade ago, "*All that glisters is not gold*", and it should be borne in mind that common testis gene transcripts are not always what they seem.[108] Furthermore, simply determining gene expression or protein levels may not be meaningful. The way in which genes or proteins interact with other genes/proteins in response to internal or external signals remains a key issue. Microarray profiling experiments bridge the gap between DNA sequence annotation data and information on protein structure, function and network interaction.[109] They do so by providing data on mRNA levels and exon composition in different cell types, at different developmental stages. In the near future, it should be possible, using novel all-exon and tiling arrays covering all known exons and the complete genomes of rodents and *H. sapiens*, to determine properties of the testicular somatic and germ cell transcriptomes, including transcript length, concentration and alternative splicing patterns.[110] These experiments should also make it possible to identify novel non coding RNAs not detected by current approaches.

Proteomics has already provided important new information concerning basic somatic and germ cell function and organization within the testis and has expanded our understanding of spermatogenesis. Technological innovations, improving the sensitivity of instruments and protein quantification, and concerning posttranslational modifications, are rapidly occurring. This will no doubt attract new biologists and clinicians to this field. However, starry-eyed newcomers to proteomics technologies should proceed with caution in this field, which remains highly technical. They would be prudent to rely on expert platforms to provide them with top-quality biological material, allowing them to concentrate on the biological questions they wish to address.

References

1. Jégou B. The Sertoli-germ cell communication network in mammals. Int Rev Cytol 1993; 147:25-96.
2. Jégou B, Sharpe RM. Paracrine mechanisms in testicular control. In: de Kretser DM, ed. Molecular Biology of the Male Reproduction System. New York: Academic Press, 1993:271-310.
3. Sharpe RM. Regulation of spermatogenesis. In: Knobil E, Neill JD, eds. The Physiology of Reproduction. 2nd ed. New York: Lippincott Williams & Wilkins, 1994:1363-1436.
4. Zhao GQ, Garbers DL. Male germ cell specification and differentiation. Dev Cell 2002; 2:537-547.
5. Gnessi L, Fabbri A, Spera G. Gonadal peptides as mediators of development and functional control of the testis: An integrated system with hormones and local environment. Endocr Rev 1997; 18:541-609.
6. Jégou B, Pineau C, Dupaix A. Paracrine control of testis function. In: Wang C, ed. Male Reproductive Function. Endocrine Update Series. Berlin: Kluwer Academic, 1999:41-64.
7. Matzuk MM, Lamb DJ. Genetic dissection of mammalian fertility pathways. Nat Cell Biol 2002; 4:s41-49.
8. de Rooij DG, de Boer P. Specific arrests of spermatogenesis in genetically modified and mutant mice. Cytogenet Genome Res 2003; 103:267-276.
9. Wrobel G, Primig M. Mammalian male germ cells are fertile ground for expression profiling of sexual reproduction. Reproduction 2005; 129:1-7.
10. Huang SY, Lin JH, Chen YH et al. A reference map and identification of porcine testis proteins using 2-DE and MS. Proteomics 2005; 5:4205-4212.
11. Com E, Evrard B, Roepstorff P et al. New insights into the rat spermatogonial proteome: Identification of 156 additional proteins. Mol Cell Proteomics 2003; 2:248-261.
12. Essader AS, Cargile BJ, Bundy JL et al. A comparison of immobilized pH gradient isoelectric focusing and strong-cation-exchange chromatography as a first dimension in shotgun proteomics. Proteomics 2005; 5:24-34.

13. Rolland AD, Evrard B, Guitton N et al. Two-dimensional fluorescence difference gel electrophoresis analysis of spermatogenesis in the rat. J Proteome Res 2007; 6:683-697.
14. Wilkins MR, Sanchez JC, Gooley AA et al. Progress in proteome projects: Why all proteins expressed by a genome should be identified and how to do it. Biotechnol Genet Eng Rev 1995; 13:19-50.
15. Aebersold R, Mann M. Mass spectrometry-based proteomics. Nature 2003; 422:198-207.
16. Waterston RH, Lindblad-Toh K, Birney E et al. Initial sequencing and comparative analysis of the mouse genome. Nature 2002; 420:520-562.
17. Lander ES, Linton LM, Birren B et al. Initial sequencing and analysis of the human genome. Nature 2001; 409:860-921.
18. Venter JC, Adams MD, Myers EW et al. The sequence of the human genome. Science 2001; 291:1304-1351.
19. Hubbard TJ, Aken BL, Beal K et al. Ensembl 2007. Nucleic Acids Res 2007; 35:D610-617.
20. Modrek B, Resch A, Grasso C et al. Genome-wide detection of alternative splicing in expressed sequences of human genes. Nucleic Acids Res 2001; 29:2850-2859.
21. Johnson JM, Castle J, Garrett-Engele P et al. Genome-wide survey of human alternative pre-mRNA splicing with exon junction microarrays. Science 2003; 302:2141-2144.
22. Mann M, Jensen ON. Proteomic analysis of post-translational modifications. Nat Biotechnol 2003; 21:255-261.
23. Kettman JR, Coleclough C, Frey JR et al. Clonal proteomics: One gene—Family of proteins. Proteomics 2002; 2:624-631.
24. Humphery-Smith I. A human proteome project with a beginning and an end. Proteomics 2004; 4:2519-2521.
25. Mueller M, Martens L, Apweiler R. Annotating the human proteome: Beyond establishing a parts list. Biochim Biophys Acta 2007; 1774:175-191.
26. Conrads KA, Yi M, Simpson KA et al. A combined proteome and microarray investigation of inorganic phosphate-induced preosteoblast cells. Mol Cell Proteomics 2005; 4:1284-1296.
27. Chen G, Gharib TG, Huang CC et al. Discordant protein and mRNA expression in lung adenocarcinomas. Mol Cell Proteomics 2002; 1:304-313.
28. Gygi SP, Rochon Y, Franza BR et al. Correlation between protein and mRNA abundance in yeast. Mol Cell Biol 1999; 19:1720-1730.
29. Small CL, Shima JE, Uzumcu M et al. Profiling gene expression during the differentiation and development of the murine embryonic gonad. Biol Reprod 2005; 72:492-501.
30. Nef S, Schaad O, Stallings NR et al. Gene expression during sex determination reveals a robust female genetic program at the onset of ovarian development. Dev Biol 2005; 287:361-377.
31. Beverdam A, Koopman P. Expression profiling of purified mouse gonadal somatic cells during the critical time window of sex determination reveals novel candidate genes for human sexual dysgenesis syndromes. Hum Mol Genet 2006; 15:417-431.
32. Wilhelm D, Huang E, Svingen T et al. Comparative proteomic analysis to study molecular events during gonad development in mice. Genesis 2006; 44:168-176.
33. Han BK, Kim JN, Shin JH et al. Proteome analysis of chicken embryonic gonads: Identification of major proteins from cultured gonadal primordial germ cells. Mol Reprod Dev 2005; 72:521-529.
34. Guillaume E, Dupaix A, Moertz E et al. Proteome analysis of spermatogonia: Identification of a first set of 53 spermatogonial proteins. Proteome 2000, in press.
35. Ito T, Chiba T, Ozawa R et al. A comprehensive two-hybrid analysis to explore the yeast protein interactome. Proc Natl Acad Sci USA 2001; 98:4569-4574.
36. Hamra FK, Schultz N, Chapman KM et al. Defining the spermatogonial stem cell. Dev Biol 2004; 269:393-410.
37. Oatley JM, Avarbock MR, Telaranta AI et al. Identifying genes important for spermatogonial stem cell self-renewal and survival. Proc Natl Acad Sci USA 2006; 103:9524-9529.
38. Costoya JA, Hobbs RM, Barna M et al. Essential role of Plzf in maintenance of spermatogonial stem cells. Nat Genet 2004; 36:653-659.
39. Chen C, Ouyang W, Grigura V et al. ERM is required for transcriptional control of the spermatogonial stem cell niche. Nature 2005; 436:1030-1034.
40. Hofmann MC, Braydich-Stolle L, Dym M. Isolation of male germ-line stem cells; influence of GDNF. Dev Biol 2005; 279:114-124.
41. Chu DS, Liu H, Nix P et al. Sperm chromatin proteomics identifies evolutionarily conserved fertility factors. Nature 2006; 443:101-105.
42. Govin J, Caron C, Escoffier E et al. Post-meiotic shifts in HSPA2/HSP70.2 chaperone activity during mouse spermatogenesis. J Biol Chem 2006; 281:37888-37892.

43. Zhu YF, Cui YG, Guo XJ et al. Proteomic analysis of effect of hyperthermia on spermatogenesis in adult male mice. J Proteome Res 2006; 5:2217-2225.
44. Reinke V, Smith HE, Nance J et al. A global profile of germline gene expression in C. elegans. Mol Cell 2000; 6:605-616.
45. Divina P, Vlcek C, Strnad P et al. Global transcriptome analysis of the C57BL/6J mouse testis by SAGE: Evidence for nonrandom gene order. BMC Genomics 2005; 6:29.
46. Yao J, Chiba T, Sakai J et al. Mouse testis transcriptome revealed using serial analysis of gene expression. Mamm Genome 2004; 15:433-451.
47. Fox MS, Ares VX, Turek PJ et al. Feasibility of global gene expression analysis in testicular biopsies from infertile men. Mol Reprod Dev 2003; 66:403-421.
48. Wu SM, Baxendale V, Chen Y et al. Analysis of mouse germ-cell transcriptome at different stages of spermatogenesis by SAGE: Biological significance. Genomics 2004; 84:971-981.
49. Shima JE, McLean DJ, McCarrey JR et al. The murine testicular transcriptome: Characterizing gene expression in the testis during the progression of spermatogenesis. Biol Reprod 2004; 71:319-330.
50. Namekawa SH, Park PJ, Zhang LF et al. Postmeiotic sex chromatin in the male germline of mice. Curr Biol 2006; 16:660-667.
51. Chalmel F, Rolland AD, Niederhauser-Wiederkehr C et al. The conserved transcriptome in human and rodent male gametogenesis. Proc Natl Acad Sci USA 2007; 104:8346-8351.
52. Schlecht U, Demougin P, Koch R et al. Expression profiling of mammalian male meiosis and gametogenesis identifies novel candidate genes for roles in the regulation of fertility. Mol Biol Cell 2004; 15:1031-1043.
53. Almstrup K, Nielsen JE, Hansen MA et al. Analysis of cell-type-specific gene expression during mouse spermatogenesis. Biol Reprod 2004; 70:1751-1761.
54. Ellis PJ, Furlong RA, Wilson A et al. Modulation of the mouse testis transcriptome during postnatal development and in selected models of male infertility. Mol Hum Reprod 2004; 10:271-281.
55. Clemente EJ, Furlong RA, Loveland KL et al. Gene expression study in the juvenile mouse testis: Identification of stage-specific molecular pathways during spermatogenesis. Mamm Genome 2006; 17:956-975.
56. Schultz N, Hamra FK, Garbers DL. A multitude of genes expressed solely in meiotic or postmeiotic spermatogenic cells offers a myriad of contraceptive targets. Proc Natl Acad Sci USA 2003; 100:12201-12206.
57. O'Shaughnessy PJ, Fleming L, Baker PJ et al. Identification of developmentally regulated genes in the somatic cells of the mouse testis using serial analysis of gene expression. Biol Reprod 2003; 69:797-808.
58. Ge RS, Dong Q, Sottas CM et al. Gene expression in rat leydig cells during development from the progenitor to adult stage: A cluster analysis. Biol Reprod 2005; 72:1405-1415.
59. Ellis PJ, Clemente EJ, Ball P et al. Deletions on mouse Yq lead to upregulation of multiple X- and Y-linked transcripts in spermatids. Hum Mol Genet 2005; 14:2705-2715.
60. Toure A, Clemente EJ, Ellis P et al. Identification of novel Y chromosome encoded transcripts by testis transcriptome analysis of mice with deletions of the Y chromosome long arm. Genome Biol 2005; 6:R102.
61. Beissbarth T, Borisevich I, Horlein A et al. Analysis of CREM-dependent gene expression during mouse spermatogenesis. Mol Cell Endocrinol 2003; 212:29-39.
62. Chaudhary J, Sadler-Riggleman I, Ague JM et al. The helix-loop-helix inhibitor of differentiation (ID) proteins induce post-mitotic terminally differentiated Sertoli cells to reenter the cell cycle and proliferate. Biol Reprod 2005; 72:1205-1217.
63. Cheng Y, Buffone MG, Kouadio M et al. Abnormal sperm in mice lacking the Taf7l gene. Mol Cell Biol 2007; 27:2582-9.
64. Cagney G, Park S, Chung C et al. Human tissue profiling with multidimensional protein identification technology. J Proteome Res 2005; 4:1757-1767.
65. Iguchi N, Tobias JW, Hecht NB. Expression profiling reveals meiotic male germ cell mRNAs that are translationally up- and down-regulated. Proc Natl Acad Sci USA 2006; 103:7712-7717.
66. Ostermeier GC, Dix DJ, Miller D et al. Spermatozoal RNA profiles of normal fertile men. Lancet 2002; 360:772-777.
67. Ostermeier GC, Goodrich RJ, Moldenhauer JS et al. A suite of novel human spermatozoal RNAs. J Androl 2005; 26:70-74.
68. Wang H, Zhou Z, Xu M et al. A spermatogenesis-related gene expression profile in human spermatozoa and its potential clinical applications. J Mol Med 2004; 82:317-324.
69. Zhao Y, Li Q, Yao C et al. Characterization and quantification of mRNA transcripts in ejaculated spermatozoa of fertile men by serial analysis of gene expression. Hum Reprod 2006; 21:1583-1590.

70. Martinez-Heredia J, Estanyol JM, Ballesca JL et al. Proteomic identification of human sperm proteins. Proteomics 2006; 6:4356-4369.
71. Johnston DS, Wooters J, Kopf GS et al. Analysis of the human sperm proteome. Ann NY Acad Sci 2005; 1061:190-202.
72. Dorus S, Busby SA, Gerike U et al. Genomic and functional evolution of the Drosophila melanogaster sperm proteome. Nat Genet 2006; 38:1440-1445.
73. Anderson NL, Anderson NG. Proteome and proteomics: New technologies, new concepts, and new words. Electrophoresis 1998; 19:1853-1861.
74. Cao W, Gerton GL, Moss SB. Proteomic profiling of accessory structures from the mouse sperm flagellum. Mol Cell Proteomics 2006; 5:801-810.
75. Kim YH, Haidl G, Schaefer M et al. Compartmentalization of a unique ADP/ATP carrier protein SFEC (Sperm Flagellar Energy Carrier, AAC4) with glycolytic enzymes in the fibrous sheath of the human sperm flagellar principal piece. Dev Biol 2007; 302:463-476.
76. Stein KK, Go JC, Lane WS et al. Proteomic analysis of sperm regions that mediate sperm-egg interactions. Proteomics 2006; 6:3533-3543.
77. Baker MA, Witherdin R, Hetherington L et al. Identification of post-translational modifications that occur during sperm maturation using difference in two-dimensional gel electrophoresis. Proteomics 2005; 5:1003-1012.
78. Sleight SB, Miranda PV, Plaskett NW et al. Isolation and proteomic analysis of mouse sperm detergent-resistant membrane fractions: Evidence for dissociation of lipid rafts during capacitation. Biol Reprod 2005; 73:721-729.
79. Ficarro S, Chertihin O, Westbrook VA et al. Phosphoproteome analysis of capacitated human sperm: Evidence of tyrosine phosphorylation of a kinase-anchoring protein 3 and valosin-containing protein/p97 during capacitation. J Biol Chem 2003; 278:11579-11589.
80. Lalancette C, Faure RL, Leclerc P. Identification of the proteins present in the bull sperm cytosolic fraction enriched in tyrosine kinase activity: A proteomic approach. Proteomics 2006; 6:4523-4540.
81. Bohring C, Krause E, Habermann B et al. Isolation and identification of sperm membrane antigens recognized by antisperm antibodies, and their possible role in immunological infertility disease. Mol Hum Reprod 2001; 7:113-118.
82. Bohring C, Krause W. Characterization of spermatozoa surface antigens by antisperm antibodies and its influence on acrosomal exocytosis. Am J Reprod Immunol 2003; 50:411-419.
83. Paradowska A, Bohring C, Krause E et al. Identification of evolutionary conserved mouse sperm surface antigens by human antisperm antibodies (ASA) from infertile patients. Am J Reprod Immunol 2006; 55:321-330.
84. Fijak M, Iosub R, Schneider E et al. Identification of immunodominant autoantigens in rat autoimmune orchitis. J Pathol 2005; 207:127-138.
85. McLean DJ, Friel PJ, Pouchnik D et al. Oligonucleotide microarray analysis of gene expression in follicle-stimulating hormone-treated rat Sertoli cells. Mol Endocrinol 2002; 16:2780-2792.
86. Sadate-Ngatchou PI, Pouchnik DJ, Griswold MD. Follicle-stimulating hormone induced changes in gene expression of murine testis. Mol Endocrinol 2004; 18:2805-2816.
87. Meachem SJ, Ruwanpura SM, Ziolkowski J et al. Developmentally distinct in vivo effects of FSH on proliferation and apoptosis during testis maturation. J Endocrinol 2005; 186:429-446.
88. Sadate-Ngatchou PI, Pouchnik DJ, Griswold MD. Identification of testosterone-regulated genes in testes of hypogonadal mice using oligonucleotide microarray. Mol Endocrinol 2004; 18:422-433.
89. Zhou Q, Shima JE, Nie R et al. Androgen-regulated transcripts in the neonatal mouse testis as determined through microarray analysis. Biol Reprod 2005; 72:1010-1019.
90. Petrusz P, Jeyaraj DA, Grossman G. Microarray analysis of androgen-regulated gene expression in testis: The use of the androgen-binding protein (ABP)-transgenic mouse as a model. Reprod Biol Endocrinol 2005; 3:70.
91. Meng J, Holdcraft RW, Shima JE et al. Androgens regulate the permeability of the blood-testis barrier. Proc Natl Acad Sci USA 2005; 102:16696-16700.
92. Eacker SM, Shima JE, Connolly CM et al. Transcriptional profiling of androgen receptor (AR) mutants suggests instructive and permissive roles of AR signaling in germ cell development. Mol Endocrinol 2007; 21:895-907.
93. Denolet E, De Gendt K, Allemeersch J et al. The effect of a sertoli cell-selective knockout of the androgen receptor on testicular gene expression in prepubertal mice. Mol Endocrinol 2006; 20:321-334.
94. Khaitovich P, Hellmann I, Enard W et al. Parallel patterns of evolution in the genomes and transcriptomes of humans and chimpanzees. Science 2005; 309:1850-1854.
95. Voolstra C, Tautz D, Farbrother P et al. Contrasting evolution of expression differences in the testis between species and subspecies of the house mouse. Genome Res 2007; 17:42-49.

96. Kan Z, Garrett-Engele PW, Johnson JM et al. Evolutionarily conserved and diverged alternative splicing events show different expression and functional profiles. Nucleic Acids Res 2005; 33:5659-5666.
97. Xu Q, Modrek B, Lee C. Genome-wide detection of tissue-specific alternative splicing in the human transcriptome. Nucleic Acids Res 2002; 30:3754-3766.
98. Yeo G, Holste D, Kreiman G et al. Variation in alternative splicing across human tissues. Genome Biol 2004; 5:R74.
99. Khil PP, Smirnova NA, Romanienko PJ et al. The mouse X chromosome is enriched for sex-biased genes not subject to selection by meiotic sex chromosome inactivation. Nat Genet 2004; 36:642-646.
100. Li Q, Lee BT, Zhang L. Genome-scale analysis of positional clustering of mouse testis-specific genes. BMC Genomics 2005; 6:7.
101. Boutanaev AM, Kalmykova AI, Shevelyov YY et al. Large clusters of coexpressed genes in the Drosophila genome. Nature 2002; 420:666-669.
102. Harris MA. The Gene Ontology (GO) project in 2006. Nucleic Acids Res 2006; 34:D322-326.
103. Chalmel F, Lardenois A, Primig M. Towards understanding the core meiotic transcriptome in mammals and its implications for somatic cancer. Ann NY Acad Sci 2007; 2:2.
104. Liu D, Brockman JM, Dass B et al. Systematic variation in mRNA 3'-processing signals during mouse spermatogenesis. Nucleic Acids Res 2007; 35:234-246.
105. Birney E. The ENCODE (ENCyclopedia Of DNA Elements) project. Science 2004; 306:636-640.
106. Birney E, Stamatoyannopoulos JA, Dutta A et al. Identification and analysis of functional elements in 1% of the human genome by the ENCODE pilot project. Nature 2007; 447:799-816.
107. Primig M, Wiederkehr C, Basavaraj R et al. GermOnline, a new cross-species community annotation database on germ-line development and gametogenesis. Nat Genet 2003; 35:291-292.
108. Ivell R. 'All that glitters is not gold'—Common testis gene transcripts are not always what they seem. Int J Androl 1992; 15:85-92.
109. Gandhi TK, Zhong J, Mathivanan S et al. Analysis of the human protein interactome and comparison with yeast, worm and fly interaction datasets. Nat Genet 2006; 38:285-293.
110. Cheng J, Kapranov P, Drenkow J et al. Transcriptional maps of 10 human chromosomes at 5-nucleotide resolution. Science 2005; 308:1149-1154.
111. Com E, Rolland A, Guerrois M et al. Identification, molecular cloning and cellular distribution of the rat homologue of Minichromosome maintenance protein 7 (MCM7) in the rat testis. Mol Reprod Dev 2006; 73:866-877.
112. Leblond CP, Clermont Y. Definition of the stages of the cycle of the seminiferous epithelium in the rat. Ann NY Acad Aci 1952; 55:548-573.

CHAPTER 3

Estrogens and Spermatogenesis

Chandrima Shaha*

Introduction

For many years androgens were thought to be the primary hormones required for proper functioning of the male reproductive system, and testes were shown to be the major producers of the hormone. In the 1970s it was recognized that in addition to androgens testes were also a source of estrogens, and the intratesticular concentration of estrogens was higher than levels present in the serum of females of reproductive age.[1,2] Since then there has been an interest in the study of the role of estrogens in the male. However, in recent years a great interest has been regenerated to decipher the role of estrogens in the control of male fertility because of various developments. For example, discovery of the estrogen receptor β (ERβ) in the male[3] was an important development ,and the evidence emerging from mice with targeted disruption of estrogen receptors showing defects in male fertility[4] was another provocative evidence of the importance of estrogens in male reproduction. In addition, the description of reduction in sperm counts and increase in the incidence of testicular tumors in men to which environmental estrogens were causally linked[5] were also important observations on pathology-inducing effects of estrogens. It is now established that estrogens are involved in numerous physiological processes in the male, for example, bone turnover, behavior and the cardiovascular system, but controversy exists as to whether male fertility over the past five decades has truly shown a decline[6] due to the relatively low levels of estrogens in the environment that humans are exposed to.[7] As a result of this renewed interest, the role of estrogens in male reproductive physiology is rapidly being redefined. It is therefore pertinent that a comprehensive evaluation of the data on the role of estrogens in the male is made. However, because of the ambiguity in the definition of precise function of the estrogens in the male, extensive research into the effects of the hormone on the male reproductive system is warranted.[8]

The most direct studies on effects of estrogens have been through administration of estrogens to animals and investigating their reproductive potential. For these studies, variations in doses have been shown to demonstrate diverse effects. Administration of estrogens and xenoestrogens during fetal and neonatal development has been reported to be associated with a series of male reproductive disturbances, such as impairment of sperm production, cryptorchidism, epididymal defects, weakened fertility, and an increased incidence of testicular cancer.[9-13] When the gene knockout technology was developed, it was shown that mice lacking a functional estrogen receptor α (ERα) receptor gene were infertile and this was the first definitive demonstration of the importance of estrogen in male fertility.[14-16] The cause of infertility in these mice were primarily due to a defect in efferent ductule development and function.[17] In addition, mice lacking a functional aromatase gene (aromatase knockout, ArKO), aromatase being the enzyme necessary for the conversion of testosterone to estrogens were, reported to be

*Chandrima Shaha—Cell Death and Differentiation Laboratory, National Institute of Immunology, Aruna Asaf Ali Marg, New Delhi 110067, India. Email: cshaha@nii.res.in

Molecular Mechanisms in Spermatogenesis, edited by C. Yan Cheng.

infertile.[18] Thus, lessons provided by knock-out (KO) mice for ERα and/or estrogen receptor β (ERβ) as well as aromatase, provided compelling evidence for a role of estrogens in spermatogenesis and male fertility. In this chapter, a review of current knowledge on estrogen production in the testis, estrogen receptors and the effects of estrogens in the testis is discussed.

Estrogens and Antiestrogens

Estrogenic activity is a property shared by a number of polycyclic compounds containing, in most cases, a phenolic ring and another oxygenated cycle located at the opposite end of the molecule (Fig. 1A). There is a large internal hydrocarbon moiety that contributes to an optimal orientation of these two polar functions for selective H-bonding with specific amino acid residues of the ligand-binding pocket of estrogen receptor (ER). Other than steroid hormones, flavones, isoflavones and coumestanes also are potent estrogens.[19] All these chemicals are linear, planar molecules. The planar feature of the estrogens gives a closed conformation to the receptor upon binding.[20] This structural property distinguishes these strong ER agonists from a variety of angular ligands, *gem*-diphenylethylenes, triphenylethylenes, diarylimidazolines and diarylpiperazines,[21,22] which maintain the ligand-binding pocket in an open conformation.[23] Linear, planar molecules are currently referred to as type I estrogens, while angular molecules are categorized as type II estrogens (Fig. 1A,B). Grafting of a reactive group, i.e., amido (ICI 164,384) or sulfoxide (ICI 182,780; RU 58,668) via a long alkyl side chain onto estradiol at positions of 7α and 11α totally abrogates its estrogenicity and converts it into a "pure" antiestrogen (Fig. 1C). Selective estrogen receptor modulators or SERMs are synthetic compounds mainly derived from type II estrogens. The large majority of SERMs contains a dialkylaminoethyl side chain (Fig. 1D) which is responsible for their antagonistic activity.[24,25] Like the long alkyl side chain characterizing pure antiestrogens described above, dialkylaminoethyl side chains of SERMs protrude from the binding pocket,[26] allowing for interactions with critical amino acid residues in the receptor.

Overview of Spermatogenesis

Spermatogenesis is a complex process of male germ cell proliferation and maturation from diploid spermatogonia through meiosis to mature haploid spermatozoa.[27] Spermatogonia arise from the primordial germ cells, which migrate into the genital ridge during fetal life.[28] Under the influence of the Y-chromosome-bearing stromal cells of the developing gonad, they differentiate into gonocytes, the male germ cell precursors and undergo mitotic arrest.[29] After birth, they are reactivated and differentiate into spermatogonia that go through a cycle of division and differentiation with cellular apoptosis keeping the number of cells in check.[29,30,31] Spermatogenesis in the adult takes place within the seminiferous tubules of the testis which consist of the seminiferous epithelium, comprising of germ cells and supportive somatic Sertoli cells that stand on the basement membrane which is surrounded by the peritubular myoid cells. The interstitial tissue between the seminiferous tubules contain androgen-producing Leydig cells and interstitial macrophages. Developing germ cells in different stages of differentiation form intimate associations with the Sertoli cells. The germ cells are arranged in defined cellular associations that constitute the cycle of the seminiferous epithelium, and each particular association of germ cells is referred to as a stage.[32] The cycle of the seminiferous epithelium is the time interval between the appearance of the same stage at a certain point of the tubule.[33-35] Spermatogonia, the stem germ cells in the testis include type A spermatogonia, and type B spermatogonia. Spermatogonia undergo continuous mitoses to produce a large number of germ cells available for entry into meiosis. After the last mitosis of type B spermatogonia, preleptotene primary spermatocytes are formed and these cells initiate meiotic division. After completion of the meiotic division, the differentiation of round spermatids into the mature elongated spermatid take place through the process of spermiogenesis. This process involves formation and development of the acrosome and flagellum, condensation of the chromatin, change in shape of the nucleus, and removal of the cytoplasm before release of the spermatid during spermiation.[32]

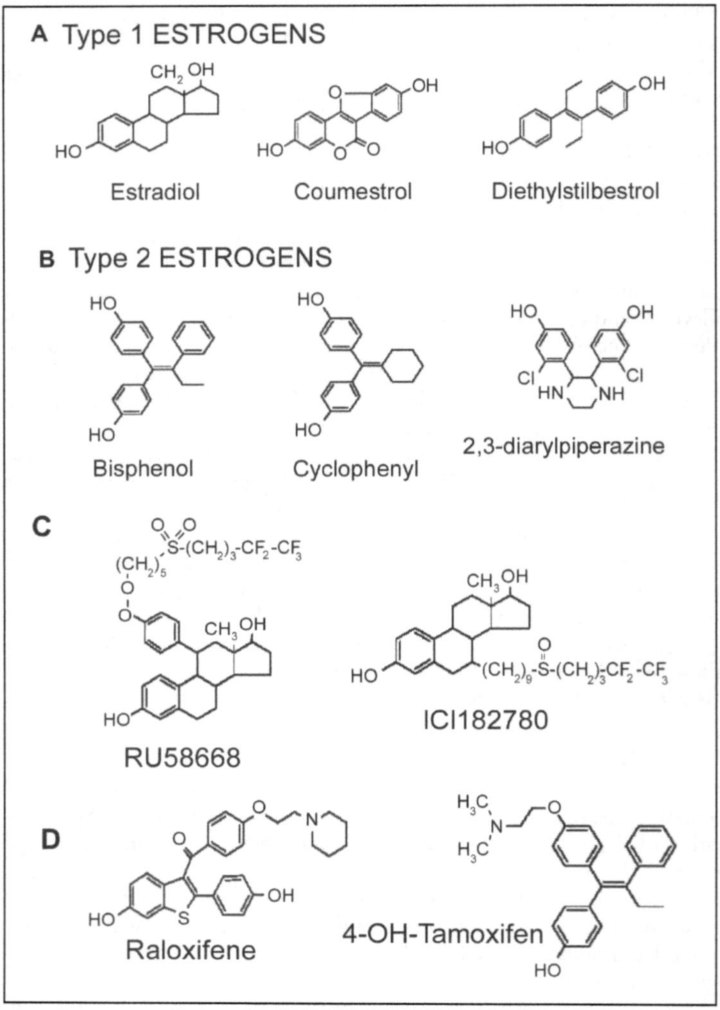

Figure 1. Structures of estrogens and antiestrogens. A) Structures of type I estrogens which are linear, planar molecules that include estradiol, coumestrol and diethylstilbestrol. B) Structures of type II estrogens which are angular molecules that includes bisphenol A, Cyclophenyl and 2,3-diarylpiperazine. C) Structures of pure antiestrogens, RU58668 and ICI 182,780. Grafting of a reactive group, i.e., sulfoxide (ICI 182,780; RU 58,668) via a long alkyl side chain ("spacer") onto estradiol at 7α or 11β totally abrogates its estrogenicity and converts it into a "pure" antiestrogen. D) Structure of Selective Estrogen Receptor Modulators, namely raloxifene and 4-hydroxytamoxifen. These are synthetic compounds mainly derived from type II estrogens. The large majority of Selective Estrogen Receptor Modulators contains a dialkylaminoethyl side chain which is responsible for their antagonistic activity.

The Gonadotropins and the Hypothalamic-Pituitary Gonadal Axis

Gonadotropins are the major endocrine regulators of spermatogenesis.[36-38] Luteinizing hormone (LH) acts on the Leydig cell to stimulate the secretion of androgens, namely testosterone, which in turn acts on androgen receptors in the seminiferous epithelium to control spermatogenesis. Follicle stimulating hormone (FSH) receptors on the Sertoli cells react to FSH and regulate spermatogenesis by stimulating the production of numerous Sertoli cell factors. The role of androgens is very well demonstrated in the hypogonadal (*hpg*) mouse where the androgens have been shown to fuel all phases of germ cell development.[39] Transgenic mice with targeted disruptions of the FSH receptor gene[40] or the FSH β-subunit gene[41] are fertile and display all stages of germ cell development, suggesting that FSH is not an absolute requirement for fertility. However, in these mice testes are smaller and less sperm are produced with many defective spermatozoa.[42] Therefore, full fertility relies on the delicate balance of the hypothalamic-pituitary-testis axis. It is important to understand the functioning of the hypothalamic-pituitary gonadal axis in the context of estrogens because estrogens provide the feedback stimulus along with androgens (Fig. 2). The reproductive hormonal axis consists of three main components: (A) the hypothalamus, (B) the pituitary gland, (C) the testis. This axis functions in a strongly regulated manner to produce optimal concentrations of circulating steroids required for normal male sexual development, sexual function and fertility.

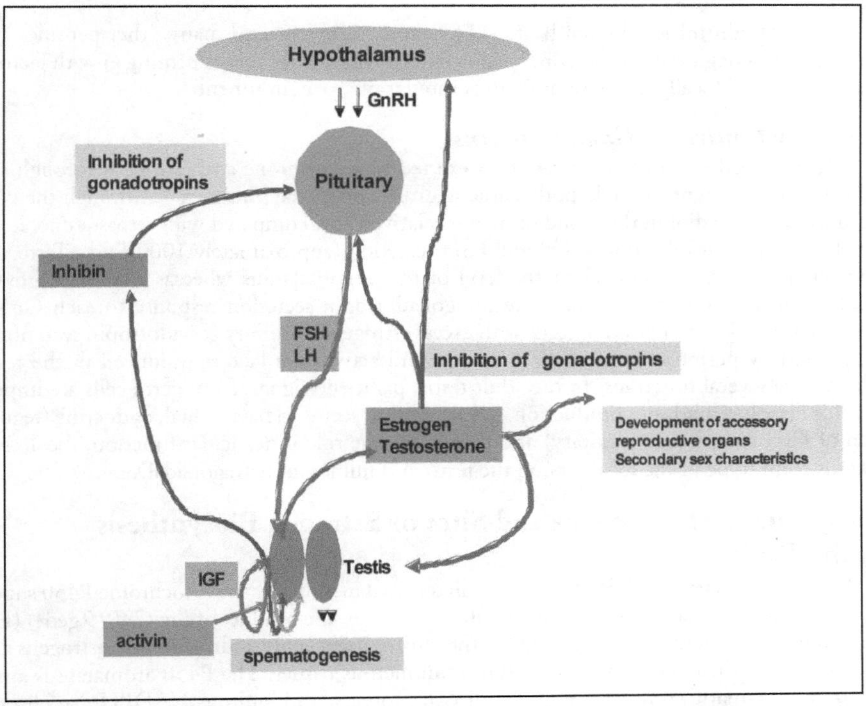

Figure 2. The hypothalamic-pituitary axis. A diagram illustrating the orientation of the hypothalamic-pituitary axis and the feedback loops with inhibin and the steroid hormones secreted by the testis. The paracrine routes in the testis are also indicated. The cell types expressing ERα and ERβ are indicated as well.

Hypothalamus

The integrating center of the reproductive hormonal axis is the hypothalamus (Fig. 2) that is the site of production of the peptide hormone gonadotropin-releasing hormone (GnRH) which is delivered to the adenohypophysis of the pituitary gland by a short portal venous system where it stimulates the synthesis and release of gonadotropic hormones LH and FSH.[7] The release of GnRH is seasonal (peaks in the spring), circadian (highest testosterone levels are in the a.m.) and pulsatile (peaks occur every 90-120 minutes). The GnRH production from hypothalamus is under feedback control from gonadal hormones.

Pituitary

LH and FSH are glycopeptides consisting of two peptide chains (α and β) synthesized by the pituitary cells and are secreted into the general circulation thereby transporting to the testis.[43] LH and FSH share a common α peptide chain (α chain) with thyroid-stimulating hormone and human chorionic gonadotropin and differ from each other by the presence of a specific β chain, the latter providing specificity of biologic action.[44] The pituitary also secretes prolactin which affects testicular function indirectly by inhibiting GnRH release from the hypothalamus and therefore LH and FSH secretion from the pituitary. Prolactin also directly inhibits pituitary gonadotrophic cells and the Leydig cells of the testes.

Testis

Testicular control is achieved by LH, FSH and androgens and many other peptides and growth factors (e.g., inhibin, activin, insulin-like growth factor 1, transforming growth factors) that are secreted locally in the seminiferous tubular microenvironment.[45]

Feedback Control of Gonadotropins

Negative-feedback of GnRH release is exerted by testosterone and estrogens through steroid receptors present in the hypothalamic neurons and in the pituitary.[46] Although the concentration of estradiol in the blood of men is relatively low compared with testosterone, it is a much more potent inhibitor of LH and FSH secretion (approximately 1000-fold). Testosterone acts primarily to feedback at the level of the hypothalamus whereas estrogens provide feedback to the pituitary to modulate the gonadotropin secretion response to each GnRH surge. Several disease states can occur with excess estrogens. Pituitary gonadotropin secretion is suppressed by peripheral estrogens.[47] Inhibin and activin are factors produced in the testis which have several functions. In the adult testis, paracrine signals from germ cells are important for Sertoli cell inhibin production. While inhibin seems to have a dual, endocrine (regulation of FSH secretion in pituitary) and para/autocrine role in testicular function, the activin actions seem to be of the local type in the testis and numerous extragonadal sites.[48,49]

Biosynthesis of Estrogens and Sites of Estrogen Biosynthesis in the Testis

Estrogen biosynthesis is catalyzed by a microsomal member of the cytochrome P450 superfamily, namely aromatase cytochrome P450 (P450arom, the product of the *CYP19* gene) (Fig. 3). Aromatase is a terminal enzyme which transforms irreversibly androgens into estrogens and it is present in the endoplasmic reticulum of numerous tissues. The P450 aromatase is a microsomal enzymatic complex composed of two proteins: a ubiquitous NADPH-cytochrome P450 reductase and a cytochrome P450 aromatase, which contains the heme and the steroid binding pocket. Six isoforms of cytochrome-dependent mono-oxygenases (CYP) are involved in the biosynthesis of various steroid hormones, starting from cholesterol—CYP11A, CYP17, CYP19, CYP11B1, CYP21B, and CYP11B2.[50] The rate-limiting step in all steroid hormone biosynthesis is the cleavage of the side chain of cholesterol by CYP11A to form the C21 steroids, pregnenolone and progesterone (Fig. 3). Hydroxylation and subsequent cleavage of the two-carbon side chain of the C21 steroids by the CYP17 (17-α hydroxylase activity/C17-20

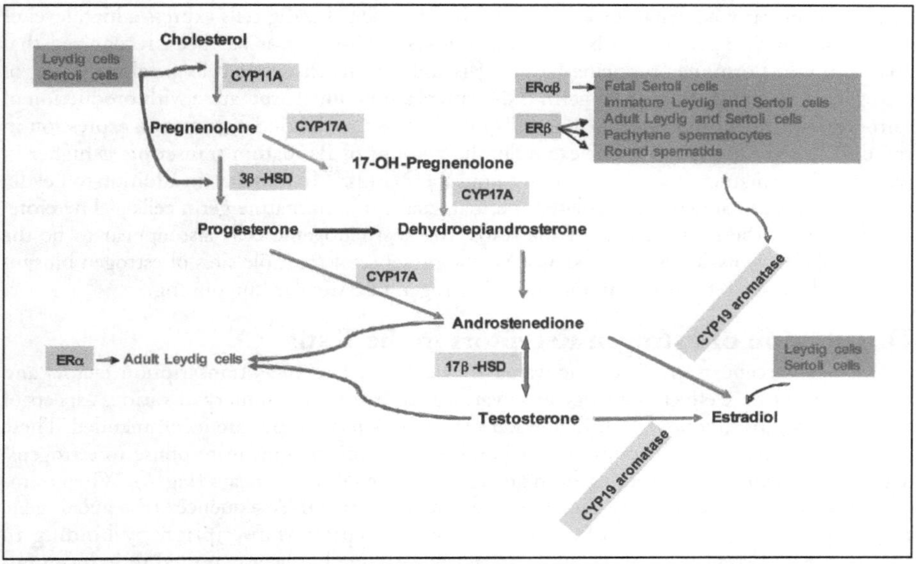

Figure 3. Synthesis of estradiol. Figure shows the primary routes of estrogen biosynthesis in the testis. The first and rate-limiting step in the synthesis of all steroid hormones is conversion of cholesterol to pregnenolone that involves the cleavage of a 6-carbon group from cholesterol. CYP 11A, the cholesterol side chain cleavage cytochrome P450 is used for the purpose. Pregnenolone is converted to progesterone through the use of 3 β-hydroxysteroid dehydrogenase. Hydroxylation and subsequent cleavage of the two-carbon side chain of the C21 steroids by the CYP17 (17-α hydroxylase activity/C17-20 lyase activity) yields the C19 steroids, androstenedione and dehydroepiandrosterone. Testosterone is formed from the precursor, androstenedione and estrogens are ultimately formed by aromatization of androstenedione and testosterone, catalyzed by the CYP19 (aromatase).

lyase activity) yields the C19 steroids, androstenedione and dehydroepiandrosterone. While testosterone is formed from the precursor, androstenedione,[51] estrogens are ultimately formed by aromatization of androstenedione and testosterone, catalyzed by the CYP19 (aromatase).[52] In addition to the cytochrome P450, a series of hydroxysteroid dehydrogenases (3β-HSD and 17β -HSD) participate in the biosynthesis of the steroid hormones. The 3β -HSD converts pregnenolone to progesterone, whereas the 17β-HSD converts androstenedione to testosterone. 17β- HSD type 1 and CYP19 catalyze the end steps in 17β-estradiol biosynthesis through androstenedione (Fig. 3). Estrogens are extensively metabolized by a number of oxidative and conjugative reactions that can lead to their deactivation and subsequent elimination. Alternatively, oxidation and conjugation reactions of estrogens may generate metabolites that have distinct biological activities, including altered hormonal properties; genotoxicity, through the formation of reactive species that modify cellular DNA and protein or chemotherapeutic properties as anti-estrogens. They are also potentially anti-angiogenic.

The identification of sites for estrogen biosynthesis is done by identifying aromatase activity and this activity is even visible in embryonic testes. For example, aromatase activity is present in the fetal rat testis around day 19 of gestation.[53] At this stage of development, basal aromatase activity is found in both the immature Leydig cells and Sertoli cells.[54,55] In fact in the neonates, the Sertoli cells are more active in producing estrogens than Leydig cells suggesting that these cells are an important source of estrogen in the postnatal testis.[56] It is during this time that FSH receptors first appear on the Sertoli cells but germ cells do not contain detectable aromatase activity at the early neonatal stage.[57] By adulthood, rodent Leydig cells express a high level of aromatase which is stimulated by LH and steroids.[58] However, it has been recognized that apart from the hormone producing Leydig cells and Sertoli cells, germ cells are also a source of estrogen in the adult. Mature rat germ cells express a functional aromatase with production of estrogens equivalent to that of Leydig cells but there is a variation in aromatase expression in the different germ cell types. For example, the amount of P450arom transcripts is higher in pachytene spermatocytes as compared to round spermatids.[59] In humans, in addition to Leydig cells, aromatase is present in ejaculated spermatozoa and in immature germ cells.[59] Therefore, in addition to the somatic cells of the testis, the spermatogenic cells also appear to be the sources of estrogens. Thus, the evidence for the presence of multiple sites of estrogen biosynthesis in the testis reflects the importance of estrogen in testicular functioning.

Distribution of Estrogen Receptors in the Testis

Estrogen receptors are ligand activated molecules that serve as transcription factors and mediate pleiotropic effect of estrogens on various tissues. For a summary of various aspects of estrogen receptor functioning, several other reviews (see refs. 60-62) are recommended. These receptors orchestrate both transcriptional and nongenomic actions in response to estrogens, xenoestrogens and signals coming from growth factor signaling pathways (Fig. 4). When estrogen binds to its receptors they dimerize and interact with DNA sequences to regulate gene transcription.[63,64] Estrogens can also stimulate or repress transcription by binding to DNA-associated transcription factors.[65] Recently, estrogen has been reported to induce multiple cytosolic signaling processes, such as activation of Src, Ras, Raf, protein kinase C (PKC), protein kinase A (PKA), potassium channels, intracellular calcium levels and nitric oxide (for reviews, see refs. 66-69). Since activation of these signaling molecules depends on cell types studied and the conditions used, the precise nongenomic signaling pathways of estrogen and their functional significance are still controversial.[70-73]

Two types of distinct receptors are expressed, namely, ERα and ERβ.[74] ERs are members of the steroid hormone superfamily of nuclear receptors, which share a common structural architecture and consist of three independent functional domains: the N-terminal or A/B domains, the C or DNA-binding domain, and the D/E/F or ligand-binding domain. Binding of a ligand to the ER causes a series of downstream events, including receptor dimerization, receptor-DNA interactions mediated by EREs present in the promoter region of target genes, recruitment of and interaction with transcription factors, and the formation of a preinitiation complex. Ligand-receptor interactions ultimately cause changes in target gene expression. The N-terminal domain of nuclear receptors encodes an activation function called AF-1, which mediates protein-protein interactions to induce transcriptional activity. The C-terminal or ligand-binding domain contains the AF-2 interacting surface that mediates ligand binding and receptor dimerization to stimulate transcriptional activity.[75] Thus, AF-1 and AF-2 are both involved in mediating the transcriptional activation function of ERs. The most conserved region of the α and β forms of ER is the DNA-binding domain; the positions of the cysteine residues that coordinate the two zinc fingers of the C domain are conserved in both (ERα and ERβ). There is general agreement that ERs function as dimers, and coexpression of ERα and ERβ in the same cell causes the formation of homodimers (ERα/ERα and ERβ/ERβ) or heterodimers (ERα/ERβ), which affect ligand-specificity. The relative amounts of ERα and ERβ in a given tissue are key determinants of cellular responses to estrogen and other ER agonists and antagonists.[76] The interactions between ERs and EREs are mediated by other factors, including the ability of ERβ to modulate ERα transcriptional activity and recruitment of several protein coactivators and repressors by both ER subtypes. The effects could also occur through nontranscriptional mechanisms mediated by protein-protein interactions occurring between ERs and growth factors e.g., IGF-1 and EGF.[77,78] As mentioned earlier, there is evidence for the presence of a small pool of ERs localized to the plasma membrane. For example, BSA-conjugated estradiol, which is unable to gain entry into the cytosol and acts at the plasma membrane, decreases testicular

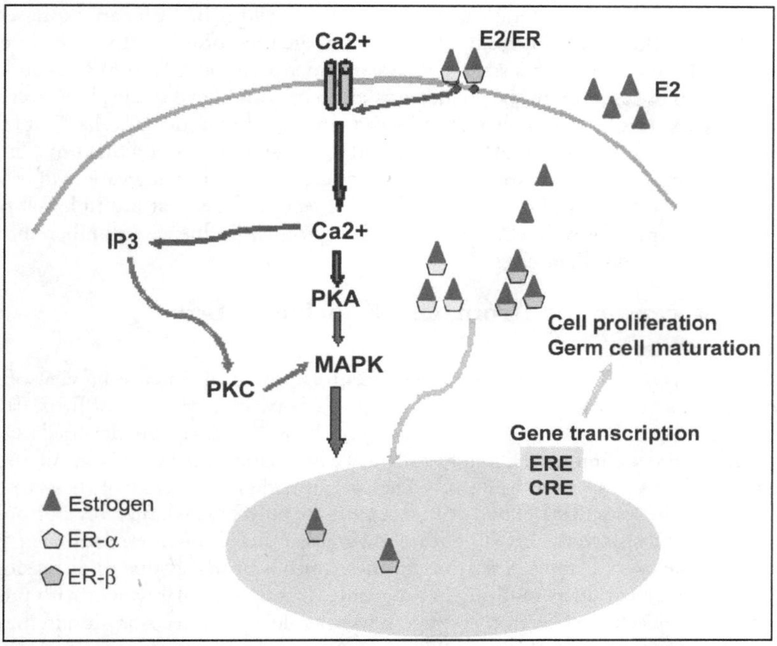

Figure 4. Estrogen induced signaling pathways in the testis. This figure is a schematic representation of signaling pathways operative in estrogen responsive cells. ERs respond to a wide variety of extracellular signals including steroid hormones, growth factors and xenoestrogens. ER mediated transcription in the nucleus is coordinated through complex reversible phosphorylation events while rapid nongenomic signaling is mediated through Ca^{2+} mobilization.

androgen production in vitro.[79] Membrane ER is thought to signal mainly by coupling to GTP-activating proteins and through pathways involving second messengers (e.g., calcium) and kinase cascades.[80] The integration of several pathways implies that estrogen action in any particular tissue and organ is the result of activities mediated by both the genomic and nongenomic pathways.

An overview of the distribution of estrogen receptors in the testis provides information on the cells that are potentially capable of responding to estrogen. Both types of estrogen receptors ERα and ERβ are present in the testis. While ERα dominates in some specific tissues and is mainly involved in reproductive events, ERβ is the more generally expressed estrogen receptor.[81] In the testis, ERβ is the more abundant receptor and is typically found in nearly every cell type of the interstitium and the seminiferous tubule, except for the elongated spermatids. ERβ is expressed in the Sertoli cells, Leydig cells, and germ cells, as well as in the epididymis, prostate, and seminal vesicles. ERα is present predominantly in the Leydig cells, rete testis, efferent ducts and epididymis of rats and monkeys.[82] ERα is primarily present in the efferent ducts that transport spermatozoa suspended in the fluid secreted by the Sertoli cells from the testis to the epididymis. Although there are reported differences in ERα localization in the epididymis of various species, its presence in efferent ductule epithelium has remained constant across species. ERα protein is abundant in epithelial cells of the efferent ductule with intense immunohistochemical staining of the nonciliated cell nucleus and the ciliated cells showing considerable variability in staining. ERα protein is also present in the fetal testis. Immunohistochemical studies show the presence of ERα in the mouse undifferentiated gonad between days 10-12 after birth, suggesting that estrogen may have a role very early in the differentiation process.[83]

Leydig cells within the rodent fetal testis contain ERα until birth.[84] ERs are expressed in the Leydig cells at a stage in development when the androgen receptor is not yet expressed highlighting a role for estrogen at this stage.[85] There is evidence for both ERβ mRNA and protein as early as day 16 of gestation in the gonocytes, Sertoli cells and Leydig cells. However, it is the gonocytes that express ERβ in higher abundance than the other testicular cells.[86] At birth, the testis expresses both ERα and ERβ that is localized to the seminiferous epithelium, Sertoli cells and developing germ cells.[86] As we have seen in the earlier section that a variety of cells in the testis synthesize estrogen, studies represented in this section show that multiple cell types express estrogen receptors as well which indicates that estrogens influence a number of cell types including the germ cells themselves.

Estrogen Receptor and Aromatase Knockout Mice and Their Phenotypes

Mice with targeted disruption of estrogen receptors provide us interesting view of the role of estrogens in the males and there is a great difference between disruption of ERα, ERβ and a combination of both. For example, ERα disruption (ERKO mice) cause increased plasma testosterone levels and are infertile. Upon histological examination they show seminiferous tubular swelling and loss of spermatogenesis.[87] The sperm made in the testes of these animals are nonfunctional. The testicular LH and FSH receptors are up-regulated, but gonadotropin levels are normal. ERβ persists in the ERKO mice, showing that there is no interrelationship between expressions of the two ER types. Infertility in these mice is primarily due to distension of the rete testis and excurrent ducts resulting in progressive loss of testicular weight with prominent exfoliation of germ cells.[87] Therefore, estrogens have a role in fluid reabsorption in the efferent ducts and the initial segment of the epididymis.[87] As regards sexual behavior, the ERKO mice have normal amount of mountings with lesser levels of aggression and lower number of intromissions and ejaculations.[88]

ERβ knockout (BERKO) mice were first generated by inserting a neomycin resistance gene into exon 3 of the coding gene, using homologous recombination in embryonic stem cells.[89] BERKO mice exhibit phenotypes distinctly different than those of αERKO mice.[89] They develop normally and as young adults, they are indistinguishable grossly and histologically from their littermates. Unlike males lacking ERα, male BERKO mice are fully fertile and reproduce normally. The mice exhibit no major alterations in the function of the male reproductive system. Therefore, it appears that ERβ is not essential for normal testicular functioning.[89]

The reproductive phenotype of αβ-ERKO mice is very close to that of α-ERKO mice and it is characterized by infertility and enlarged seminiferous tubules.[4,90] ArKO mouse lacks aromatase products (namely, estradiol and estrone). At around 18 week of age these mice show a specific postmeiotic defect coinciding with an elevation in apoptosis and a reduction in fertility.[18] The ArKO mice also present with a significant reduction in copulatory behavior in adulthood, reiterating the importance of estrogen in male reproduction.[18]

The mechanisms involved in the development of infertility is different in α-ERKO male mice if compared with ArKO, because reduced fluid reabsorbion occurs in α-ERKO male mice and in ArKO mice early arrest of spermatogenesis suggests a failure in germ cell differentiation probably due to the lack of estrogens in the testicular environment. It appears that estrogen activity in the male reproductive tract differs with regard to both the types of ERs involved in the pathway of estrogenic action, and the site of action through the male reproductive tract because β-ERKO male mice are fully fertile[89] as compared to the other two. Accordingly, in ArKO male mice, the failure of germ cell differentiation that is probably related to the lack of estrogen action on seminiferous epithelium while ERα disruption and related arrest of fluid reabsorption take place in the efferent ductules of α-ERKO mice.[90,91] Spermatogenesis is conserved in very young ArKO mice because a small quantity of estrogens, from external sources, probably is sufficient to promote germ cell maturation for a brief period, and therefore, the degree of infertility is less severe in ArKO mice than in α-ERKO. Later, the continuous lack of estrogens causes sperm abnormalities with advancing age in ArKO mice, since estradiol is probably necessary to maintain spermatogenesis and promote normal sperm maturation, both in the seminiferous epithelium and through the reproductive tract.[92] Therefore, ERα appears to be the most important component for estrogens action in male reproduction because α-ERKO mice are infertile while the β-ERKO mice are fertile.

Effects of Estrogen Administration on Testicular Function

Estrogen administration in animals has provided a substantial amount of literature on how estrogens affect the different cellular components of the testis and what are the functional consequences. The confusion about the involvement of estrogen in spermatogenesis is due to the fact that estrogen action is important at numerous levels in male reproductive physiology including effects on the hypothalamic-pituitary-testis axis, Leydig cells, Sertoli cells, germ cells, and epididymal function. Thus the extensive range of effects that estrogens have in the male reproductive tract, cause difficulties in the interpretation of experimental findings. The following section discusses the effects of estrogen administration and deprivation on processes that are required for normal spermatogenesis and fertility.

Estrogen Exposure and Spermatogenesis

A major component of the negative feedback action of androgens on gonadotropin secretion is mediated by estrogen. Studies in humans show that administration of estradiol enhance gonadotropin suppression induced by a testosterone-based contraceptive,[6] indicating estrogen's role as a negative feedback regulator of gonadotropin secretion that disrupts spermatogenesis. Neonatal exposure to either estrogens or estrogen-like compounds promotes changes in gonadotropin secretion in rodents.[93,94] Neonatal estrogen exposure can have important long-term effects on the hypothalamic-pituitary-testis axis and thus spermatogenesis. A single high dose of estradiol benzoate to 1-day-old male rats causes a reduction in both GnRH secretion and pituitary responsiveness to GnRH.[95] In male hamsters, neonatal exposure to diethylstilbestrol (DES), a synthetic estrogen during neonatal period impairs the action of androgens on target organs.[96] In rats neonatal administration of DES delays the establishment of the blood-testis barrier affecting spermatogenesis.[97] It has also been shown that neonatal exposure of rats to low levels of estrogens can advance the first wave of spermatogenesis at puberty and also affect the development of excurrent ducts of the rat testis.[98,99] Other than germ cells, neonatal estrogen treatment results in dose-dependent alterations in Sertoli cell numbers, efficiency of spermatogenesis, and germ cell apoptosis in adulthood.[99] Therefore, the above studies show that neonatal exposure to estrogen affects spermatogenesis but depending on the time and dose of exposure this effect can be reversible.

Given that the appropriate concentrations of LH and FSH as well as a tightly regulated onset of secretion during the neonatal and pubertal periods, is fundamental to whether normal spermatogenesis proceeds,[100] neonatal estrogen exposure can have important long-term effects on the hypothalamic-pituitary-testis axis and thus spermatogenesis. Interestingly, whether or not estrogen administration to juvenile mice will interfere with the hypothalamo-pituitary-gonadal axis appears to be strain-dependent,[101] which could lead to confusion when interpreting the literature on the interaction between estrogen, the regulation of pituitary hormone production, and fertility.

Adult monkeys treated with an aromatase inhibitor show a decrease in the conversion of round to elongated spermatids and a decrease in sperm output from the testis, also suggesting that estrogen is important for spermatid differentiation in the primates.[102] A different scenario appears to be relevant in boars. It has been shown that boars treated with aromatase inhibitors show a delayed lumen formation, lower testicular weight, fewer detergent resistant spermatids, and fewer Sertoli cells, but by 7 to 8 months, these boars recover and show larger testes with more Sertoli cells. Total Leydig cell volume increases in proportion to testis size. Therefore, reducing endogenous estrogen is consistent with a delay in testicular maturation/puberty that allows for a longer window for the proliferation of Sertoli cells and maturation of Leydig cells, resulting in larger testes and higher spermatid production.[103]

Effects of Estrogens on Sertoli Cells

Through the development of the testis, estrogen has varied effects on the Sertoli cells. The proliferation of Sertoli cells occur from day 16 of fetal life in the rat and at birth, there are 1 million cells and around 15 days there are about 40 million cells. After postnatal day 15, proliferation ceases,[104] differentiation commences and the number of the Sertoli cells in the testis remains stable throughout adulthood.[105] During this period, Sertoli cells produce considerable amounts of estrogen, leading to the suggestion that estrogen is involved in the division of the Sertoli cells. Aromatase activity is highest in Sertoli cells from prepubertal rats, declines as Sertoli cells mature, and is hormonally regulated, principally by FSH. The data show that estrogen has a stimulatory effect on Sertoli cell division yet a negative effect on Sertoli cell differentiation and development, because, estrogen production is high in proliferating Sertoli cells but lower in differentiated cells[106] and FSH-induced aromatase activity starts to decline towards the end of division. The ability of Leydig cells to produce testosterone increases from about day 14 after birth,[107] which inhibits Sertoli cell aromatase activity,[108] suggesting that androgens from the maturing Leydig cells may participate in the down-regulation of aromatase during the switch from Sertoli cell division to differentiation. Germ cells which are starting to develop during the switch between Sertoli cell division and differentiation, induce a decrease Sertoli cell aromatase activity.[109]

Effects of Estrogen on Germ Cells

The presence of estrogen receptors during various stages of germ cell development indicates that there could be a direct effect of estrogens on germ cells. For details on expression of estrogen receptors in germ cell a review by ref. 110 is referred to. The presence of aromatase in germ cells demonstrate the capability of these cells to synthesize estrogens that could be affecting the same cells in an autocrine mode. In a study aimed at investigating the effect of estradiol and diethylstilbestrol on the testis from 14.5-day-old rat fetuses in culture, alterations in the germ cells in terms of changes in viability occurred after estradiol and DES exposure.[111] In the human testis, estradiol appears to be a potent germ cell survival factor when studied in in vitro cultures.[112] Studies using rat gonocytes in culture show that estrogen stimulates gonocyte proliferation.[113] The high aromatase activity in the Sertoli cells during proliferation of gonocytes is an indication of estrogen action where differentiating spermatogonia during the early neonatal period have been shown to contain ERβ.[114]

Estrogens and Spermatozoa

In the last stage of mammalian spermiogenesis, the bulk of spermatid cytoplasm is extruded in tubular lumen while a small cytoplasmic mass is retained around the sperm mid-piece as cytoplasmic droplet. This droplet moves to the end of the tail and finally sheds from mature spermatozoa.[115] Human ejaculate can contain spermatozoa with excess residual cytoplasm which has been retained around the sperm mid-piece due to an incomplete maturation process. Both estrogen receptors are found in the excess residual cytoplasm of immature sperm, while sperm tails show only ERα.[116] It has been shown that specific allelic combinations of the ERα, which confer a stronger estrogen effect, may negatively influence human spermatogenesis.[117] Concomitant expression of ERβ and ERα in human ejaculated spermatozoa has been reported showing a differential distribution of the two ER subtypes, the former being prevalently located in the midpiece, but the latter being in the tail. In the same study, ERα was shown to interact with the p55 regulatory subunit of PI3K, whereas ERβ interacts with Akt1.[118] Additional studies have also demonstrated presence of ERβ on sperm.[119] Interestingly, while possessing estrogen receptors, human ejaculated spermatozoa also express cytochrome P450 aromatase indicating the cell could also serve as a source of estrogen.[120] ERβ contains two silent polymorphisms, RsaI (G1082A) and

AluI (G1730A), the frequency of the heterozygous RsaI AG-genotype is three times higher in infertile men showing that ERβ may have modulating effects on human spermatogenesis.[121]

Studies on Xenoestrogens

Synthetic estrogens, also called xenoestrogens, are a diverse group of compounds in the environment that mimic the action of the natural hormone 17β-estradiol in estrogen-dependent tissues. There is considerable controversy as to whether environmental chemicals that mimic estrogens can adversely affect the endocrine and reproductive systems. Evidence has accumulated over several decades now that estrogen is essential for spermatogenesis and that intratesticular concentrations of estrogen are very high.[82] It has also been realized that estrogen like chemicals present in the environment adversely affects male reproductive function. The compounds thought to be responsible for such changes include industrial chemicals (e.g., polychlorobiphenyls, alkyphenols, pesticides (e.g., DDT derivatives, methoxychlor, kepone), pharmaceutical agents (e.g., DES, tamoxifen, raloxifene), phthalates (e.g., di-2-ethylhexylphthalate, di-*n*-butyl phthalate), and phytoestrogens (e.g., genistein, daidzen).[122,123] The extent of exposure to these chemicals on members of a population differs as occupations in agriculture, petrochemicals and the construction industry entails higher exposure. Since estrogen receptors are present in the pituitary and spermatogenic cells,[82] estrogen like chemicals can act as agonists or antagonists for the hormone and interfere with spermatogenesis. Therefore, agents able to mimic estrogens can potentially alter the action of the hormone on spermatogenic cells leading to functional impairment of the male gamete. Reports of impaired spermatogenesis as a consequence of exposure to agents with estrogenic activity termed as endocrine disruptors are well documented in rats.[124] In addition to such examples, it is well established that estrogen administration to experimental animals during adulthood can impair sperm production and maturation.[125] The mechanism by which these xenoestrogens exert their action on the cell could occur by either agonistic or antagonistic actions on ERα and ERβ[126] resulting in changes in steroid hormone receptor gene expression, altered steroid hormone metabolism, change in cross-talk between ERs and other signaling systems.[127]

Exposure of neonatal testis, populated by fetal-type Leydig cells to endocrine-active compounds may have far-reaching consequences. Fetal rat testis shows inhibition of development of spermatogonia, Leydig cells and Sertoli cells on estrogen exposure.[111,128] Bisphenol A (BPA), [2,2-(4,4-dihydroxydiphenol)propane] is an estrogenic compound that is widely used in the manufacture of polycarbonate plastics, which serve as containers for foods and beverages and as a constituent of dental sealants. The core structure of BPA resembles that of the natural estrogen, consisting of two phenolic rings joined by a bridging carbon. Exposure of the human population to BPA is significant given its widespread use in consumer products. BPA and its metabolites have been measured in the blood of normal men.[129] Administration of low doses of the industrial and estrogenic chemical BPA reduces spermatogenesis in mice[130] and suppresses androgen biosynthesis by mature rat Leydig cells. In mice, neonatal exposure to a relatively large dose of BPA causes damage to the motility and morphology of sperm.[131] BPA induces apoptosis in Sertoli cell cultures isolated from 18-day-old rats.[132] 4-tert-octylphenol is an environmental pollutant with estrogenic activity and is directly toxic to cultured rat spermatogenic cells and Sertoli cells.[133] Therefore, BPA, a xenoestrogen appears to have the potential to affect multiple cell types in the testis. Chronic exposures of mice to 0.5 or 50 μg/ml bisphenol A decreases ERβ and increases ERα gene expression in germ cells[134] but a single injection of estradiol benzoate at high doses (500 μg) causes the opposite effect in prepubertal rats, i.e., decreased ERα mRNA levels and increased ERβ expression.[135] Parabens are p-hydroxybenzoic acid ester compounds widely used as preservatives in foods, cosmetics, toiletries and pharmaceuticals. These compounds exert a weak estrogenic activity as determined by in vitro estrogen receptor assay and in vivo uterotrophic assay. In mice, a decrease in daily sperm production occurs when treated with the above compound.[136]

Tumors of germ cell origin comprise about 95% of all testis cancers. Interaction between genetic and environmental factors, including inappropriate exposures to endocrine-active chemicals can lead to hypospadias, testicular cancer, abnormal spermatogenesis and undescended testis.[137,138] Exposure to estrogens early in life can lead to defects in tissue differentiation in the fetal period.[139] Although the effects of exposures to environmental chemicals in adulthood are typically transient, chemical exposures that alter gene activity during development disrupt differentiated function in hormone-responsive tissues of the adult. Testicular cancer incidence is highest in younger men (20-40 years old), and the etiology of this disease could be related to estrogen exposure during the prenatal period.[140] For example, in a study of young adult twins in England, the overall risk of testicular cancer was higher for dizygotic than for monozygotic twins.[141] These observations support a role for estrogens in the etiology of this disease, which has been increasing in most countries.[142] The possibility that xenoestrogens may cause adverse effects in the reproductive tract was first highlighted by reports on adolescent sons born to pregnant women who had taken the highly potent synthetic estrogen DES. These individuals developed a variety of testicular and epididymal abnormalities in adulthood.[143,144]

Phytoestrogens are plant-derived compounds with estrogenic activity. They are common in both human and animal diets, particularly through soy-based foods. Adult male rats, fed a high phytoestrogen diet for 3 days, demonstrate significantly reduced fecundity which is reversible. In these instances, the expression of ERα increases in the initial segment of the epididymis, but decreases in the cauda epididymis following 3 days on the high phytoestrogen diet.[145] Therefore, phytoestrogens can also affect estrogen receptors on spermatozoa and eventually fertility.

Estrogen Deprivation and Spermatogenesis

The functional consequences of estrogen deprivation in adulthood have also been investigated by the administration of the anti-estrogens. For example, Faslodex (ICI 182,870) compound binds to both ERα and ERβ and reduces the stability of ERα in vitro.[146] Rats and mice treated with Faslodex (2 to 150 days) shows efferent duct dilation, a progressive decrease in testis weight, decreased sperm concentration and decreased fertility indicating massive effects of antiestrogens in germ cells.[147-149] These changes are similar to those observed in the ERαKO mice where they occur after a reduction in expression of ERα with no change in expression of ERβ.[147]

Estrogens and Germ Cell Apoptosis

The physiological significance of the spontaneous germ cell apoptosis that occurs during spermatogenesis is possibly related to maintenance of the proper number of germ cells per Sertoli cells because these cells are terminally differentiated cells with no capacity for renewal, and are able to support only a certain number of germ cells. Therefore, germ cell death during development is to limit the number of germ cells to match the supportive capacity of the Sertoli cells.[150] Apoptosis may also serve to eliminate germ cells with mutations in the DNA. In meiotic spermatocytes, there appears to be a quality-control system or checkpoint for monitoring chromosome synapsis. This control system is thought to recognize unrepaired double-strand DNA breaks in unsynapsed chromosomes during meiotic metaphase and to induce apoptosis of the affected cell.[151,152] During prepubertal development, a wave of extensive germ cell apoptosis occurs in the rodent testis.[153] This early germ cell apoptosis, which mainly affects spermatogonia and spermatocytes, appears to be essential for functional spermatogenesis in adulthood. In the adult testis, spermatogenesis is accompanied by spontaneous germ cell degeneration resulting in the loss of up to 75% of the potential number of mature spermatozoa.[154-156] In the human testis, spontaneous germ cell apoptosis involves all three classes of germ cell, i.e., spermatogonia, spermatocytes, and spermatids.[157] Various apoptotic signaling pathways are operative in the testis. The Fas system has been suggested to play a role both in maintaining the immune-privileged nature of the testis and in regulating testicular germ cell apoptosis. FasL has been found in mouse, rat, and human Sertoli cells[158-161] and is generally assumed to be constitutively expressed by the Sertoli cells. Some reports have shown FasL presence in germ cells also.[125,174] Fas expression, in turn has been demonstrated in the germ cells of the rat and human testes[125,162] and in some reports Fas presence has also been shown in the Sertoli cells.[163]

Estrogen exerts different effects in specific cell types, for example, in estrogen receptor positive MCF-7 human breast cancer cells, estrogen strongly stimulates cell proliferation and does not induce cell death.[164] In contrast, for several cell types, stably transfected with ER, estrogen is highly toxic and induces cell death.[165,166] Recent studies demonstrate that estrogens also exert nongenomic effects[167] possibly related to its ability to activate signaling pathways such as nitric-oxide synthase in endothelial cells.[168] Estrogens have been linked to apoptosis in a variety of cell lines[168,169,170] but studies on spermatogenic cell apoptosis in response to estrogens are relatively few and consequently very little information is available on estrogen induced changes. Apoptosis is of great relevance for successful production of spermatogenic cells as excess cells need to be removed for the proper maintenance of testicular homeostasis.[171] As in other tissues, selection of the apoptotic pathway depends on the physiological and pathological state of the spermatogenic cells and members of the Bcl-2 family of proteins have been implicated in apoptosis induced by certain agents along with activation of the Fas-FasL system under various conditions.[125,172,173] While earlier studies implicated FasL from Sertoli cells for engaging Fas receptor on spermatogenic cells during apoptosis, later studies provided evidence in support of both Fas and FasL being expressed in spermatogenic cells as well.[125,174] Estradiol given subcutaneously to adult male rats for 10 days show a decrease in apoptosis of germ cells.[175] Similarly, low concentrations of 17β-estradiol (10^{-9} and 10^{-10} mol/L) effectively inhibits male germ cell apoptosis induced by deprivation of survival factors to human seminiferous tubules in culture.[176] A study of the effect of estradiol on testicular function in *hpg* mice with slow-release estradiol implants, which achieved circulating estradiol concentrations of approximately 40 pg/ml show full qualitatively normal spermatogenesis after 70 days of treatment illustrating that spermatogenesis could be restored in the hpg mice with estradiol.[177] Studies from our laboratory show a distinct increase in Fas-FasL expression in rat spermatogenic cells upon exposure to DES leading to germ cell death. This increase was confined to the spermatid population, which correlated with increased apoptosis seen in the haploid cells. Testosterone supplementation was able to prevent DES-induced Fas-FasL up-regulation and apoptosis in the spermatogenic cells. DES-induced germ cell apoptosis did not occur in Fas-deficient *lpr/lpr* mice.[125] Subsequently, using an in vitro model we provided evidence for the amplification of the death-inducing signals through mitochondria resulting in cytochrome c release. The activation of the apoptotic pathway occurred through estrogen receptors because estrogen antagonists prevented the activation of apoptosis. Since a part of this study was done with germ cell cultures independent of Sertoli cells, the importance of the independent capability of cells of the spermatogenic lineage to respond to estrogens was established.[178] For the role of Fas/FasL in the testis, a review by ref. 179 is recommended. Estradiol treatment increases germ-cell apoptosis mainly at stages IV-X of the spermatogenic cycle, rather than at stage VII when apoptotic germ-cell death is triggered by gonadotrophin withdrawal in adult rats.[180] Testis regression in Syrian hamsters is associated with an important increase of apoptosis 3 days post DES administration primarily affecting spermatocytes and, to a much lesser extent, spermatogonia.[181] A combined regimen of gossypol plus methyltestosterone and ethinylestradiol as a contraceptive induces germ cell apoptosis in rats.[182] In another model of seasonally breeding bank vole testis, males treated with a high dose of estradiol or its antagonist ICI 182,780, disruption of testicular structure and tubular atrophy showed increased apoptosis of germ cells.[183] Zearalenone, a non-steroidal estrogenic mycotoxin induces testicular germ cell apoptosis in a time-dependent and stage-specific pattern, peak frequency of apoptosis gradually progressing at stages I-VI of seminiferous tubules with time after dosing, suggesting that the damaged germ cells, especially spermatogonia and spermatocytes, gradually underwent the processes leading to apoptosis.[184]

Future Directions

There are many important questions regarding the role of estrogens in male fertility that are still to be completely answered. For example, is there a physiological role for estrogen in male reproduction through the pituitary-gonadal axis or is there a local effect? Can exposure to low doses of estrogen or estrogenic substances interfere with spermatogenesis and male fertility? What kind of estrogen receptors is most important for testicular function and in which cell types? It is also necessary to identify putative causal agents by the systematic screening of environmental chemicals and chemicals present in human foods to assess their ability to disrupt the endocrine system. In addition, it will be necessary to develop methods to measure cumulative exposure to estrogen mimics.

Sperm counts in Western countries might have fallen by approximately 50% since the 1930s to 1940s[185] and was an issue about environmental effects on the male. The initial study by Carlsen and colleagues was subjected to much criticism and reanalysis.[186-190] Independent reanalysis reached exactly the same conclusions as had the original study, and a relatively recent updated analysis[191] that included semen analysis data up to 1996 (101 studies in all) again confirmed the trends and conclusions of the original study. However, these studies are all based on meta-analyses of retrospective data, and therefore, fresh systematic studies are needed to readdress the questions of sperm count and environmental exposure to estrogenic chemicals.

It is known that disorders of sexual differentiation, a hormonally mediated process that occur in the fetus in utero are associated with a high risk of developing testis cancer in young adulthood.[192] In utero DES exposure has been linked to testis cancer.[193] Estrogen exposure in the first trimester of pregnancy is particularly important as it is associated with a small but significant increase in risk of developing testis cancer.[5] However, this view has been contradicted.[194-196] In general, it seems fair to conclude that exposure to *exogenous* estrogens in early pregnancy results in only a modest increase in risk of developing testis cancer. It has also been speculated that increased risk of testis cancer might stem from increased exposure to *endogenous* (maternal) estrogens. The premalignant germ cells, the carcinoma in situ cells[197,198] from which testis cancer arises, have their origins in fetal life. Subnormal androgen exposure and increased estrogen exposure can be the potential stimulus for these cells to be predisposed towards cancerous growth later in life.[197-200] Few reviews recommended for readings on endocrine disruption and male reproduction see refs. 201-206.

Therefore, it is substantiated by literature that there is a strong possibility of estrogens being responsible for several reproductive disorders. To conclusively prove the role of estrogens where different doses play different roles under different cellular conditions further research is necessary with specific goals. With our increased understanding of the role of estrogens in male fertility, we should be able to design small molecule modulators of estrogen action to interfere with deleterious effects of estrogens.

List of Abbreviations

ArKO, aromatase knockout; ERα, estrogen receptor α; ERβ, estrogen receptor β; ER, estrogen receptor; SERMs, Selective estrogen receptor modulators; *hpg*, hypogonadal; GnRH, gonadotropin-releasing hormone; FSH, Follicle stimulating hormone; LH, Luteinizing hormone; P450arom, aromatase cytochrome P450; HSD, hydroxysteroid dehydrogenases; PKC, protein kinase C; PKA, protein kinase A; ERKO, ERα knockout; BERKO, ERβ knockout; DES, diethylstilbestrol; BPA, Bisphenol A.

Acknowledgements

Part of our work was supported Indo-US collaboration on "Contraceptive and Reproductive Health Research" USA and Department of Biotechnology, India.

References

1. Kelch RP, Jenner MR, Weinstein R et al. Estradiol and testosterone secretion by human, simian, and canine testes, in males with hypogonadism and in male pseudohermaphrodites with the feminizing testes syndrome. J Clin Invest 1972; 51:824-830.
2. Payne AH, Kelch RP, Musich SS et al. Intratesticular site of aromatization in the human. J Clin Endocrinol Metab 1976; 42:1081-1087.
3. Kuiper GG, Carlsson B, Grandien K et al. Comparison of the ligand binding specificity and transcript tissue distribution of estrogen receptors α and β. Endocrinology 1997; 138:863-870.
4. Couse JF, Korach KS. Estrogen receptor null mice: What have we learned and where will they lead us? Endocr Rev 1999; 20:358-417.
5. Toppari J, Larsen JC, Christiansen P et al. Male reproductive health and environmental xenoestrogens. Environ Health Perspect 1996; 104(Suppl 4):741-803.
6. Handelsman DJ. Estrogens and falling sperm counts. Reprod Fertil Dev 2001; 13:317-324.
7. Akingbemi BT. Estrogen regulation of testicular function. Reprod Biol Endocrinol 2005; 3:51.
8. Sonnenschein C, Soto AM. An updated review of environmental estrogen and androgen mimics and antagonists. J Steroid Biochem Mol Biol 1998; 65:143-150.
9. Jensen TK, Toppari J, Keiding N et al. Do environmental estrogens contribute to the decline in male reproductive health? Clin Chem 1995; 41:1896-1901.
10. McLachlan JA. Commentary: Prenatal exposure to diethylstilbestrol (DES): A continuing story. Int J Epidemiol 2006; 35:868-870.
11. Gill WB, Schumacher GF, Bibbo M et al. Association of diethylstilbestrol exposure in utero with cryptorchidism, testicular hypoplasia and semen abnormalities. J Urol 1979; 122:36-39.
12. Steinberger E, Duckett GE. Effect of estrogen or testosterone on initiation and maintenance of spermatogenesis in the rat. Endocrinology 1965; 76:1184-1189.
13. Meistrich ML, Hughes TH, Bruce WR. Alteration of epididymal sperm transport and maturation in mice by oestrogen and testosterone. Nature 1975; 258:145-147.
14. Lubahn DB, Moyer JS, Golding TS et al. Alteration of reproductive function but not prenatal sexual development after insertional disruption of the mouse estrogen receptor gene. Proc Natl Acad Sci USA 1993; 90:11162-11166.
15. Korach KS. Insights from the study of animals lacking functional estrogen receptor. Science 1994; 266:1524-1527.
16. Eddy EM, Washburn TF, Bunch DO et al. Targeted disruption of the estrogen receptor gene in male mice causes alteration of spermatogenesis and infertility. Endocrinology 1996; 137:4796-4805.
17. Hess RA, Bunick D, Lee KH et al. A role for oestrogens in the male reproductive system. Nature 1997; 390:509-512.
18. Robertson KM, O'Donnell L, Jones ME et al. Impairment of spermatogenesis in mice lacking a functional aromatase (cyp 19) gene. Proc Natl Acad Sci USA 1999; 96:7986-799.
19. Jacquot Y, Rojas C, Refouvelet B et al. Recent advances in the development of phytoestrogens and derivatives: An update of the promising perspectives in the prevention of postmenopausal diseases. Mini Rev Med Chem 2003; 3:387-400.
20. Brzozowski AM, Pike AC, Dauter Z et al. Molecular basis of agonism and antagonism in the oestrogen receptor. Nature 1997; 389:753-758.
21. Fink BE, Mortensen DS, Stauffer SR et al. Novel structural templates for estrogen-receptor ligands and prospects for combinatorial synthesis of estrogens. Chem Biol 1999; 6:205-219.
22. Gust R, Keilitz R, Schmidt K. Synthesis, structural evaluation, and estrogen receptor interaction of 2,3-diarylpiperazines. J Med Chem 2002; 45:2325-2337.
23. Shiau AK, Barstad D, Loria PM et al. The structural basis of estrogen receptor/coactivator recognition and the antagonism of this interaction by tamoxifen. Cell 1998; 95:927-937.
24. Jordan VC. Biochemical pharmacology of antiestrogen action. Pharmacol Rev 1984; 36:245-276
25. Robertson DW, Katzenellenbogen JA, Hayes JR et al. Antiestrogen basicity—Activity relationships: A comparison of the estrogen receptor binding and antiuterotrophic potencies of several analogues of (Z)-1,2-diphenyl-1-[4-[2-(dimethylamino)ethoxy]phenyl]-1-butene (tamoxifen, Nolvadex) having altered basicity. J Med Chem 1982; 25:167-171.
26. Kekenes-Huskey PM, Muegge I, von Rauch M et al. A molecular docking study of estrogenically active compounds with 1,2-diarylethane and 1,2-diarylethene pharmacophores. Bioorg Med Chem 2004; 12:6527-6537.
27. de Kretser DM, Loveland KL, Meinhardt A et al. Spermatogenesis. Hum Reprod 1998; 13(Suppl 1):1-8.
28. Meachem S, von S, V, Schlatt S. Spermatogonia: Stem cells with a great perspective. Reproduction 2001; 121:825-834.

29. Print CG, Loveland KL. Germ cell suicide: New insights into apoptosis during spermatogenesis. Bioessays 2000; 22:423-430.
30. Sutton KA. Molecular mechanisms involved in the differentiation of spermatogenic stem cells. Rev Reprod 2000; 5:93-98.
31. de Rooij DG. Proliferation and differentiation of spermatogonial stem cells. Reproduction 2001; 121:347-354.
32. Toppari J, Kangasniemi M, Kaipia A et al. Stage- and cell-specific gene expression and hormone regulation of the seminiferous epithelium. J Electron Microsc Tech 1991; 19:203-214.
33. Parvinen M. Regulation of the seminiferous epithelium. Endocr Rev 1982; 3:404-417.
34. Russell LD, Ettlin RA, Sinha Hikkim AP et al. The classification and timing of spermatogenesis. In: Russell LD, Ettlin RA, Sinha Hikkim AP, et al, eds. Histological and Histopathological Evaluation of the Testis. Clearwater: Cache River Press, 1990:41-57.
35. Hess RA, Schaeffer DJ, Eroschenko VP et al. Frequency of the stages in the cycle of the seminiferous epithelium in the rat. Biol Reprod 1990; 43:517-524.
36. Weinbauer GF, Nieschlag E. Gonadotrophin control of testicular germ cell development. Adv Exp Med Biol 1995; 377:55-65.
37. Amory JK, Bremner WJ. Regulation of testicular function in men: Implications for male hormonal contraceptive development. J Steroid Biochem Mol Biol 2003; 85:357-361.
38. Luetjens CM, Weinbauer GF, Wistuba J. Primate spermatogenesis: New insights into comparative testicular organisation, spermatogenic efficiency and endocrine control. Biol Rev Camb Philos Soc 2005; 80:475-488.
39. Singh J, O'Neill C, Handelsman DJ. Induction of spermatogenesis by androgens in gonadotropin-deficient (hpg) mice. Endocrinology 1995; 136:5311-5321.
40. Dierich A, Sairam MR, Monaco L et al. Impairing follicle-stimulating hormone (FSH) signaling in vivo: Targeted disruption of the FSH receptor leads to aberrant gametogenesis and hormonal imbalance. Proc Natl Acad Sci USA 1998; 95:13612-13617.
41. Kumar TR, Wang Y, Lu N et al. Follicle stimulating hormone is required for ovarian follicle maturation but not male fertility. Nat Genet 1997; 15:201-204.
42. Krishnamurthy H, Danilovich N, Morales CR et al. Qualitative and quantitative decline in spermatogenesis of the follicle-stimulating hormone receptor knockout (FORKO) mouse. Biol Reprod 2000; 62:1146-1159.
43. Steinberger E. Hormonal control of mammalian spermatogenesis. Physiol Rev 1971; 51:1-22.
44. Boime I, Ben Menahem D. Glycoprotein hormone structure-function and analog design. Recent Prog Horm Res 1999; 54:271-288.
45. Jegou B, Sharpe RM. Paracrine mechanisms in testicular control. In: De Kretser D, ed. Molecular Biology of the Male Reproductive System. New York: Academic Press, 1993:271-310.
46. Franchimont P, Chari S, Demoulin A. Hypothalamus-pituitary-testis interaction. J Reprod Fertil 1975; 44:335-350
47. Burger HG. Physiological principles of endocrine replacement: Estrogen Horm Res 2001; 56(Suppl 1):82-85.
48. Anderson RA, Sharpe RM. Regulation of inhibin production in the human male and its clinical applications. Int J Androl 2000; 23:136-144.
49. Risbridger GP, Cancilla B. Role of activins in the male reproductive tract. Rev Reprod 2000; 5:99-104.
50. Omura T, Morohashi K. Gene regulation of steroidogenesis. J Steroid Biochem Mol Biol 1995; 53:19-25.
51. Payne AH. Hormonal regulation of cytochrome P450 enzymes, cholesterol side-chain cleavage and 17 alpha-hydroxylase/C17-20 lyase in Leydig cells. Biol Reprod 1990; 42:399-404.
52. Kelloff GJ, Lubet RA, Lieberman R et al. Aromatase inhibitors as potential cancer chemopreventives. Cancer Epidemiol Biomarkers Prev 1998; 7:65-78.
53. Weniger JP. Aromatase activity in fetal gonads of mammals. J Dev Physiol 1990; 14:303-306.
54. Papadopoulos V, Carreau S, Szerman-Joly E et al. Rat testis 17 β-estradiol: Identification by gas chromatography-mass spectrometry and age related cellular distribution. J Steroid Biochem 1986; 24:1211-1216.
55. Tsai-Morris CH, Aquilano DR, Dufau ML. Cellular localization of rat testicular aromatase activity during development. Endocrinology 1985; 116:38-46.
56. Rommerts FF, de Jong FH, Brinkmann AO et al. Development and cellular localization of rat testicular aromatase activity. J Reprod Fertil 1982; 65:281-288.
57. Kurosumi M, Ishimura K, Fujita H et al. Immunocytochemical localization of aromatase in rat testis. Histochemistry 1985; 83:401-404.

58. Levallet J, Bilinska B, Mittre H et al. Expression and immunolocalization of functional cytochrome P450 aromatase in mature rat testicular cells. Biol Reprod 1998; 58:919-926.
59. Carreau S, Delalande C, Silandre D et al. Aromatase and estrogen receptors in male reproduction. Mol Cell Endocrinol 2006; 246:65-68.
60. Moggs JG, Orphanides G. Estrogen receptors: Orchestrators of pleiotropic cellular responses. EMBO Rep 2001; 2:775-781.
61. Dechering K, Boersma C, Mosselman S. Estrogen receptors α and β: Two receptors of a kind? Curr Med Chem 2000; 7:561-576.
62. Pettersson K, Gustafsson JA. Role of estrogen receptor α in estrogen action. Annu Rev Physiol 2001; 63:165-192.
63. Beato M, Klug J. Steroid hormone receptors: An update. Hum Reprod Update 2000; 6:225-236.
64. Mangelsdorf DJ, Thummel C, Beato M et al. The nuclear receptor superfamily: The second decade. Cell 1995; 83:835-839.
65. Hermanson O, Glass CK, Rosenfeld MG. Nuclear receptor coregulators: Multiple modes of modification. Trends Endocrinol Metab 2002; 13:55-60.
66. Manavathi B, Kumar R. Steering estrogen signals from the plasma membrane to the nucleus: Two sides of the coin. J Cell Physiol 2006; 207:594-604.
67. Kelly MJ, Levin ER. Rapid actions of plasma membrane estrogen receptors. Trends Endocrinol Metab 2001; 12:152-156.
68. Migliaccio A, Di Domenico M, Castoria G et al. Tyrosine kinase/p21Ras/MAP-kinase pathway activation by estradiol-receptor complex in MCF-7 cells. EMBO J 1996; 15:1292-1300.
69. Segars JH, Driggers PH. Estrogen action and cytoplasmic signaling cascades. Part I: Membrane-associated signaling complexes. Trends Endocrinol Metab 2002; 13:349-354.
70. Collins P, Webb C. Estrogen hits the surface. Nat Med 1999; 5:1130-1131.
71. Falkenstein E, Tillmann HC, Christ M et al. Multiple actions of steroid hormones—A focus on rapid, nongenomic effects. Pharmacol Rev 2000; 52:513-556.
72. Foster JS, Wimalasena J. Estrogen regulates activity of cyclin-dependent kinases and retinoblastoma protein phosphorylation in breast cancer cells. Mol Endocrinol 1996; 10:488-498.
73. Revelli A, Massobrio M, Tesarik J. Nongenomic actions of steroid hormones in reproductive tissues. Endocr Rev 1998; 19:3-17.
74. Enmark E, Gustafsson JA. Oestrogen receptors—An overview. J Intern Med 1999; 246:133-138.
75. Lavery DN, McEwan IJ. Structure and function of steroid receptor AF1 transactivation domains: Induction of active conformations. Biochem J 2005; 391:449-464.
76. Hall JM, McDonnell DP. The estrogen receptor β-isoform (ERβ) of the human estrogen receptor modulates ERalpha transcriptional activity and is a key regulator of the cellular response to estrogens and antiestrogens. Endocrinology 1999; 140:5566-5578.
77. Hewitt SC, Korach KS. Estrogen receptors: Structure, mechanisms and function. Rev Endocr Metab Disord 2002; 3:193-200.
78. Bjornstrom L, Sjoberg M. Mechanisms of estrogen receptor signaling: Convergence of genomic and nongenomic actions on target genes. Mol Endocrinol 2005; 19:833-842.
79. Loomis AK, Thomas P. Effects of estrogens and xenoestrogens on androgen production by Atlantic croaker testes in vitro: Evidence for a nongenomic action mediated by an estrogen membrane receptor. Biol Reprod 2000; 62:995-1004.
80. Razandi M, Pedram A, Merchenthaler I et al. Plasma membrane estrogen receptors exist and functions as dimers. Mol Endocrinol 2004; 18:2854-2865.
81. Gustafsson JA. Estrogen receptor β—A new dimension in estrogen mechanism of action. J Endocrinol 1999; 163:379-383.
82. Hess RA. Estrogen in the adult male reproductive tract: A review. Reprod Biol Endocrinol 2003; 1:52.
83. O'Donnell L, Robertson KM, Jones ME et al. Estrogen and spermatogenesis. Endocr Rev 2001; 22:289-318.
84. Greco TL, Furlow JD, Duello TM et al. Immunodetection of estrogen receptors in fetal and neonatal male mouse reproductive tracts. Endocrinology 1992; 130:421-429.
85. Fisher JS, Millar MR, Majdic G et al. Immunolocalisation of oestrogen receptor-alpha within the testis and excurrent ducts of the rat and marmoset monkey from perinatal life to adulthood. J Endocrinol 1997; 153:485-495.
86. van Pelt AM, de Rooij DG, van der BB et al. Ontogeny of estrogen receptor-β expression in rat testis. Endocrinology 1999; 140:478-483.
87. Hess RA, Bunick D, Lubahn DB et al. Morphologic changes in efferent ductules and epididymis in estrogen receptor-α knockout mice. J Androl 2000; 21:107-121.

88. Ogawa S, Chester AE, Hewitt SC et al. Abolition of male sexual behaviors in mice lacking estrogen receptors α and β (α β ERKO). Proc Natl Acad Sci USA 2000; 97:14737-14741.
89. Krege JH, Hodgin JB, Couse JF et al. Generation and reproductive phenotypes of mice lacking estrogen receptor β. Proc Natl Acad Sci USA 1998; 95:15677-15682.
90. Toda K, Okada T, Takeda K et al. Oestrogen at the neonatal stage is critical for the reproductive ability of male mice as revealed by supplementation with 17β-oestradiol to aromatase gene (Cyp19) knockout mice. J Endocrinol 2001; 168:455-463.
91. Robertson KM, Simpson ER, Lacham-Kaplan O et al. Characterization of the fertility of male aromatase knockout mice. J Androl 2001; 22:825-830.
92. Murata Y, Robertson KM, Jones ME et al. Effect of estrogen deficiency in the male: The ArKO mouse model. Mol Cell Endocrinol 2002; 193:7-12.
93. Sharpe RM, Atanassova N, McKinnell C et al. Abnormalities in functional development of the Sertoli cells in rats treated neonatally with diethylstilbestrol: A possible role for estrogens in Sertoli cell development. Biol Reprod 1998; 59:1084-1094.
94. Atanassova N, McKinnell C, Turner KJ et al. Comparative effects of neonatal exposure of male rats to potent and weak (environmental) estrogens on spermatogenesis at puberty and the relationship to adult testis size and fertility: Evidence for stimulatory effects of low estrogen levels. Endocrinology 2000; 141:3898-3907.
95. Pinilla L, Garnelo P, Gaytan F et al. Hypothalamic-pituitary function in neonatally oestrogen-treated male rats. J Endocrinol 1992; 134:279-286.
96. Karri S, Johnson H, Hendry III WJ et al. Neonatal exposure to diethylstilbestrol leads to impaired action of androgens in adult male hamsters. Reprod Toxicol 2004; 19:53-63.
97. Toyama Y, Ohkawa M, Oku R et al. Neonatally administered diethylstilbestrol retards the development of the blood-testis barrier in the rat. J Androl 2001; 22:413-423.
98. Fisher JS, Turner KJ, Brown D et al. Effect of neonatal exposure to estrogenic compounds on development of the excurrent ducts of the rat testis through puberty to adulthood. Environ Health Perspect 1999; 107:397-405.
99. Atanassova N, McKinnell C, Walker M et al. Permanent effects of neonatal estrogen exposure in rats on reproductive hormone levels, Sertoli cell number, and the efficiency of spermatogenesis in adulthood. Endocrinology 1999; 140:5364-5373.
100. de Kretser DM. Endocrinology of male infertility. Br Med Bull 1979; 35:187-92.
101. Spearow JL, Doemeny P, Sera R et al. Genetic variation in susceptibility to endocrine disruption by estrogen in mice. Science 1999; 285:1259-1261.
102. Shetty G, Krishnamurthy H, Krishnamurthy HN et al. Effect of long-term treatment with aromatase inhibitor on testicular function of adult male bonnet monkeys (M. radiata). Steroids 1998; 63:414-420.
103. At-Taras EE, Berger T, McCarthy MJ et al. Reducing estrogen synthesis in developing boars increases testis size and total sperm production. J Androl 2006; 27:552-559.
104. Orth JM. Proliferation of Sertoli cells in fetal and postnatal rats: A quantitative autoradiographic study. Anat Rec 1982; 203:485-492.
105. Wang ZX, Wreford NG, De Kretser DM. Determination of Sertoli cell numbers in the developing rat testis by stereological methods. Int J Androl 1989; 12:58-64.
106. Papadopoulos V, Jia MC, Culty M et al. Rat Sertoli cell aromatase cytochrome P450: Regulation by cell culture conditions and relationship to the state of cell differentiation. In Vitro Cell Dev Biol Anim 1993; 29A:943-949.
107. Hardy MP, Gelber SJ, Zhou ZF et al. Hormonal control of Leydig cell differentiation. Ann NY Acad Sci 1991; 637:152-163.
108. Verhoeven G, Cailleau J. Prolonged exposure to androgens suppresses follicle-stimulating hormone-induced aromatase activity in rat Sertoli cell cultures. Mol Cell Endocrinol 1988; 57:61-67.
109. Le Magueresse B, Jegou B. Paracrine control of immature Sertoli cells by adult germ cells, in the rat (an in vitro study). Cell-cell interactions within the testis. Mol Cell Endocrinol 1988; 58:65-72.
110. Sierens JE, Sneddon SF, Collins F et al. Estrogens in testis biology. Ann NY Acad Sci 2005; 1061:65-76.
111. Lassurguere J, Livera G, Habert R et al. Time- and dose-related effects of estradiol and diethylstilbestrol on the morphology and function of the fetal rat testis in culture. Toxicol Sci 2003; 73:160-169.
112. Carreau S. Estrogens—Male hormones? Folia Histochem Cytobiol 2003; 41:107-111.
113. Li H, Papadopoulos V, Vidic B et al. Regulation of rat testis gonocyte proliferation by platelet-derived growth factor and estradiol: Identification of signaling mechanisms involved. Endocrinology 1997; 138:1289-1298.

114. Jefferson WN, Couse JF, Banks EP et al. Expression of estrogen receptor β is developmentally regulated in reproductive tissues of male and female mice. Biol Reprod 2000; 62:310-317.
115. Cooper TG. Cytoplasmic droplets: The good, the bad or just confusing? Hum Reprod 2005; 20:9-11.
116. Rago V, Siciliano L, Aquila S et al. Detection of estrogen receptors ER-α and ER-β in human ejaculated immature spermatozoa with excess residual cytoplasm. Reprod Biol Endocrinol 2006; 4:36.
117. Guarducci E, Nuti F, Becherini L et al. Estrogen receptor α promoter polymorphism: Stronger estrogen action is coupled with lower sperm count. Hum Reprod 2006; 21:994-1001.
118. Aquila S, Sisci D, Gentile M et al. Estrogen receptor (ER)α and ER β are both expressed in human ejaculated spermatozoa: Evidence of their direct interaction with phosphatidylinositol-3-OH kinase/Akt pathway. J Clin Endocrinol Metab 2004; 89:1443-1451.
119. Solakidi S, Psarra AM, Nikolaropoulos S et al. Estrogen receptors α and β (ERα and ERβ) and androgen receptor (AR) in human sperm: Localization of ERβ and AR in mitochondria of the midpiece. Hum Reprod 2005; 20:3481-3487.
120. Lambard S, Galeraud-Denis I, Saunders PT et al. Human immature germ cells and ejaculated spermatozoa contain aromatase and oestrogen receptors. J Mol Endocrinol 2004; 32:279-289.
121. Aschim EL, Giwercman A, Stahl O et al. The RsaI polymorphism in the estrogen receptor-beta gene is associated with male infertility. J Clin Endocrinol Metab 2005; 90:5343.
122. Witorsch RJ. Endocrine disruptors: Can biological effects and environmental risks be predicted? Regul Toxicol Pharmacol 2002; 36:118-130.
123. Akingbemi BT, Hardy MP. Oestrogenic and antiandrogenic chemicals in the environment: Effects on male reproductive health. Ann Med 2001; 33:391-403.
124. Boockfor FR, Blake CA. Chronic administration of 4-tert-octylphenol to adult male rats causes shrinkage of the testes and male accessory sex organs, disrupts spermatogenesis, and increases the incidence of sperm deformities. Biol Reprod 1997; 57:267-277.
125. Nair R, Shaha C. Diethylstilbestrol induces rat spermatogenic cell apoptosis in vivo through increased expression of spermatogenic cell Fas/FasL system. J Biol Chem 2003; 278:6470-6481.
126. Soto AM, Sonnenschein C, Chung KL et al. The E-SCREEN assay as a tool to identify estrogens: An update on estrogenic environmental pollutants. Environ Health Perspect 1995; 103(Suppl 7):113-122.
127. Hess-Wilson JK, Boldison J, Weaver KE et al. Xenoestrogen action in breast cancer: Impact on ER-dependent transcription and mitogenesis. Breast Cancer Res Treat 2006; 96:279-292.
128. Williams K, McKinnell C, Saunders PT et al. Neonatal exposure to potent and environmental oestrogens and abnormalities of the male reproductive system in the rat: Evidence for importance of the androgen-oestrogen balance and assessment of the relevance to man. Hum Reprod Update 2001; 7:236-247.
129. Akingbemi BT, Sottas CM, Koulova AI et al. Inhibition of testicular steroidogenesis by the xenoestrogen bisphenol A is associated with reduced pituitary luteinizing hormone secretion and decreased steroidogenic enzyme gene expression in rat Leydig cells. Endocrinology 2004; 145:592-603.
130. Toyama Y, Yuasa S. Effects of neonatal administration of 17β-estradiol, β-estradiol 3-benzoate, or bisphenol A on mouse and rat spermatogenesis. Reprod Toxicol 2004; 19:181-188.
131. Aikawa H, Koyama S, Matsuda M et al. Relief effect of vitamin A on the decreased motility of sperm and the increased incidence of malformed sperm in mice exposed neonatally to bisphenol A. Cell Tissue Res 2004; 315:119-124.
132. Iida H, Maehara K, Doiguchi M et al. Bisphenol A-induced apoptosis of cultured rat Sertoli cells. Reprod Toxicol 2003; 17:457-464.
133. Raychoudhury SS, Blake CA, Millette CF. Toxic effects of octylphenol on cultured rat spermatogenic cells and Sertoli cells. Toxicol Appl Pharmacol 1999; 157:192-202.
134. Takao T, Nanamiya W, Nazarloo HP et al. Exposure to the environmental estrogen bisphenol A differentially modulated estrogen receptor-α and -β immunoreactivity and mRNA in male mouse testis. Life Sci 2003; 72:1159-1169.
135. Tena-Sempere M, Navarro J, Pinilla L et al. Neonatal exposure to estrogen differentially alters estrogen receptor α and β mRNA expression in rat testis during postnatal development. J Endocrinol 2000; 165:345-357.
136. Oishi S. Effects of propyl paraben on the male reproductive system. Food Chem Toxicol 2002; 40:1807-1813.
137. Skakkebaek NE. Testicular dysgenesis syndrome: New epidemiological evidence. Int J Androl 2004; 27:189-191.

138. Virtanen HE, Rajpert-De Meyts E, Main KM et al. Testicular dysgenesis syndrome and the development and occurrence of male reproductive disorders. Toxicol Appl Pharmacol 2005; 207:501-505.
139. Leffers H, Naesby M, Vendelbo B et al. Oestrogenic potencies of Zeranol, oestradiol, diethylstilboestrol, Bisphenol-A and genistein: Implications for exposure assessment of potential endocrine disrupters. Hum Reprod 2001; 16:1037-1045.
140. Depue RH, Pike MC, Henderson BE. Estrogen exposure during gestation and risk of testicular cancer. J Natl Cancer Inst 1983; 71:1151-1155.
141. Swerdlow AJ, De Stavola BL, Swanwick MA et al. Risks of breast and testicular cancers in young adult twins in England and Wales: Evidence on prenatal and genetic aetiology. Lancet 1997; 350:1723-1728.
142. Adami HO, Bergstrom R, Mohner M et al. Testicular cancer in nine northern European countries. Int J Cancer 1994; 59:33-38.
143. Wilcox AJ, Baird DD, Weinberg CR et al. Fertility in men exposed prenatally to diethylstilbestrol. N Engl J Med 1995; 332:1411-1416.
144. Gill WB, Schumacher GF, Bibbo M. Structural and functional abnormalities in the sex organs of male offspring of mothers treated with diethylstilbestrol (DES). J Reprod Med 1976; 16:147-153.
145. Glover A, Assinder SJ. Acute exposure of adult male rats to dietary phytoestrogens reduces fecundity and alters epididymal steroid hormone receptor expression. J Endocrinol 2006; 189:565-573.
146. van den Bemd GJ, Kuiper GG, Pols HA et al. Distinct effects on the conformation of estrogen receptor α and β by both the antiestrogens ICI 164,384 and ICI 182,780 leading to opposite effects on receptor stability. Biochem Biophys Res Commun 1999; 261:1-5.
147. Oliveira CA, Nie R, Carnes K et al. The antiestrogen ICI 182,780 decreases the expression of estrogen receptor-α but has no effect on estrogen receptor-β and androgen receptor in rat efferent ductules. Reprod Biol Endocrinol 2003; 1:75.
148. Oliveira CA, Zhou Q, Carnes K et al. ER function in the adult male rat: Short- and long-term effects of the antiestrogen ICI 182,780 on the testis and efferent ductules, without changes in testosterone. Endocrinology 2002; 143:2399-2409.
149. Cho HW, Nie R, Carnes K et al. The antiestrogen ICI 182,780 induces early effects on the adult male mouse reproductive tract and long-term decreased fertility without testicular atrophy. Reprod Biol Endocrinol 2003; 1:57.
150. Richburg JH. The relevance of spontaneous- and chemically-induced alterations in testicular germ cell apoptosis to toxicology. Toxicol Lett 2000; 112-113:79-86.
151. Barchi M, Mahadevaiah S, Di Giacomo M et al. Surveillance of different recombination defects in mouse spermatocytes yields distinct responses despite elimination at an identical developmental stage. Mol Cell Biol 2005; 25:7203-7215.
152. Odorisio T, Rodriguez TA, Evans EP et al. The meiotic checkpoint monitoring synapsis eliminates spermatocytes via p53-independent apoptosis. Nat Genet 1998; 18:257-261.
153. Yan W, Suominen J, Samson M et al. Involvement of Bcl-2 family proteins in germ cell apoptosis during testicular development in the rat and pro-survival effect of stem cell factor on germ cells in vitro. Mol Cell Endocrinol 2000; 165:115-129.
154. Bartke A. Apoptosis of male germ cells, a generalized or a cell type-specific phenomenon? Endocrinology 1995; 136:3-4.
155. Clermont Y. The cycle of the seminiferous epithelium in man. Am J Anat 1963; 112:35-51.
156. Huckins C, Oakberg EF. Morphological and quantitative analysis of spermatogonia in mouse testes using whole mounted seminiferous tubules. II. The irradiated testes. Anat Rec 1978; 192:529-542.
157. Sinha Hikim AP, Swerdloff RS. Hormonal and genetic control of germ cell apoptosis in the testis. Rev Reprod 1999; 4:38-47.
158. Woolveridge I, Bryden AA, Taylor MF et al. Apoptosis and expression of apoptotic regulators in the human testis following short- and long-term anti-androgen treatment. Mol Hum Reprod 1998; 4:701-707.
159. Lee J, Richburg JH, Shipp EB et al. The Fas system, a regulator of testicular germ cell apoptosis, is differentially up-regulated in Sertoli cell versus germ cell injury of the testis. Endocrinology 1999; 140:852-858.
160. Sugihara A, Saiki S, Tsuji M et al. Expression of Fas and Fas ligand in the testes and testicular germ cell tumors: An immunohistochemical study. Anticancer Res 1997; 17:3861-3865.
161. Xerri L, Devilard E, Hassoun J et al. Fas ligand is not only expressed in immune privileged human organs but is also coexpressed with Fas in various epithelial tissues. Mol Pathol 1997; 50:87-91.
162. Lee J, Richburg JH, Younkin SC et al. The Fas system is a key regulator of germ cell apoptosis in the testis. Endocrinology 1997; 138:2081-2088.
163. Riccioli A, Starace D, D'Alessio A et al. TNF-α and IFN-γ regulate expression and function of the Fas system in the seminiferous epithelium. J Immunol 2000; 165:743-749.

164. Liu H, Lee ES, Gajdos C et al. Apoptotic action of 17beta-estradiol in raloxifene-resistant MCF-7 cells in vitro and in vivo. J Natl Cancer Inst 2003; 95:1586-1597.
165. Jiang SY, Langan-Fahey SM, Stella AL et al. Point mutation of estrogen receptor (ER) in the ligand-binding domain changes the pharmacology of antiestrogens in ER-negative breast cancer cells stably expressing complementary DNAs for ER. Mol Endocrinol 1992; 6:2167-2174.
166. Jiang SY, Jordan VC. A molecular strategy to control tamoxifen resistant breast cancer. Cancer Surv 1992; 14:55-70.
167. Pedram A, Razandi M, Aitkenhead M et al. Integration of the nongenomic and genomic actions of estrogen. Membrane-initiated signaling by steroid to transcription and cell biology. J Biol Chem 2002; 277:50768-50775.
168. Chen Z, Yuhanna IS, Galcheva-Gargova Z et al. Estrogen receptor α mediates the nongenomic activation of endothelial nitric oxide synthase by estrogen. J Clin Invest 1999; 103:401-406.
169. Marino M, Galluzzo P, Leone S et al. Nitric oxide impairs the 17beta-estradiol-induced apoptosis in human colon adenocarcinoma cells. Endocr Relat Cancer 2006; 13:559-569.
170. Song RX, Santen RJ. Apoptotic action of estrogen. Apoptosis 2003; 8:55-60.
171. Sinha Hikim AP, Lue Y, Diaz-Romero M et al. Deciphering the pathways of germ cell apoptosis in the testis. J Steroid Biochem Mol Biol 2003; 85:175-182.
172. Koji T, Hishikawa Y. Germ cell apoptosis and its molecular trigger in mouse testes. Arch Histol Cytol 2003; 66:1-16.
173. Sasagawa I, Yazawa H, Suzuki Y et al. Stress and testicular germ cell apoptosis. Arch Androl 2001; 47:211-216.
174. D'Alessio A, Riccioli A, Lauretti P et al. Testicular FasL is expressed by sperm cells. Proc Natl Acad Sci USA 2001; 98:3316-3321.
175. D'Souza R, Gill-Sharma MK, Pathak S et al. Effect of high intratesticular estrogen on the seminiferous epithelium in adult male rats. Mol Cell Endocrinol 2005; 241:41-48.
176. Pentikainen V, Erkkila K, Suomalainen L et al. Estradiol acts as a germ cell survival factor in the human testis in vitro. J Clin Endocrinol Metab 2000; 85:2057-2067.
177. Ebling FJ, Brooks AN, Cronin AS et al. Estrogenic induction of spermatogenesis in the hypogonadal mouse. Endocrinology 2000; 141:2861-2869.
178. Mishra DP, Shaha C. Estrogen-induced spermatogenic cell apoptosis occurs via the mitochondrial pathway: Role of superoxide and nitric oxide. J Biol Chem 2005; 280:6181-6196.
179. Koji T. Male germ cell death in mouse testes: Possible involvement of Fas and Fas ligand. Med Electron Microsc 2001; 34:213-222.
180. Blanco-Rodriguez J, Martinez-Garcia C. Apoptosis pattern elicited by oestradiol treatment of the seminiferous epithelium of the adult rat. J Reprod Fertil 1997; 110:61-70.
181. Nonclercq D, Reverse D, Toubeau G et al. In situ demonstration of germinal cell apoptosis during diethylstilbestrol-induced testis regression in adult male Syrian hamsters. Biol Reprod 1996; 55:1368-1376.
182. Cui GH, Xu ZL, Yang ZJ et al. A combined regimen of gossypol plus methyltestosterone and ethinylestradiol as a contraceptive induces germ cell apoptosis and expression of its related genes in rats. Contraception 2004; 70:335-342.
183. Gancarczyk M, Paziewska-Hejmej A, Carreau S et al. Dose- and photoperiod-dependent effects of 17β-estradiol and the anti-estrogen ICI 182,780 on testicular structure, acceleration of spermatogenesis, and aromatase immunoexpression in immature bank voles. Acta Histochem 2004; 106:269-278.
184. Kim IH, Son HY, Cho SW et al. Zearalenone induces male germ cell apoptosis in rats. Toxicol Lett 2003; 138:185-192.
185. Carlsen E, Giwercman A, Keiding N et al. Evidence for decreasing quality of semen during past 50 years. BMJ 1992; 305:609-613.
186. Sharpe RM, Turner KJ, Sumpter JP. Endocrine disruptors and testis development. Environ Health Perspect 1998; 106:A220-A221.
187. Sharpe RM, Martin B, Morris K et al. Infant feeding with soy formula milk: Effects on the testis and on blood testosterone levels in marmoset monkeys during the period of neonatal testicular activity. Hum Reprod 2002; 17:1692-1703.
188. Irvine DS. Declining sperm quality: A review of facts and hypotheses. Baillieres Clin Obstet Gynaecol 1997; 11:655-671.
189. Jégou B, Auger J, Multigner L et al. In: Gagnon C, ed. The MaleGamete: From Basic Science to Clinical Applications. Clearwater: Cache River Press, 1999:446-454.
190. Swan MA. Improved preservation of ultrastructural morphology in human spermatozoa using betaine in the primary fixative. Int J Androl 1997; 20:45-54.

191. Swan SH, Elkin EP, Fenster L. The question of declining sperm density revisited: An analysis of 101 studies published 1934-1996. Environ Health Perspect 2000; 108:961-966.
192. Savage MO, Lowe DG. Gonadal neoplasia and abnormal sexual differentiation. Clin Endocrinol (Oxf) 1990; 32:519-533.
193. Henderson BE, Ross R, Bernstein L. Estrogens as a cause of human cancer: The Richard and Hinda Rosenthal Foundation award lecture. Cancer Res 1988; 48:246-253.
194. Dieckmann KP, Classen J, Souchon R et al. Management of testicular intraepithelial neoplasia (TIN)—A review based on the principles of evidence-based medicine. Wien Klin Wochenschr 2001; 113:7-14.
195. Weir HK, Marrett LD, Kreiger N et al. Prenatal and peri-natal exposures and risk of testicular germ-cell cancer. Int J Cancer 2000; 87:438-443.
196. Strohsnitter WC, Noller KL, Hoover RN et al. Cancer risk in men exposed in utero to diethylstilbestrol. J Natl Cancer Inst 2001; 93:545-551.
197. Skakkebaek NE, Berthelsen JG, Giwercman A et al. Carcinoma-in-situ of the testis: Possible origin from gonocytes and precursor of all types of germ cell tumours except spermatocytoma. Int J Androl 1987; 10:19-28.
198. Dieckmann KP, Skakkebaek NE. Carcinoma in situ of the testis: Review of biological and clinical features. Int J Cancer 1999; 83:815-822.
199. Rajpert-De Meyts E, Jorgensen N, Brondum-Nielsen K et al. Developmental arrest of germ cells in the pathogenesis of germ cell neoplasia. APMIS 1998; 106:198-204.
200. Slowikowska-Hilczer J, Walczak-Jedrzejowska R, Kula K. Immunohistochemical diagnosis of preinvasive germ cell cancer of the testis. Folia Histochem Cytobiol 2001; 39:67-72.
201. Jones ME, Simpson ER. Oestrogens in male reproduction. Baillieres Best Pract Res Clin Endocrinol Metab 2000; 14:505-516.
202. Lombardi G, Zarrilli S, Colao A et al. Estrogens and health in males. Mol Cell Endocrinol 2001; 178:51-55.
203. Safe S. Clinical correlates of environmental endocrine disruptors. Trends Endocrinol Metab 2005; 16:139-144.
204. Moggs JG. Molecular responses to xenoestrogens: Mechanistic insights from toxicogenomics. Toxicology 2005; 213:177-193.
205. Tabb MM, Blumberg B. New modes of action for endocrine-disrupting chemicals. Mol Endocrinol 2006; 20:475-482.
206. Sharpe RM. Pathways of endocrine disruption during male sexual differentiation and masculinization. Best Pract Res Clin Endocrinol Metab 2006; 20:91-110.

Chapter 4

Selenium, a Key Element in Spermatogenesis and Male Fertility

Carla Boitani* and Rossella Puglisi

Abstract

Selenium is essential for normal spermatogenesis of mammals and its critical role is mainly mediated by two selenoproteins, namely phospholipid hydroperoxide glutathione peroxidase (PHGPx/GPx4) and Selenoprotein P. PHGPx/GPx4 is the major selenoprotein expressed by germ cells in the testis, having multiple functions and representing the pivotal link between selenium, sperm quality and male fertility. Selenoprotein P is a plasma protein that is required for selenium supply to the testis. In the last years, nutritional studies and experimental animal models lacking/overexpressing a specific PHGPx isoform and selenoprotein P have highly expanded our understanding on how the male reproductive system depends on selenium. The focus of this review is to report and discuss the most relevant and recent findings in this field. Clinical data have pointed to a correlation between abnormal PHGPx content in sperm and disturbance of human male fertility. However, additional evidence is still required to draw any definitive conclusions about therapeutical strategies for improving fertility by selenium administration.

Introduction

Selenium (Se) is an essential trace element that plays an important role in a number of physiological processes in animals and humans. This element is incorporated into proteins as selenocysteine (Sec, the 21st amino acid), thanks to a peculiar translation reprogramming that allows mRNA UGA codon to be specifically recognized by the selenocysteinyl-tRNA, instead of canonically functioning as stop signal. One or more Sec residues are consistently found in the primary structure of all selenoproteins and they are essential catalytic site components in a variety of selenoenzymes.

The testis represents a specific and privileged target of Se. This element, in fact, appears to be essential for maintaining a normal spermatogenesis and for male fertility. In case of Se deficiency, regulatory mechanisms strive to maintain an adequate level of this element in the male gonad and, when selenium is administered again, the Se is supplied to the testis with priority over other tissues.[1] Given the strict dependence of normal sperm production on Se, a particular interest has been addressed to selenoprotein P (SEPP1), a plasma and extracellular selenoprotein predominantly produced by liver, that carries Se to male germ cells.[2] In the mammalian testis, almost the entire Se content is associated with the enzyme phospholipid hydroperoxide glutathione peroxidase (PHGPx/GPx4), a member of the large subfamily of the glutathione peroxidases (GPx) selenoproteins, most of which are antioxidant enzymes that

*Corresponding Author: Carla Boitani—Department of Histology and Medical Embryology, "Sapienza" University of Rome, Rome, Italy. Email: carla.boitani@uniroma1.it

Molecular Mechanisms in Spermatogenesis, edited by C. Yan Cheng. ©2008 Landes Bioscience and Springer Science+Business Media.

reduce hydroperoxides at the expense of glutathione (GSH). However, PHGPx has a number of unique features compared to other family members, making the role of this enzyme in the testis worth of particular interest.

In this review, we provide a brief overview of the importance of selenium and selenoproteins in mammalian spermatogenesis and male fertility, and report the most relevant findings in this field.

The Selenoproteins of the Male Gonad

A comprehensive and comparative analysis of all known members of the selenoprotein family has recently been performed in the mouse testis by real-time PCR.[3] As mentioned above, PHGPx/GPx4mRNA is by far the most abundant among those coding for selenoproteins and large evidence has recently highlighted the different roles this gene plays in the male gonad. Other selenoprotein transcripts approximate levels that are 10fold lower than that of PHGPx. Among these, the protein product of the *Thioredoxin/Glutathione Reductase* (TGR) gene, a member of the thioredoxin reductase (TR) family, is expressed in post-puberal testis and is particularly abundant in elongating spermatids at the site of mitochondrial sheat formation, while it is absent in mature sperm. It was recently proposed that TGR cooperates with PHGPx by acting as a novel disulfide bond formation system at the level of structural protein components of the sperm.[4] As for Selenoprotein V (Sel V), Northern blot and in situ hybridisation analyses showed a low, yet testis-specific, expression of this molecule restricted to the seminiferous tubules,[5] the physiological function of which is still unknown. Low abundancy transcripts for Selenoprotein W, Selenoprotein K, Selenoprotein 15 and Selenoprotein S also appear in the testis; however, the specific roles of these proteins have not been characterized yet. SEPP1, a tipically plasma selenoprotein and also synthesized in the testis, only in the Leydig cells,[6] was recently shown to be required for sperm development by the sterility phenotype of the male *Sepp1* knock out mice.[7] In addition, a number of selenoprotein-synthesis key factors are also expressed in the testis, including the Selenocysteine Lyase, an enzyme (not containing Se) that specifically catalyzes Sec decomposition to alanine and elemental Se, and the Selenophosphate Synthetase (SPS2), allowing Se utilization in selenoprotein biosynthesis.[8] Table 1 lists the selenoproteins expressed in the mouse testis.

Table 1. Selenoproteins in the testis

Selenoprotein	mRNA	Protein	Function
PHGPx/GPx4	+ + + +	+ + + +	-Antioxidant -Structural protein of sperm midpiece mitochondrial sheath -Involved in sperm chromatin condensation
TGR	+	+	-Disulfide bond formation
SEPP1	+	+	-Selenium delivery and antioxidant
Sel V	+	n.d.	n.d.
Sel W	+	+	n.d.
Sel K	+ +	n.d.	n.d.
Sep 15	+	n.d.	n.d.
Sel S	+	n.d.	n.d.
SPS 2	+	n.d.	-Selenium donor in selenoprotein biosynthesis

n.d., Not determined. Relative abundance: + + + +, very high; + +, modest; +, low.

PHGPx/GPx4

Expression of PHGPx in the Testis

The selenoprotein phospholipid hydroperoxide glutathione peroxidase (PHGPx), first purified from pig liver by Ursini and coworkers in 1982, was included among peroxidases, with particular reference to GSH-peroxidases superfamily, because of its ability to reduce phosphatidylcholine hydroperoxides.[9] Nowdays we know that this enzyme has unique properties compared with other members of the family, including the ability to reduce the intracellular membrane phospholipid hydroperoxides and to use the thiol groups of proteins as substrates, besides those of GSH,[10] particularly when the GSH intracellular level is low.

The *Phgpx* gene encodes for three isoforms having specific subcellular localization in mitochondria, cytosol and nucleus, respectively, and differing on their N-terminal amino acid sequence. The N-termini of the mitochondrial (mPHGPx) and cytosolic (cPHGPx) variants derive from the same exon 1a by different translation sites, whereas the N-terminus of the nuclear isoform (nPHGPx) is generated by the alternative exon 1b, which in turn is driven by another promoter located in the first intron of the gene.[11]

It is interesting to note that the testis exhibits the highest specific activity of PHGPx so far measured in mammalian tissues, being almost two orders of magnitude higher than that of brain and liver.[11,12] Based on this observation, the interest in the presence and function of different variants of this enzyme in the testis has rapidly increased. During mouse embryogenesis, both mitochondrial and cytosolic PHGPx mRNAs are expressed at higher levels with respect to that of the nuclear isoform. However, the expression of both nuclear and mitochondrial PHGPx is down-regulated between E15.5 and E17.5.[13] During postnatal life, PHGPx expression in the testis is initiated at puberty and is hormone-dependent. In both hypophysectomized rats and testosterone-deprived rats, in fact, testicular PHGPx activity and mRNA appeared to significantly decrease and were partially restored by treatment with hCG and testosterone, resepctively. [14,15] Our group has studied the cellular distribution of different PHGPx isoforms within the male gonad in both rat and mouse. We investigated the patterns of mPHGPx and nPHGPx expression during male germ cell differentiation at both mRNA level and protein level, using highly enriched fractions of pachytene spermatocyte germ cells, as well as fractions of steps 1-8 round spermatids. We demonstrated that nPHGPx is switched on in the post-meiotic phase and that, by contrast, mPHGPx is expressed from mid-late pachytene spermatocytes onwards.[16] Moreover, we also observed the presence of abundant catalytic activity of PHGPx and/or nPHGPx in purified populations of pachytene spermatocytes and round spermatids, the haploid cells showing the highest activity.[16] The presence of PHGPx was also demonstrated in elongated spermatids as well as epididymal spermatozoa by immunohistochemistry with antibodies recognizing the three isoforms.[10,17]

In spite of PHGPx abundance in the testis, still very little is known about mechanism(s) underlying the massive up-regulation of the gene in this tissue. The existence of two distinct promoters resulting in alternative transcription of mPHGPx/cPHGPx and nPHGPx was conclusively demonstrated by reporter gene analysis.[11] Functional cis-regulatory elements were identified within the proximal promoter region of nPHGPx.[18] By using highly purified rat spermatid cells, Tramer et al[19] were able to demonstrate that nPHGPx expression is mediated by the transcription factor CREM-t, binding a genetic element localized in the first intron of *Phgpx* gene. In addition, reporter gene assays carried on in a somatic cell line showed that CREM-t expression activates the promoter region of *Phgpx* intron1a.[19]

Evidence for More Than One Function for PHGPx in the Testis

The high expression of PHGPx in the testis underlines the relevance of this gene to spermatogenesis. All three isoforms of this enzyme efficiently catalyze the reduction of phospholipid hydroperoxides by oxidation of glutathione, clearly indicating that they are involved in germ cell protection against oxidative damage. In particular sperm cells, which are provided of a very special membrane enrichment in phospholipids with polyunsaturated fatty acids (PUFA), depend on several scavenging systems, including PHGPx, for protection from oxidative stress.[20] Consistent with this idea, spermatozoa contain a large amount of PHGPx.[10] On the other hand, both in vitro and in vivo evidence has been accumulating in the last years, pointing to other roles for PHGPx beyond the classical antioxidant one. Both mPHGPx and cPHGPx represent almost 50% of the capsule material embedding the spermatozoa mitochondrial helix, where these molecules are apparently enzymatically inactive and form protein aggregates by disulfide bridge cross-linking.[21] The role of PHGPx as structural protein may explain the impairment of sperm motility associated with morphological alterations of sperm midpiece that was observed in Se-deficient animals.[22] In line with this conclusion, spermatozoa of infertile men with asthenozoospermia showed a significant, albeit controversial, decrease of rescued PHGPx specific activity and expression,[23-25] thus emphasizing the clinical relevance of PHGPx enzyme(s).

As for the nuclear variant, it was proposed to be involved in the stabilization of condensed chromatin during sperm maturation.[26] Indeed, knock-out mice specifically lacking nPHGPx, although viable and fertile, displayed defective chromatin condensation in caput epididymis sperm. This defect was apparently overcome during subsequent epididymal sperm maturation, suggesting that nPHGPx is dispensable for the maintenance of male fertility in the mouse.[26] In agreement with this, the sperm of Se-deficient mice displayed abnormal heads.[27,28] In addition, nPHGPx is expressed is concomitance with the chromatin remodelling process in haploid cells.[16] This complex event is paralleled by loss of glutathione[29,30] and the thiol-oxidase activity of PHGPx is preferentially addressed to protamines, the nuclear proteins required for sperm head condensation.[10] In contrast, the deletion of all exons of the *Phgpx* gene results in embryonic lethality between 7.5 and 8.5 dpc of homozygous mice, pinpointing the vital relevance of this gene.[31,32] Functional silencing of the different PHGPx isoforms during in vitro embryogenesis by short interfering RNA technology, provided a possible explanation for the early intrauterine death of *Phgpx*-deficient mice.[13] In fact, targeted knockdown of mPHGPx strongly impaired hindbrain development and induced cerebral apoptosis, whereas a silenced expression of the nuclear isoform led to a delayed heart development. These data suggest that mPHGPx and/or cPHGPx are more important for murine embryogenesis than nPHGPx.

Gain-of-function approaches were used to study the protective role of PHGPx against oxidative stress in vivo. Indeed, transgenic mice overexpressing PHGPx in all tissues were more resistant to diquat-induced liver damage, due to the decrease in lipid peroxidation compared to wild-type animals. In line with this finding, mice having a single copy of *Phgpx* gene displayed an increased sensitivity to oxidative stress produced by gamma irradiation, paraquat and hydrogen peroxide.[32] However, more informative models to investigate specific PHGPx functions in spermatogenesis in vivo consist in conditioned knock-out and /or transgenic animal models that lack/overexpress a specific isoform in a cell/stage-specific manner. In this direction, we investigated the physiological effects of mPHGPx overexpression during early male germ cell differentiation by generating transgenic mice bearing the rat *mPhgpx* coding sequence driven by the mouse Synaptonemal Complex Protein 1 promoter. This strategy allows the transgene to be specifically activated in the testis from the zygotene to diplotene stages of the first meiotic division.[33] Because endogenous mPHGPx transcripts first appear at the middle-late pachytene stage, the expression of the mPHGPX transgene was not only increased in amount, but also developmentally anticipated.[34] Transgenic mice were fully viable and developed normally, indicating that mPHGPx overexpression did not affect embryogenesis and postnatal life and ruling out the possibility of nonspecific effects due to transgene insertion per se. Interestingly, primary spermatocytes specifically underwent an increase in apoptosis frequency, according to testis- and stage-specific expression of the transgene, which eventually resulted in a severe loss of haploid germ cells and tubular epithelium disorganization. In line with these features, adult transgenic male mice also displayed a reduction in fertility. This study thus suggested that mPHGPx expression is tightly regulated in pachytene spermatocytes and that any spatial-temporal increase in mPHGPx expression results in a damage to spermatogenesis and eventual loss of haploid cells.[34]

Selenoprotein P

Selenoprotein P (SEPP1) is a peculiar selenoproteome member, differing from other selenoproteins because of its unique content of several Sec residues (up to 17, depending on the species). SEPP1 is an extracellular protein that is tipically found in the plasma and that is mainly secreted by liver, even though it is also produced by other tissues, including testis.[6] The hypothesis of SPP1 function as Se transportation/distribution protein was conclusively demonstrated by studies of *Sepp1* gene inactivation in mice.[35,36] In fact, *Sepp1* knockout mice exhibited a decreased tissue distribution of Se within the organism, being the brain the most affected organ and followed by kidney and testis. In agreement with these findings, these mice had a number of neurological and sterility problems similar to those of mice bearing a specific deletion of the Se-rich C-terminal domain of SEPP1,[37] pinpointing testis and brain as the most Se-sensitive tissues. Consistent with this feature, the expression of selenoproteins, including PHGPx and Sel W, appeared to be significantly decreased in brain and testis, when *Seep1* gene was deleted.[3] The *Sepp1* knockout mouse model has provided further insight into the mechanisms of Se importance to spermatogenesis. Indeed, mature spermatozoa of these mice displayed a number of flagellar structure defects, including truncated mitochondrial sheath, extrusion of axonemal microtubules and outer dense fibers from principal piece, as well as a hairpin-like bend formation at the midpiece-principal piece junction.[7,38] Sperm defects of *Sepp1*-null mice were indistinguishable from those of wild-type males that had been fed with a low selenium diet (see also next section). However, sperm defects of Se-deficient wild-type mice were reverted by a normal Se diet, whereas in the case of *Sepp1* knockout mice, dietary Se supplementation had no effect on sperm phenotype and did not restore fertility,[7] reinforcing the notion that the testis strictly depends on Se supply by circulating SEPP1. Accordingly, it was very recently shown that a liver-specific expression of a transgene coding for human SEPP1 in *Sepp1* knockout mice can rescue the abnormal testicular phenotype and fertility of these animals, provided they are maintained under normal Se diet.[39]

It is currently accepted that preferential Se delivery to testis by SEPP1 is mediated by apolipoprotein E receptor 2 (ApoER2), a receptor expressed in the testis, exclusively by Sertoli cells.[40] Interestingly, Sertoli cells display a SEPP1 localization at the level of vesicle-like structures at the basal region suggesting SEPP1 internalization via receptor-mediated endocytosis. Moreover, coimmunoprecipitation analysis demonstrated an interaction of testicular ApoER2 with SEPP1. These morphological and biochemical findings are also supported by the genetic evidence that ApoER2-null mice display reduced levels of testis, but not liver, Se, defective spermatozoa and male infertility.[40,41] Thus, both SEPP1 and ApoER2 are essential for maintaining normal Se levels in the testis and are functionally linked with each other in the pathway(s) providing Se to male germ cells. However, it is still not known how the SE conten of SEPP1 is delivered to spermatogenic cells. In addition, SEPP1 may also be produced in the testis itself. In fact, selenoprotein P mRNA was found to be expressed in rat male gonads, only in Leydig cells.[6] However, the physiological function of SEPP1 in this cell type still remains to be elucidated. Another function of SEPP1 is to serve as oxidant defense agent. In fact, it was reported that injections of Se into Se-deficient rats resulted in the appearance of SEPP1 in plasma, correlating closely with an increase in protection against the diquat-induced liver necrosis and lipid peroxidation.[42,43]

Nutritional Considerations

The nutritional importance of Se for male reproduction has been known for decades and thoroughly assessed by feeding rats with a Se-deficient diet, eliciting the appearance of a number of reproductive disorders, including reduced fertility, sperm impaired motility and abnormal tail morphology.[22,44] When a low Se diet was administered for several generations, severe testicular atrophy that could be reversed by a Se-adequate diet was observed.[45] As mentioned above, morphological studies of spermatids and epididymal spermatozoa have pinpointed the sperm flagellum as the major target of Se deficiency,[38] as well as altered shape of spermatozoa head,[27] associated with incomplete chromatin condensation.[28]

The effect of Se-deficient, Se-adequate and Se-excess diets on spermatogenesis has extensively been investigated in a series of studies in the mouse, conclusively showing that either a Se deficiency or excess in the diet resulted in an increase in oxidative stress that negatively affected male germ cell number and differentiation and fertility,[46-49] such effect being modulated by the redox-sensitive and cell proliferation controlling transcription factors, NFkappaB and AP1.[47,48,50] It thus appears that abnormal Se levels in the diet, namely either deficiency or excess, are both detrimental to animal health and fertility. Moreover, the idea that high levels of antioxidants impair the progression of male germ cell differentiation is also strengthened by the finding of increased germ cell apoptosis in male transgenic mice that specifically overexpressed mitochondrial PHGPx in male meiotic cells.[34] Consistent with this finding, the dietary administration of a mixture of the anti-oxidant agents vitamins C and E to mice increased the occurrence of sperm head abnormalities and caused a reduction in sperm production.[51] Unfortunately, however, the alteration of male reproductive potential by increased/decreased Se does not give a clear-cut insight on this issue, in light of the very large number of selenoprotein-coding genes and the multiple body districts where these genes are expressed.[52]

Clinical Implications

In contrast to experimental animals, the impact of dietary Se on male fertility in man is not proven yet. A study performed in Scotland reported a sperm motility increase in patients that had received an oral Se supplementation, although a positive response to treatment vs. placebo was only observed in 56% of them.[53] However, owing the very limited tolerance to both a defective and an exceeding dietary Se level in mammals, including humans, any therapeutical strategy of improving fertility by Se administration in man requires that the Se status is accurately assessed before the treatment is initiated.

In light of the structural role that mPHGPx plays on sperm flagellum in the rat, the possibility that a reduction in sperm mPHGPx impairs fertilization in men was thoroughly addressed by several authors. Interestingly, sperm from infertile patients with oligoasthenozoospermia displayed a dramatic decrease in the level of mPHGPx expression, which was also associated with reduced sperm motility and defects in mitochondrial morphology and function.[23] In additon, Foresta et al,[24] studying sperm PHGPx activity after a reducing "rescuing" procedure in patients with different etiologies of infertility, found that these patients consistently had a lower level of enzymatic activity than healthy controls. They thus proposed that PHGPx is included among clinical tests for infertility diagnosis. In contrast, no significant difference in PHGPx activity was observed between normo- and hypo-motile human sperm when the enzyme activity was assayed under native conditions.[25] PHGPx activity may also depend on the genetic background. This issue was addressed by analyzing the whole *Phgpx* gene for polymorphisms in groups of infertile and fertile men and discovering the presence of 11 variant sites in 5 out of 42 infertile patients.[54] The majority of these variant sites, however, was likely irrelevant to fertility, because they were located in introns, and only 1 of exon variants actually led to an Ala93-Thr exchange that reduced PHGPx activity in the porcine *gpx-4* homologue. A more recent study[55] did not find any correlation between a low level of sperm PHGPx and the presence of *Phgpx* gene variants in oligoasthenozoospermic patients. Therefore, even though the possibility that *Phgpx* polymorphism seldom represents an actual cause of infertility cannot be ruled out, the actual relationship between quantitative/qualitative PHGPx alteration and infertility in man still remains to be further investigated.

References

1. Behne D, Hofer T, Berswordt-Wallrabe R et al. Selenium in the testis of the rat: Studies on its regulation and its importance for the organism. J Nutr 1982; 112(9):1682-1687.
2. Burk RF, Hill KE, Motley AK. Selenoprotein metabolism and function: Evidence for more than one function for selenoprotein P. J Nutr 2003; 133(5 Suppl 1):1517S-1520S.
3. Hoffmann PR, Hoge SC, Li PA et al. The selenoproteome exhibits widely varying, tissue-specific dependence on selenoprotein P for selenium supply. Nucleic Acids Res 2007; 35(12):3963-3973.
4. Su D, Novoselov SV, Sun QA et al. Mammalian selenoprotein thioredoxin-glutathione reductase: Roles in disulfide bond formation and sperm maturation. J Biol Chem 2005; 280(28):26491-26498.
5. Kryukov GV, Castellano S, Novoselov SV et al. Characterization of mammalian selenoproteomes. Science 2003; 300(5624):1439-1443.
6. Koga M, Tanaka H, Yomogida K et al. Expression of selenoprotein-P messenger ribonucleic acid in the rat testis. Biol Reprod 1998; 58(1):261-265.
7. Olson GE, Winfrey VP, Nagdas SK et al. Selenoprotein P is required for mouse sperm development. Biol Reprod 2005; 73(1):201-211.
8. Mihara H, Kurihara T, Watanabe T et al. cDNA cloning, purification, and characterization of mouse liver selenocysteine lyase: Candidate for selenium delivery protein in selenoprotein synthesis. J Biol Chem 2000; 275(9):6195-6200.
9. Ursini F, Maiorino M, Valente M et al. Purification from pig liver of a protein which protects liposomes and biomembranes from peroxidative degradation and exhibits glutathione peroxidase activity on phosphatidylcholine hydroperoxides. Biochim Biophys Acta 1982; 710(2):197-211.
10. Godeas C, Tramer F, Micali F et al. Distribution and possible novel role of phospholipid hydroperoxide glutathione peroxidase in rat epididymal spermatozoa. Biol Reprod 1997; 57(6):1502-1508.
11. Maiorino M, Scapin M, Ursini F et al. Distinct promoters determine alternative transcription of gpx-4 into phospholipid-hydroperoxide glutathione peroxidase variants. J Biol Chem 2003; 278(36):34286-34290.
12. Ursini F, Maiorino M, Brigelius-Flohe R et al. Diversity of glutathione peroxidases. Methods Enzymol 1995; 252:38-53.
13. Borchert A, Wang CC, Ufer C et al. The role of phospholipid hydroperoxide glutathione peroxidase isoforms in murine embryogenesis. J Biol Chem 2006; 281(28):19655-19664.
14. Roveri A, Casasco A, Maiorino M et al. Phospholipid hydroperoxide glutathione peroxidase of rat testis. Gonadotropin dependence and immunocytochemical identification. J Biol Chem 1992; 267(9):6142-6146.
15. Maiorino M, Wissing JB, Brigelius-Flohe R et al. Testosterone mediates expression of the selenoprotein PHGPx by induction of spermatogenesis and not by direct transcriptional gene activation. FASEB J 1998; 12(13):1359-1370.
16. Puglisi R, Tramer F, Panfili E et al. Differential splicing of the phospholipid hydroperoxide glutathione peroxidase gene in diploid and haploid male germ cells in the rat. Biol Reprod 2003; 68(2):405-411.
17. Tramer F, Micali F, Sandri G et al. Enzymatic and immunochemical evaluation of phospholipid hydroperoxide glutathione peroxidase (PHGPx) in testes and epididymal spermatozoa of rats of different ages. Int J Androl 2002; 25(2):72-83.
18. Borchert A, Savaskan NE, Kuhn H. Regulation of expression of the phospholipid hydroperoxide/sperm nucleus glutathione peroxidase gene. Tissue-specific expression pattern and identification of functional cis- and trans-regulatory elements. J Biol Chem 2003; 278(4):2571-2580.
19. Tramer F, Vetere A, Martinelli M et al. cAMP-response element modulator-tau activates a distinct promoter element for the expression of the phospholipid hydroperoxide/sperm nucleus glutathione peroxidase gene. Biochem J 2004; 383(Pt 1):179-185.
20. Lenzi A, Gandini L, Picardo M et al. Lipoperoxidation damage of spermatozoa polyunsaturated fatty acids (PUFA): Scavenger mechanisms and possible scavenger therapies. Front Biosci 2000; 5:E1-E15.
21. Ursini F, Heim S, Kiess M et al. Dual function of the selenoprotein PHGPx during sperm maturation. Science 1999; 285(5432):1393-1396.
22. Wu AS, Oldfield JE, Shull LR et al. Specific effect of selenium deficiency on rat sperm. Biol Reprod 1979; 20(4):793-798.
23. Imai H, Suzuki K, Ishizaka K et al. Failure of the expression of phospholipid hydroperoxide glutathione peroxidase in the spermatozoa of human infertile males. Biol Reprod 2001; 64(2):674-683.
24. Foresta C, Flohe L, Garolla A et al. Male fertility is linked to the selenoprotein phospholipid hydroperoxide glutathione peroxidase. Biol Reprod 2002; 67(3):967-971.

25. Tramer F, Caponecchia L, Sgro P et al. Native specific activity of glutathione peroxidase (GPx-1), phospholipid hydroperoxide glutathione peroxidase (PHGPx) and glutathione reductase (GR) does not differ between normo- and hypomotile human sperm samples. Int J Androl 2004; 27(2):88-93.
26. Conrad M, Moreno SG, Sinowatz F et al. The nuclear form of phospholipid hydroperoxide glutathione peroxidase is a protein thiol peroxidase contributing to sperm chromatin stability. Mol Cell Biol 2005; 25(17):7637-7644.
27. Watanabe T, Endo A. Effects of selenium deficiency on sperm morphology and spermatocyte chromosomes in mice. Mutat Res 1991; 262(2):93-99.
28. Pfeifer H, Conrad M, Roethlein D et al. Identification of a specific sperm nuclei selenoenzyme necessary for protamine thiol cross-linking during sperm maturation. FASEB J 2001; 15(7):1236-1238.
29. Shalgi R, Seligman J, Kosower NS. Dynamics of the thiol status of rat spermatozoa during maturation: Analysis with the fluorescent labeling agent monobromobimane. Biol Reprod 1989; 40(5):1037-1045.
30. Seligman J, Newton GL, Fahey RC et al. Nonprotein thiols and disulfides in rat epididymal spermatozoa and epididymal fluid: Role of gamma-glutamyl-transpeptidase in sperm maturation. J Androl 2005; 26(5):629-637.
31. Imai H, Hirao F, Sakamoto T et al. Early embryonic lethality caused by targeted disruption of the mouse PHGPx gene. Biochem Biophys Res Commun 2003; 305(2):278-286.
32. Yant LJ, Ran Q, Rao L et al. The selenoprotein GPX4 is essential for mouse development and protects from radiation and oxidative damage insults. Free Radic Biol Med 2003; 34(4):496-502.
33. Sage J, Martin L, Meuwissen R et al. Temporal and spatial control of the Sycp1 gene transcription in the mouse meiosis: Regulatory elements active in the male are not sufficient for expression in the female gonad. Mech Dev 1999; 80(1):29-39.
34. Puglisi R, Bevilacqua A, Carlomagno G et al. Mice overexpressing the mitochondrial phospholipid hydroperoxide glutathione peroxidase in male germ cells show abnormal spermatogenesis and reduced fertility. Endocrinology 2007; 148(9):4302-4309.
35. Hill KE, Zhou J, McMahan WJ et al. Deletion of selenoprotein P alters distribution of selenium in the mouse. J Biol Chem 2003; 278(16):13640-13646.
36. Schomburg L, Schweizer U, Holtmann B et al. Gene disruption discloses role of selenoprotein P in selenium delivery to target tissues. Biochem J 2003; 370(Pt 2):397-402.
37. Hill KE, Zhou J, Austin LM et al. The selenium-rich C-terminal domain of mouse selenoprotein P is necessary for the supply of selenium to brain and testis but not for the maintenance of whole body selenium. J Biol Chem 2007; 282(15):10972-10980.
38. Olson GE, Winfrey VP, Hill KE et al. Sequential development of flagellar defects in spermatids and epididymal spermatozoa of selenium-deficient rats. Reproduction 2004; 127(3):335-342.
39. Renko K, Werner M, Renner-Muller I et al. Hepatic selenoprotein P (Sepp) expression restores selenium transport and prevents infertility and motor-incoordination in Sepp-knockout mice. Biochem J 2007.
40. Olson GE, Winfrey VP, Nagdas SK et al. Apolipoprotein E receptor-2 (ApoER2) mediates selenium uptake from selenoprotein P by the mouse testis. J Biol Chem 2007; 282(16):12290-12297.
41. Andersen OM, Yeung CH, Vorum H et al. Essential role of the apolipoprotein E receptor-2 in sperm development. J Biol Chem 2003; 278(26):23989-23995.
42. Atkinson JB, Hill KE, Burk RF. Centrilobular endothelial cell injury by diquat in the selenium-deficient rat liver. Lab Invest 2001; 81(2):193-200.
43. Burk RF, Hill KE, Awad JA et al. Pathogenesis of diquat-induced liver necrosis in selenium-deficient rats: Assessment of the roles of lipid peroxidation and selenoprotein P. Hepatology 1995; 21(2):561-569.
44. Wu SH, Oldfield JE, Whanger PD et al. Effect of selenium, vitamin E, and antioxidants on testicular function in rats. Biol Reprod 1973; 8(5):625-629.
45. Behne D, Weiler H, Kyriakopoulos A. Effects of selenium deficiency on testicular morphology and function in rats. J Reprod Fertil 1996; 106(2):291-297.
46. Shalini S, Bansal MP. Dietary selenium deficiency as well as excess supplementation induces multiple defects in mouse epididymal spermatozoa: Understanding the role of selenium in male fertility. Int J Androl 2007.
47. Shalini S, Bansal MP. Alterations in selenium status influences reproductive potential of male mice by modulation of transcription factor NFkappaB. Biometals 2007; 20(1):49-59.
48. Shalini S, Bansal MP. Role of selenium in regulation of spermatogenesis: Involvement of activator protein 1. Biofactors 2005; 23(3):151-162.
49. Kaur P, Bansal MP. Effect of selenium-induced oxidative stress on the cell kinetics in testis and reproductive ability of male mice. Nutrition 2005; 21(3):351-357.

50. Brigelius-Flohe R. Glutathione peroxidases and redox-regulated transcription factors. Biol Chem 2006; 387(10-11):1329-1335.
51. Ten J, Vendrell FJ, Cano A et al. Dietary antioxidant supplementation did not affect declining sperm function with age in the mouse but did increase head abnormalities and reduced sperm production. Reprod Nutr Dev 1997; 37(5):481-492.
52. Kohrle J, Jakob F, Contempre B et al. Selenium, the thyroid, and the endocrine system. Endocr Rev 2005; 26(7):944-984.
53. Scott R, MacPherson A, Yates RW et al. The effect of oral selenium supplementation on human sperm motility. Br J Urol 1998; 82(1):76-80.
54. Maiorino M, Bosello V, Ursini F et al. Genetic variations of gpx-4 and male infertility in humans. Biol Reprod 2003; 68(4):1134-1141.
55. Diaconu M, Tangat Y, Bohm D et al. Failure of phospholipid hydroperoxide glutathione peroxidase expression in oligoasthenozoospermia and mutations in the PHGPx gene. Andrologia 2006; 38(4):152-157.

Chapter 5

Extracellular Matrix and Its Role in Spermatogenesis

Michelle K.Y. Siu* and C. Yan Cheng

Abstract

In adult mammalian testes, such as rats, Sertoli and germ cells at different stages of their development in the seminiferous epithelium are in close contact with the basement membrane, a modified form of extracellular matrix (ECM). In essence, Sertoli and germ cells in particular spermatogonia are "resting" on the basement membrane at different stages of the seminiferous epithelial cycle, relying on its structural and hormonal supports. Thus, it is not entirely unexpected that ECM plays a significant role in regulating spermatogenesis, particularly spermatogonia and Sertoli cells, and the blood-testis barrier (BTB) constituted by Sertoli cells since these cells are in physical contact with the basement membrane. Additionally, the basement membrane is also in close contact with the underlying collagen network and the myoid cell layers, which together with the lymphatic network, constitute the tunica propria. The seminiferous epithelium and the tunica propria, in turn, constitute the seminiferous tubule, which is the functional unit that produces spermatozoa via its interaction with Leydig cells in the interstitium. In short, the basement membrane and the underlying collagen network that create the acellular zone of the tunica propria may even facilitate cross-talk between the seminiferous epithelium, the myoid cells and cells in the interstitium. Recent studies in the field have illustrated the crucial role of ECM in supporting Sertoli and germ cell function in the seminiferous epithelium, including the BTB dynamics. In this chapter, we summarize some of the latest findings in the field regarding the functional role of ECM in spermatogenesis using the adult rat testis as a model. We also highlight specific areas of research that deserve attention for investigators in the field.

Introduction

Spermatogenesis is a precisely regulated process by which one spermatogonium (diploid, 2n) divides and differentiates into 256 spermatids (haploid, 1n) via 14 stages of the seminiferous epithelial cycle with six mitotic and two meiotic divisions in adult rat testes.[1] In order to complete these intriguingly regulated events, there are extensive junction restructuring in the seminiferous epithelium at both the blood-testis barrier (BTB; note: BTB is a testis-specific structure composed of side-by-side arranged tight junctions [TJ], the basal ectoplasmic specialization [ES], the basal tubulobulbar complexes [TBC], both are testis-specific adherens junction [AJ] types, and the desmosome-like junctions [DJ]) between adjacent Sertoli cells; and anchoring junctions, such as apical ES, apical TBS, DJs and gap junctions (GJ), between Sertoli and germ cells (see Fig. 1). This thus permits developing germ cells, such as preleptotene

*Corresponding Author: Michelle K.Y. Siu—Department of Pathology, Queen Mary Hospital, University of Hong Kong, Hong Kong, China. Email: mkysiu@pathology.hku.hk

Molecular Mechanisms in Spermatogenesis, edited by C. Yan Cheng. ©2008 Landes Bioscience and Springer Science+Business Media.

and leptotene spermatocytes, traverse the BTB at stage VIII of the seminiferous epithelial cycle for further development into round, elongating, and elongated spermatids, yet these cells must remain attached to the nourishing and supporting Sertoli cells.[2,3] In light of these extensive junction restructuring events during spermatogenesis to accommodate the timely migration of germ cells across the epithelium, it is not entirely unexpected that the morphological layouts of TJ and anchoring junctions in the testis are relatively unique versus other epithelia. Furthermore, unlike other blood-tissue barriers, such as the blood-brain and the blood-retina barriers, which are constituted by endothelial TJs of the microvessels in the corresponding organs namely brain and eyes, respectively, the BTB is contributed almost exclusively by adjacent Sertoli cells near the basement membrane of the seminiferous tubules, and the TJ-barrier in the microvessels in the interstitium contribute little, if any, to the BTB function. Interestingly, the peritubular myoid cell layer in rodent testes was shown to prevent the penetration of electron dense markers, such as lanthanum, colloidal carbon or thorium, into the seminiferous epithelium in almost ~85% of the tubules examined,[4,5] even though myoid cells in primate testes were much less effective to restrict the penetration of these markers across the BTB.[6] Collectively, these findings illustrate the myoid cell layer in the tunica propria contributes to the BTB integrity, at least in rodent testes.

The BTB, which physically divides the seminiferous epithelium into the basal and the adluminal (apical) compartments, segregating virtually the entire events of post-meiotic germ cell development and maturation from the systemic circulation, is located closely to the basement membrane (a modified form of extracellular matrix, ECM) (Fig. 1).[7] This morphological layout is in sharp contrast to other epithelia where TJ is located at the apical portion of the cell epithelium, to be followed by the adherens belt (composed of AJ) and desmosomes. Such physical intimacy between the BTB and the basement membrane thus illustrates the possible role of ECM on junction dynamics at the BTB in the testis.[2,3,8,9] Indeed, it was reported that infertile patients with aspermatogenesis were shown to have abnormal basement membrane structures.[10,11] Recent studies have also demonstrated the crucial role of ECM components, such as collagens and laminins, in junction dynamics since these proteins were shown to work in concert with proteases, protease inhibitors, cytokines (e.g., TNFα), and focal adhesion (FA) components found at the ES to regulate the steady-state levels of integral membrane proteins at the cell-cell interface.[12-16] In this chapter, we intend to highlight the recent advances of how ECM proteins and their partners regulate junction dynamics in the testis.

Unique Features of Extracellular Matrix (ECM) in the Testis

ECM, largely composed of glycoproteins and polysaccharides, fills the extracellular space at the cell-cell contact sites.[7] In rodent testes, a specialized form of ECM, constituted largely by type IV collagen and laminins, along with heparan sulfate proteoglycan[17] and entactin,[18] forms the basement membrane (~0.15 μm thick), which encloses each seminiferous tubule and is in contact with the base of Sertoli cells and spermatogonia (Fig. 1). One interesting feature of the basement membrane is that it is adjacent to the blood-testis barrier (BTB),[2,3] where tight junctions (TJ) coexist with adherens junctions (AJ) (Fig. 1), such as basal ectoplasmic specialization (ES) and basal tubulobulbar complex (TBC),[19-21] and desmosome-like junctions (DS);[22] unlike other blood-tissue barriers (e.g., blood-brain barrier and blood-retina barrier) where TJs are furthest away from the ECM, and are localized to the apical portion of the epithelium/endothelium, to be followed by AJ, desmosomes and gap junctions.[23]

Functions of the Blood-Testis Barrier (BTB)

The BTB divides the seminiferous epithelium into the basal and adluminal compartments and thus creates a unique microenvironment for spermatogenesis (Fig. 1). It maintains an immunological barrier by sequestering post-meiotic germ cell development from the systemic circulation, regulates the passage of molecules into the adluminal compartment or vice versa and confers cell polarity.[2,3,24] As such, developing germ cells depend exclusively on Sertoli cells

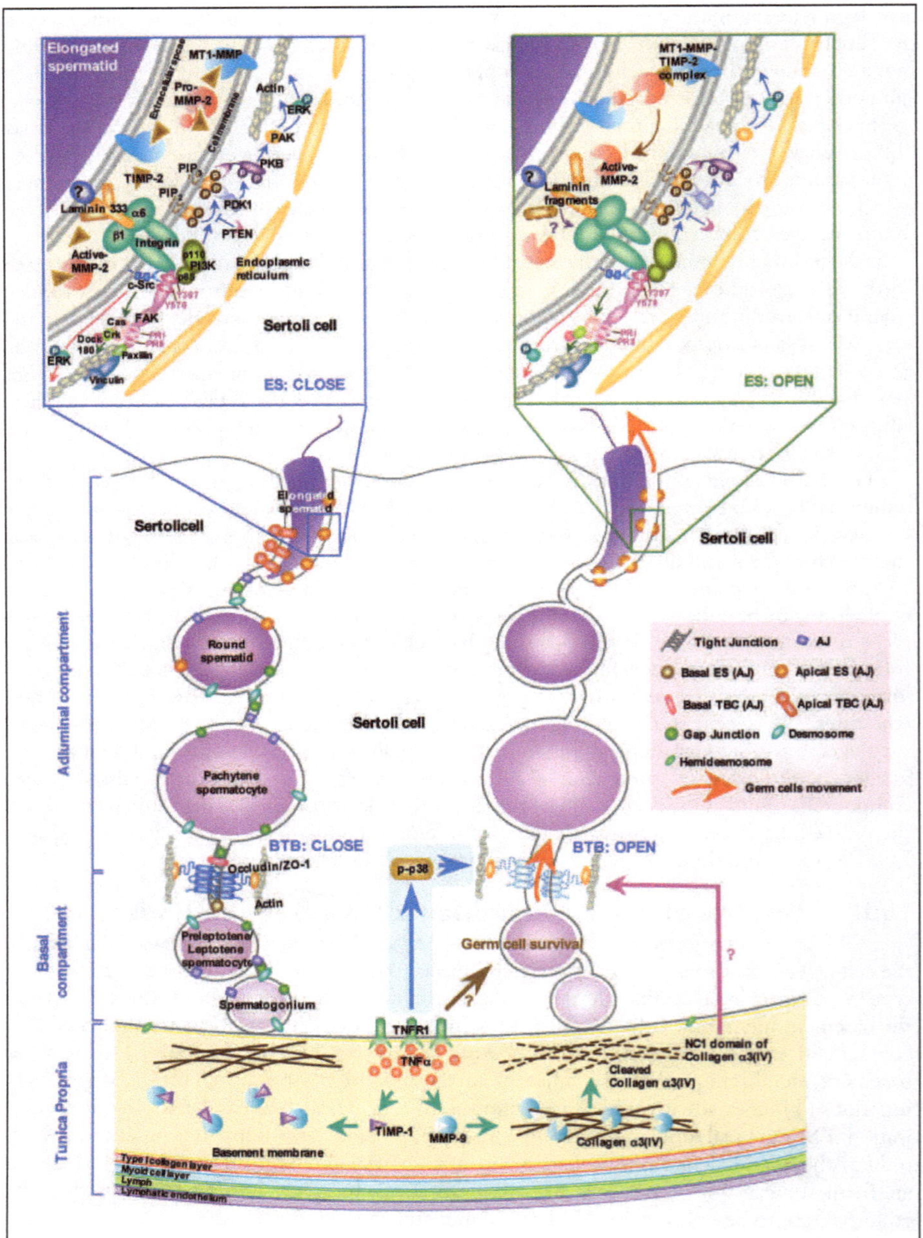

Figure 1. A schematic drawing illustrating the latest model on the regulation of junction dynamics in adult rat testes, including the blood-testis barrier (BTB) and the ectoplasmic specialization (ES). For instance, junction restructuring events that occur at the blood-testis barrier (BTB) and the apical ectoplasmic specialization (apical ES) in the seminiferous epithelium during spermatogenesis apparently are regulated via intriguing interactions between cytokines (e.g., TNFα), proteases (MMP-2, MMP-9, MT1-MMP), protease inhibitors (TIMP-1, TIMP-2), collagens, laminins, adaptors, kinases and phosphatases. Legend continues on following page.

Figure 1, continued from previous page. As described in the text, TNFα regulates the homeostasis of the proteases and protease inhibitors in the basement membrane, which in turn affects the collagen ultrastructural network, perhaps forming biologically active fragments that regulate BTB and/or ES dynamics. However, it remains to be shown if NC1 domain of collagen α3(IV) is indeed responsible for the transient "opening" of the BTB to accommodate preleptotene spermatocyte migration across the barrier that occurs at stage VIII of the seminiferous epithelial cycle, which should be vigorously examined in future studies. Recent studies have shown that similar mechanism(s) is also operating at the apical ES to regulate the transient opening and/or closing of the apical ES to facilitate spermatid movement during spermatogenesis and perhaps also the cellular events that occur at spermiation at late stage VIII of the epithelial cycle, which also involve the participation of proteases and protease inhibitors. This figure was prepared based on recent findings in the field as described in the text.

for structural, anchoring and nutrient supports. Although BTB confers one of the tightest blood-tissue barriers in mammalian body, it is highly dynamic in nature since it must 'open' (or 'disassemble') at stage VIII of the epithelial cycle in adult rat testes on the apical portion of the migrating preleptotene and leptotene spermatocytes and then 'close' (or 'reassemble') at the basal portion of the cell to facilitate cell migration while maintaining the barrier integrity.[24] Without this, spermatogenesis cannot complete. At present, the mechanism(s) governing this timely BTB restructuring is not entirely clear. However, recent studies have shown that ECM components, such as collgen IV, are working in concert with proteases, protease inhibitors and cytokines (e.g., TNFα) to regulate TJ dynamics in the testis.[8,9,14]

Collagen IV

Its Expression and Localization in the Testis

Type IV collagen and laminins are the building blocks of the basement membrane in the testis.[7,23,25] Type IV collagen network is formed by the association of monomer, which is a triple helical structure composed of three α chains.[25,26] Each monomer is characterized by an N-terminus noncollagenous 7S domain (~15 amino acid residues), a middle collagenous domain (~1400 residues of Gly-Xaa-Yaa repeats) and a carboxyl terminal noncollagenous (NC1) domain (~230 residues). There are six genetically distinct α chains including ubiquitous α1(IV) and α2(IV) chains and more restricted α3(IV)-α6(IV) chains.[26,27] α1(IV)-α5(IV) chains are present in rodent testes.[28-30] Moreover, α3(IV) and α4(IV) chains are the major (~80%) collagen chains found in the basement membrane of bovine testes,[31] implicating the unique structural and/or functional role of α3(IV) and α4(IV) chains in the seminiferous tubule basement membrane in the testis. Collagen α1(IV) and α2(IV) chains are products of Sertoli and myoid cells,[28,32,33] whereas α3(IV) is a product of Sertoli and germ cells in the rat.[34]

Roles in TJ Dynamics

There is mounting evidence that collagen functions perhaps not just as a scaffolding protein.[23] For instance, recent studies have shown that Sertoli cell TJ-barrier assembly in vitro was associated with a transient but significant increase in collagen α3(IV) indicating de novo synthesis of collagens is associated with TJ assembly, suggesting the involvement of collagen α3(IV) in TJ dynamics.[14] Furthermore, the presence of an anti-collagen antibody in Sertoli cell cultures during TJ-barrier assembly reversibly disrupted the TJ-barrier, further supporting that the interference of an ECM function affects TJ dynamics. Although the underlying mechanism is presently unclear, subsequent studies have shown that these effects were mediated, at least in part, by cytokines, such as TNF-α, which regulate ECM homeostasis via proteolysis.[14]

TNFα

TNFα and its Receptor and Testicular Function

ECM harbors a pool of cytokines, such as TNFα, which can be released when ECM proteins, such as collagens, are degraded.[7] TNFα (a ~50 kDa trimeric protein, consisting of three identical subunits of 17 kDa each) is produced mainly by activated monocytes and macrophages in the systemic circulation, and is crucial to inflammation, cell proliferation and apoptosis.[35] In the testis, TNFα is a product of germ cells (e.g., round and elongating spermatids), macrophages, and Sertoli cells.[14] Its receptors, p55 and p75, are two structurally related, but functionally distinct receptors found in epithelial cells, including Sertoli cells;[36] however, the p55 TNFα receptor (TNFR p55) in Sertoli cells is the main receptor for TNF signaling.[12,37] In the testis, TNFα plays a crucial role in regulating germ cell apoptosis,[38] Leydig cell steroidogenesis[39] as well as junction dynamics (Fig. 1). For instance, it is now known that in adult rat testes, the number of Sertoli cells, at ~40 million cells, remain relatively stable throughout the adulthood[40,41] since by day 15 post-partum, Sertoli cells cease to divide.[40] As such, these limited number of Sertoli cells cannot support an unlimited number of developing germ cells. Indeed, it has been shown that each Sertoli cells support ~40-50 developing germ cells in adult rodent testes,[42] and that as much as 75% of the developing germ cells undergo apoptosis and/or spontaneous degeneration,[43,44] failing to become mature spermatozoa, which is the mechanism being used in the seminiferous epithelium to regulate the precise number of developing germ cells.[45] Interesting, TNFα was shown to reduce germ cell spontaneous degeneration in rat and human seminiferous tubules cultured in vitro,[38,46] illustrating its germ cell survival promoting effect.

Roles in TJ Dynamics

The role of TNFα on BTB dynamics has been elucidated by both recent in vitro and in vivo studies and a summary of the results on these studies are depicted in Figure 1. In a recent in vitro study, the presence of recombinant TNFα was shown to perturb the Sertoli cell TJ-permeability barrier dose-dependently and specifically since the disrupted TJ-barrier can be resealed upon its removal.[14] This in vitro effect of TNFα on the Sertoli cell TJ-barrier was also confirmed by an in vivo study.[12] In this study, transient and reversible BTB disruption was shown when adult rats were treated with 2 μg recombinant TNFα per testis, which is comparable to its endogenous intratesticular level (~0.5 μg per testis when estimated by a solid-phase immunoblot assay), via an intratesticular injection and assessed by electron microscopy, fluorescent microscopy and a functional assay that monitors the diffusion of a fluorescent dye (fluorescein thioisocyanate, FITC, Mr 389) from the systemic circulation to the seminiferous epithelium behind the BTB.[12] These in vitro and in vivo studies, along with the observations that the expression of TNFα is stage-specific, being highest at stages VII-VIII,[14] coinciding with the events of preleptotene and leptotene spermatocyte migration across the BTB, further support the hypothesis that TNFα secreted by Sertoli and germ cells into the microenvironment at the BTB at stage VIII contributes to the transient BTB "opening" to assist preleptotene spermatocyte migration. This effect of TNFα in "opening" the BTB perhaps is working in concert with its germ cell survival promoting ability so that the migrating preleptotene spermatocytes that likely to take place in "clones" would not undergo spontaneous degeneration. For instance, it is known that germ cell maturation and development occur in "clones" via inter-cellular bridges as they traverse the seminiferous epithelium.[47,48] Perhaps it is important in future studies to design functional experiments to assess if the level of TNFα at the BTB microenvironment is sufficient to induce BTB restructuring while promoting germ cell survival.

Regulation of TJ Dynamics: Effects on TJ-Proteins and ECM Proteins

Furthermore, TNFα apparently exerts its effects on the Sertoli cell TJ-permeability barrier function by regulating the expression of TJ-proteins (e.g., occludin) as illustrated by both in vitro and in vivo studies,[12,14] thereby determining the steady-state protein levels of the integral membrane proteins at the BTB. Besides regulating TJ-proteins, TNFα was shown to induce Sertoli cell collagen α3(IV), matrix metalloprotease (MMP)-9 and tissue-inhibitor of metalloproteases (TIMP)-1, and to promote the activation of pro-MMP-9 to proteolytically active MMP-9.[14] MMPs and TIMPs are proteases and protease inhibitors respectively, that work synergistically to regulate ECM remodeling.[49] As such, these results suggest that the activated MMP-9 induced by TNF-α may be used to breakdown the existing collagen network by cleaving collagen IV, separating the middle collagenous domain from the N-terminal 7S and the COOH-terminal NCI domains in the ECM. Such cleavage process possibly affects the scaffolding function of ECM,[49] thus inducing a loss of other basement membrane proteins (e.g., laminins) and cytokines (e.g., TNFα and TGF-β), which, in turn, contributes to TJ disruption and BTB restructuring because Sertoli cells can no longer attach to an intact ECM. Furthermore, the released biologically active fragments, the NC1 domains, can bind to the middle collagenous domain, inhibit the assembly of intact collagen IV network.[50] Also, these biologically active fragments can have a negative feedback effect that inhibits collagenase production and thus affecting collagen degradation.[51] As such, the induced collagen α3(IV) and TIMP-1 by TNFα may be a negative feedback mediated by the biologically active fragments, so as to replenish the collagen network in the disrupted TJ-barrier and limit the activity of MMP-9. Obviously, this hypothesis must be vigorously examined in future studies. In short, the following question must be address. First, can the collagen α3(IV) NC1 synthetic peptides regulate Sertoli cell MMP-9 and TIMP-1 production and/or their activation using Sertoli cells cultured in vitro? If they can, can they also regulate Sertoli cell TJ-permeability barrier when administered in vitro, or perhaps in vivo? Second, can these in vitro studies be reproduced in vivo that an administration of the NC1 domain peptides intratesticularly that leads to a disruption of the BTB function by disrupting the levels of MMPs and TIMPs in the basement membrane?

After reviewing the involvement of collagen in TJ dynamics, the following section introduces the crucial role of laminin, another ECM component, in ES dynamics.

Ectoplasmic Specialization (ES)

ES is a testis-specific, actin-based adherens junction residing in the basal (defined as basal ES) and apical (defined as apical ES) compartment of the seminiferous epithelium.[3,52,53] Both basal and apical ES consist of a layer of hexagonally packed actin bundles sandwiched between the plasma membrane of the Sertoli cell and the cisternae of endoplasmic reticulum. Basal ES is localized at the Sertoli-Sertoli cell interface at the BTB, present side-by-side with TJ, desmosome-like junctions and gap junctions. Apical ES is found between the heads of developing elongating/elongate spermatids (step 8 and beyond in rat and mouse testes) and Sertoli cells which persists until replacing by apical tubulobulbar complex (apical TBC) restricted to the concave side of the elongated spermatid heads just a few hours before spermiation that occurs at late stage VIII of the seminiferous epithelial cycle in adult rat testes.[20,52]

Basal ES

Cadherins[54] and nectin-2[55] are two AJ transmembrane proteins that are currently found at the basal ES. Recent study has shown that there is an engagement/disengagement mechanism between basal ES and TJ proteins via their corresponding peripheral adaptors, catenins and ZO-1,[56] perhaps being used to reinforce the BTB conferring its barrier function, making the BTB as one of the "tightest" blood-tissue barriers in the mammalian body. Such mechanism was suggested to facilitate preleptotene/leptotene spermatocyte migrate across the BTB at stage VIII of the epithelial cycle that the TJ and basal ES proteins become "disengaged" during BTB restructuring to facilitate germ cell migration across the barrier. However, much study is needed to elucidate the intriguing cross-talk mechanism(s) between basal and apical ES since the "opening" (or restructuring) of the BTB near the basement membrane and the disruption of the apical TBC at spermiation at the luminal edge of the epithelium take place almost simultaneously and since both ultrastructures are present at the opposite ends of the Sertoli cell epithelium, it is not entirely unexpected these events are intimately regulated in the Sertoli cell. Indeed, recent studies have shown that FAK (focal adhesion kinase) is restricted to the basal ES at the BTB where its activated and phosphorylated form, pFAK, is restricted to the apical ES,[15] suggesting that protein kinases that are found at the apical and basal ES are likely play a crucial role to coordinate cross-talk between different cellular events that occur at the opposing ends of the Sertoli cell epithelium.

Apical ES: A Hybrid Cell-Matrix-Cell Junction Type

Besides cadherin·catenin, nectin·afadin protein complexes that are found at both basal and apical ES, apical ES also consists of integrin·laminin complex,[13,15,16,57] which is usually restricted to the focal contact in cell-matrix interface in other epithelia.[58] Such hybrid cell-matrix-cell junction type is suggested to be involved in the rapid junction remodeling facilitating the orientation and movement of spermatids at spermiation.[8,9] While most of the previous studies on ES were largely focus on its morphology, recent studies have shifted the focus to identify the putative components in the ES in order to explore the mechanisms that regulate ES restructuring during the epithelial cycle.[8,9,13,15,16,57,59,60] These findings will be summarized and discussed herein; in particular, recent data regarding the involvement of laminin·integrin complex and its downstream effectors in facilitating germ cell migration are discussed.

Integrin: The First FA Component Found at the Apical ES

Integrin, a heterodimeric transmembrane receptor composed of α and β subunits, is the first integral membrane protein positively identified at the ES.[61] To date, there are 18 α subunits and 8 β subunits present in mammals. Among them, α1, α3, α4, α5, α6, α9, β1, β2 and β3 integrins have been identified in testes.[8,9,61-65] α1, α3, α9, β1 subunits are detected in the basement membrane of the seminiferous epithelium, whereas α1, α4, α5, α6 and β1 subunits are found at the apical ES. When β1 integrin subunit was first detected at the ES in 1992,[61] this study first demonstrated the presence of a ECM-associated protein at the nonbasement membrane site namely the ES, since studies from other epithelia have shown that integrins are largely restricted to focal contacts and hemidesmosomes at the sites of cell-matrix anchoring junctions.[8,9,66] For instance, α6β1 integrin is a known receptor for a wide variety of ECM including collagens, fibronectin and laminin in other epithelia.[67] However, there is no ECM protein present in nonbasement membrane at the time when integrin was first reported at ES. Until recently, more than 10 years after integrin being detected at ES, laminin α3β3γ3[13,56] and other FAC component proteins[15,16,56,60] were detected and structurally linked to integrin at the apical ES. Such findings, along with the presence of proteases activity at the apical ES site,[13] illustrating that apical ES is utilizing the most efficient migration device usually restricted to cell-matrix anchoring junctions to facilitate germ cell movement across the epithelium during spermatogenesis.

Laminin 333 and α6β1 Integrin form a Bona Fide Complex at the Apical ES

Laminins are heterotrimers composed of one each of the α, β, and γ chains. To date, 5 α-subunits, 4 β-subunits, and 3 γ-subunits have been found in mammalian tissues, which can give rise to at least 16 different functional laminins.[68,69] By binding to their transmembrane receptors, integrins, at the cell/matrix anchoring junctions, also known as focal contacts constituted by focal adhesion complexes (FAC), laminins and integrins provide not only adhesion between epithelial cells and basal lamina, they also mediate signaling through the downstream effectors, the FAC, leading to cell migration during normal and in pathological conditions, such as tumor invasion.[70-72] Laminin γ3 was the first laminin subunit found at the apical ES by immunofluorescent microscopy and was shown to form a bona fide complex with β1 integrin by coimmunoprecipitation studies.[13,73] Subsequently, this γ3 chain was found to form a functional laminin protein complex with the α3 and β3 chains, known as laminin 333, which are restricted to the elongating/elongated spermatids and also interact with β1 integrin at the apical ES.[57] Perhaps the most important of all, the pivotal role of laminin 333 at the apical ES was demonstrated by the perturbed adhesion between Sertoli and germ cells (mostly spermatids), leading to germ cell loss from the epithelium following treatment of adult rat testes with the laminin blocking antibodies, including anti-laminin α3 or γ3 IgG.[57]

Proteolysis of Laminin by MMP-2 and MT1-MMP Regulate Apical ES Dynamics

At apical ES, not unlike the cell-matrix interface, proteolysis may also present to regulate its restructuring. For instance, the remodeling of laminin can occur via the effects of proteases since MMP-2, MT1-MMP (a membrane anchored metalloprotease that can activate MMP-2) and TIMP-2 were found to colocalize with laminin γ3 and β1 integrin at the apical ES in adult rat testes.[13,74] Furthermore, MMP-2 and MT1-MMP were shown to be activated when germ cells, especially spermatids, were detached from the epithelium in vivo after treating rats with Adjudin, formerly called AF-2364 [1-(2,4-dichlorobenzyl)-1H-indazole-3-carbohydrazide], which is a potential male contraceptive derived from indazole-3-carboxylic acid and has the capability to selectively disrupt adherens junction between Sertoli cells and germ cells.[75-77] Perhaps the most important of all, the use of a specific MMP-2 and MMP-9 inhibitor, (2R)-2-[(4-biphenylylsulfonyl)amino]-3-phenylpropionic acid, could effectively delay the loss of spermatids from the epithelium induced by Adjudin, indicating the potential role of proteolysis in apical ES disassembly.[13] Such proteolysis of laminin by MMPs leading to the production of laminin fragments at apical ES may be essential for spermatid movement and spermiation since laminin-5 fragments has been shown to affect migration in both breast epithelial cells and prostate cancer cells (see Fig. 1).[78-81] This possibility should be vigorously tested in future studies.

FA Complexes at the Apical ES

The laminin integrin complex at the apical ES confers its cell-matrix FA property. Such property is further confirmed by the discovery of numerous FA components (see Table 1), including βα-integrin, vinculin, c-Src, Csk, ILK, phosphatidylinositol 4,5-bisphosphate ($PI(4,5)P_2$), phospholipase C (PLC)-γ, Fyn and Keap1 in the ES site.[2,53,64,82-86] Recent findings in our laboratories further explore another vital FA component, phosphorylated focal adhesion kinase (pFAK), and its downstream effectors, the p85 subunit of phosphatidylinositol 3-kinase (P13K), protein kinase B (PKB), p21 activated kinases (PAKs) and Crk- associated substrate (CAS), at the apical ES.[15,16] FAK is a nonreceptor protein tyrosine kinase (PTK) that may be a crucial linker for β1 integrin, recruiting ES components to apical ES.[15] When FAK interacts with β1 integrin, FAK undergoes autophosphorylation at Tyr-397, creating high-affinity-binding site for multiple molecules, including (i) SH2-domain-containing molecules, such as Src family protein kinases, (ii) effector proteins, such as P13K and PLC-γ, and (iii) adaptor proteins, such as growth-factor-receptor-bound protein (Grb)7 and Nck-2.[87-89] Furthermore, the newly recruited Src-family kinases at the apical ES can further enhance FAK catalytic activity by inducing phosphorylation of FAK at Tyr-576 and Tyr-577 in the kinase domain activation loop. Two other FAK-associated proteins, CAS and paxillin, can also be phosphorylated by Src-family kinases, leading to Rho family GTPase-mediated cell motility.[87-95]

Recent studies using both in vitro and in vivo models, including Adjudin and androgen suppression models, to study ES dynamics have illustrated the involvement of several signaling pathways which are initiated by β1 integrin/pFAK during apical ES restructuring. These pathways include (i) the integrin/pFAK/c-Src/pERK,[15] (ii) the integrin/pFAK/PI3K/pPKB/PAK/pERK[16] and (iii) the integrin/pFAK/c-Src/Cas/Crk/Dock180 (Siu and Cheng, unpublished observations) (see Fig. 1). All these three pathways have the ability to modulate cell adhesion, migration, tissue remodeling and development, and tumor cell metastasis as shown in studies of other epithelia.[87-95] These signaling pathways were shown to be triggered within a few hours after treating adult male rats with a single or multiple doses of Adjudin (40-50 mg/kg b.w.)

Table 1. ECM-related proteins that are found in the ectoplasmic specialization (ES) in adult rat/mouse testes: their interacting partners, functions, properties, and phenotypes after their knock-outs in mice*

Proteins	*Mr* (kDa)	Binding Partners	Functions/ Properties	Phenotypes in Knock-Out Mice
ECM proteins				
Laminin γ3	146	β1 Integrin, $pFAK^{397}$, c-Src, MMP-2, MT1-MMP	Adhesion, signaling	n.k.
Laminin α3	165	Laminin β3, Laminin γ3	Adhesion, signaling	Neonatal lethality
Laminin β3	140	Laminin α3, Laminin γ3	Adhesion, signaling	n.k.
Transmembrane proteins				
β1 Integrin	140	Laminin γ3, α6 Integrin, $pFAK^{397}$, c-Src, PI3K, p130 Cas, paxillin, vinculin, ILK, N-cadherin, β catenin, actin	Adhesion, signaling	Embryonic lethality on E5.5
α6 Integrin	118	β1 Integrin, paxillin, actin	Adhesion, signaling	Neonatal lethality
Signaling proteins				
$pFAK^{397}$	125	β1 Integrin, PI3K, c-Src, p130 Cas, paxillin, vinculin, gelsolin	PTK	Embryonic lethality on E8.5
c-Src	60	β1 Integrin, $pFAK^{397}$, PAKs 1/2, p130 Cas, Csk, ERK2, N-cadherin, Fer kinase, zyxin, axin, WASP, MTMR2, CAR, actin	PTK	Postnatal lethality
PI3K	80	β1 Integrin, $p\text{-}FAK^{397}$, p130 Cas, paxillin, vinculin, gelsolin, CAR	PTK	Perinatal lethality (in mice lacking all isoforms of P13K p85α)
PTEN	55	Actin, α tubulin, vimentin	Lipid phosphatase	Early embryonic lethality
PKB / pPKB	60	PAK1, actin, α tubulin	Ser/Thr protein kinase	Die shortly after birth
PAKs 1/2	62-65	c-Src (both PAK 1/2), PDK1 (PAK 1 only), PKB (PAK 1 only)	Ser/Thr protein kinase	n.k.
Csk	50	c-Src	PTK	Embryonic lethality on E10

Continued on next page

Table 1. Continued

Fyn	59	Actin	PTK	Viable, fertile
ERK1/2 / pERK1/2	44/42	c-Src, vinculin	MAP kinase	Viable, fertile (in ERK1 -/- mice) Early embryonic lethality after the implantation stage (in ERK2 -/- mice)
ILK	59	β1 Integrin, vinculin, N-cadherin, β catenin	Ser/Thr protein kinase	Die at the peri-implantation stage
Adaptors				
p130 Cas	130	β1 Integrin, $pFAK^{397}$, c-Src, PI3K, Crk, Dock180, paxillin, vinculin, gelsolin	Adaptor	Died in utero
Paxillin	68	β1 Integrin, α6 integrin, FAK, p130 Cas, vinculin, $p120^{ctn}$, actin, tubulin	Adaptor, signaling	Viable, fertile
Vinculin	130	β1 Integrin, $pFAK^{397}$, p130 Cas, ERK2, paxillin, ILK, $p120^{ctn}$, espin, CAR, actin	Adaptor	Embryonic lethality on E10
Proteins pertinent to actin or microtubule remodeling				
$PI(4,5)P_2$	0.971	actin	Gelsolin Inhibitor	n.k.
PLC-γ1	148	actin	Hydrolyzes $PI(4,5)P_2$	Embryonic lethality on E9
Keap1	68	Myosin VIIa	Nrf2 regulator	Postnatal lethality
Proteins pertinent to matrix remodeling				
MMP-2	64-68	MT1-MMP, TIMP-2, laminin γ3, β1 integrin	Degrades ECM proteins	Viable, fertile
MT1-MMP	45,60-63	MMP-2, TIMP-2, laminin γ3, β1 integrin	Involves in MMP-2 activation, degrades ECM proteins	Early postnatal lethality
TIMP-2	22	MMP-2, MT1-MMP	Involves in MMP-2 activation, inhibits MMPs	Viable, fertile

Continued on next page

Table 1. Continued

*This table was prepared based on the following articles and/or reviews (1-3, 7-9, 13, 15, 16, 57, 58, 68, 69, 87). Due to the page limit, many original articles were not cited, however, these references can be found in the cited reviews and/or articles listed herein.

Abbreviations used: n.k., not known; CAR, coxsackie- and adenovirus receptor; Crk, an oncogene identified in a chicken sarcoma called chicken tumor virus number 10, encoding an activator of PTK; Csk, carboxyl-terminal Src kinase, a PTK that phosphorylates a Tyr residue in src family kinases; Dock180, CED-5 (cell death abnormal-5)/180 kDa protein downstream of chicken tumor virus number 10 (Crk); ERK2, externally regulated kinase-2, a mitogen activated protein (MAP) kinase; FAK, focal adhesion kinase; Fer kinase; the Fujinami sarcoma/feline sarcoma (*fps/fes*) proto-oncogene encoding a 94 kDa nonreceptor PTK called Fps/Fes kinase; ILK, integrin-linked kinase; MMP-2, matrix metalloprotease-2; MT1-MMP, membrane-type 1-matrix metalloprotease; MTMR2, myotubularin related protein-2; $PI(4,5)P_2$, also called $PtdIns(4,5)P_2$, phosphatidylinositol 4,5-bisphosphate; PTK, protein tyrosine kinase; PI3K, phosphoinositide (or phosphatidylinositol) 3-kinase; p130 Cas, Crk-associated protein encoded by the Crkas gene; PKB, protein kinase B, also known as Akt, a Ser/Thr protein kinase, a product of the normal gene homolog of v-*akt*,the transforming oncogene of AKT8 virus; PLC-γ1, phospholipase C-γ1; TIMP-2, tissue inhibitor of metalloproteases-2; PAK, p21-activated kinase, a Ser/Thr protein kinase;; PDK1, 3-phosphoinositide-dependent protein kinase 1; PTEN, phosphatase and tensin homolog deleted on chromosome 10, a protein tyrosine phosphatase that shares homology with tensin, and a tumor-suppressor gene located on chromosome 10q23; $p120^{ctn}$, p120 catenin; c-Src, a nonreceptor PTK of the transforming gene of Rous sarcoma virus; WASP, Wiskott-Aldrich Syndrome protein.

either via i.p. or by gavage, which also matched quite nicely with the subsequent germ cell depletion events, especially spermatids at the apical ES, at 6-8 h after treatment.[15,16] Perhaps the most important of all, pretreatment of rats with anti-β1 integrin antibody,[16] PP1(a c-Src inhibitor),[59] wortmannin (a PI3K inhibitor),[16] or U0126 (an ERK inhibitor)[96] via intratesticular injection were shown to delay the Adjudin-mediated spermatid loss from the epithelium, further confirming the involvement of these signaling pathways in the regulation of apical ES restructuring. Furthermore, the integrin/pFAK/c-Src/pERK pathway has recently been validated and expanded by another in vivo model, the androgen suppression model, in which rats were treated with androgen and estrogen implants to suppress the intratesticular androgen level, leading to the alteration of the Sertoli-germ cell apical ES function and the subsequent germ cell sloughing.[60] All of these findings thus illustrate that the cell-cell anchoring junction in the testis is indeed a hybrid cell-cell and cell-matrix junction type.

Furthermore, recent studies have also demonstrated the presence of TJ component proteins at the apical ES, which include the coxsackie and adenovirus receptor (CAR)[97-99] and JAM-C (junctional adhesion molecule-C).[100] These results thus illustrate that the apical ES is also having the structural and perhaps the functional properties of the TJ. While the precise physiology underlying these observations is not entirely clear, it is increasingly clear that the apical ES is adopting some of the best features found in AJ, focal contacts and TJ to regulate the rapid events of germ cell migration and orientation essential to facilitate the rapid junction restructuring event pertinent to spermatogenesis.

Concluding Remarks and Future Perspectives

As briefly reviewed herein, there are mounting evidence illustrating the pivotal role of the basement membrane, a modified form of ECM, on the junction restructuring events that occur at the Sertoli-Sertoli and/or Sertoli-germ cell interface at the BTB and ES, many of which are mediated via the effects of cytokines (e.g., TNFα and TGF-β3) on the steady-state levels of the integral membrane proteins at these sites. Interestingly, some of these effects are likely mediated via the homeostasis of the proteases and their endogenous inhibitors, which in turn, affects the structural and physico-chemical properties of the basement membrane and/or protein levels at the cell-cell interface. It is obvious that much new information will be added in the years to come and some of the postulates put forth here and depicted in Figure 1 schematically will be updated and/or rewritten. Perhaps it is also important that future studies should include a detailed analysis on the peritubular myoid cells and their role on the BTB function, spermatogonial stem cell renewal, and perhaps ES restructuring such as the use of Sertoli-myoid cell and Sertoli-germ-myoid cell cocultures. The recent deployment of molecular, biochemical and cellular techniques to study junction dynamics in the testis has yielded some unprecedented opportunities for investigators to identify new leads to develop male contraceptives. They also offer exciting opportunities to understand the impact of environmental toxicants on male reproductive physiology.

Acknowledgements

This work was supported in part by grants from the National Institutes of Health (NICHD, U54 HD029990, Project 5 to CYC; 5R03 HD051512 to CYC; U01 HD045908 to CYC), the CONRAD Program (CICCR CIG-01-72 to CYC), and a grant from the Committee on Research and Conference Grants from the University of Hong Kong to MKYS.

References

1. de Kretser DM, Kerr JB. The cytology of the testis. In: Knobil E, Neill J, eds. The Physiology of Reproduction. Raven Press, 1988:837-932.
2. Cheng CY, Mruk DD. Cell junction dynamics in the testis: Sertoli-germ cell interactions and male contraceptive development. Physiol Rev 2002; 82:825-874.

3. Mruk DD, Cheng CY. Sertoli-Sertoli and Sertoli-germ cell interactions and their significance in germ cell movement in the seminiferous epithelium during spermatogenesis. Endocr Rev 2004; 25:747-806.
4. Fawcett DW, Leak LV, Heidger PM. Electron microscopic observations on the structural components of the blood-testis barrier. J Reprod Fertil 1970; (Suppl 10):105-122.
5. Dym M, Fawcett DW. The blood-testis barrier in the rat and the physiological compartmentation of the seminiferous epithelium. Biol Reprod 1970; 3:308-326.
6. Dym M. The fine structure of the monkey (Macaca) Sertoli cell and its role in maintaining the blood-tesis barrier. Anat Rec 1973; 175:639-656.
7. Dym M. Basement membrane regulation of Sertoli cells. Endocr Rev 1994; 15:102-115.
8. Siu MK, Cheng CY. Dynamic cross-talk between cells and the extracellular matrix in the testis. Bioessays 2004; 26:978-992.
9. Siu MK, Cheng CY. Extracellular matrix: Recent advances on its role in junction dynamics in the seminiferous epithelium during spermatogenesis. Biol Reprod 2004; 71:375-391.
10. Lehmann D, Temminck B, Da Rugna D et al. Role of immunological factors in male infertility. Immunohistochemical and serological evidence. Lab Invest 1987; 57:21-28.
11. Salomon F, Saremaslani P, Jakob M et al. Immune complex orchitis in infertile men: Immunoelectron microscopy of abnormal basement membrane structures. Lab Invest 1982; 47:555-567.
12. Li MW, Xia W, Mruk DD et al. Tumor necrosis factor α reversibly disrupts the blood-testis barrier and impairs Sertoli-germ cell adhesion in the seminiferous epithelium of adult rat testes. J Endocrinol 2006; 190:313-329.
13. Siu MK, Cheng CY. Interactions of proteases, protease inhibitors, and the β1 integrin/laminin γ3 protein complex in the regulation of ectoplasmic specialization dynamics in the rat testis. Biol Reprod 2004; 70:945-964.
14. Siu MK, Lee WM, Cheng CY. The interplay of collagen IV, tumor necrosis factor-α, gelatinase B (matrix metalloprotease-9), and tissue inhibitor of metalloproteases-1 in the basal lamina regulates Sertoli cell-tight junction dynamics in the rat testis. Endocrinology 2003; 144:371-387.
15. Siu MK, Mruk DD, Lee WM et al. Adhering junction dynamics in the testis are regulated by an interplay of β1-integrin and focal adhesion complex-associated proteins. Endocrinology 2003; 144:2141-2163.
16. Siu MK, Wong CH, Lee WM et al. Sertoli-germ cell anchoring junction dynamics in the testis are regulated by an interplay of lipid and protein kinases. J Biol Chem 2005; 280:25029-25047.
17. Hadley MA, Dym M. Immunocytochemistry of extracellular matrix in the lamina propria of the rat testis: Electron microscopic localization. Biol Reprod 1987; 37:1283-1289.
18. Lian G, Miller KA, Enders GC. Localization and synthesis of entactin in seminiferous tubules of the mouse. Biol Reprod 1992; 47:316-325.
19. Vogl A, Pfeiffer D, Redenbach D et al. Sertoli cell cytoskeleton. In: Russell L, Griswold M, eds. The Sertoli Cell. Cache River Press, 1993:39-86.
20. Russell LD, Malone JP. A study of Sertoli-spermatid tubulobulbar complexes in selected mammals. Tissue Cell 1980; 12:263-285.
21. Guttman JA, Obinata T, Shima J et al. Non-muscle cofilin is a component of tubulobulbar complexes in the testis. Biol Reprod 2004; 70:805-812.
22. Russell L. Desmosome-like junctions between Sertoli and germ cells in the rat testis. Am J Anat 1977; 148:301-312.
23. Alberts B, Johnson A, Lewis J et al. Cell junctions, cell adhesion, and the extracellular matrix. Molecular Biology of the Cell. 4th ed. New York: Garland Science, 2002:1065-1126.
24. Pelletier R. The tight junctions in the testis, epididymis, and vas deferens. In: Cereijido M, Anderson J, eds. Tight Junctions. CRC Press, 2001:599-628.
25. Timpl R, Brown JC. Supramolecular assembly of basement membranes. Bioessays 1996; 18:123-132.
26. Hudson BG, Reeders ST, Tryggvason K. Type IV collagen: Structure, gene organization, and role in human diseases: Molecular basis of Goodpasture and Alport syndromes and diffuse leiomyomatosis. J Biol Chem 1993; 268:26033-26036.
27. Ortega N, Werb Z. New functional roles for non-collagenous domains of basement membrane collagens. J Cell Sci 2002; 115:4201-4214.
28. Davis CM, Papadopoulos V, Sommers CL et al. Differential expression of extracellular matrix components in rat Sertoli cells. Biol Reprod 1990; 43:860-869.
29. Enders GC, Kahsai TZ, Lian G et al. Developmental changes in seminiferous tubule extracellular matrix components of the mouse testis: α3(IV) collagen chain expressed at the initiation of spermatogenesis. Biol Reprod 1995; 53:1489-1499.

30. Frojdman K, Pelliniemi LJ, Virtanen I. Differential distribution of type IV collagen chains in the developing rat testis and ovary. Differentiation 1998; 63:125-130.
31. Kahsai TZ, Enders GC, Gunwar S et al. Seminiferous tubule basement membrane: Composition and organization of type IV collagen chains, and the linkage of α3(IV) and α5(IV) chains. J Biol Chem 1997; 272:17023-17032.
32. Richardson LL, Kleinman HK, Dym M. Basement membrane gene expression by Sertoli and peritubular myoid cells in vitro in the rat. Biol Reprod 1995; 52:320-330.
33. Skinner MK, Tung PS, Fritz IB. Cooperativity between Sertoli cells and testicular peritubular cells in the production and deposition of extracellular matrix components. J Cell Biol 1985; 100:1941-1947.
34. Siu MK, Lee WM, Cheng CY. The interplay of collagen IV, tumor necrosis factor-α, gelatinase B (matrix metalloprotease-9) and tissue inhibitor of metalloproteases-1 in the basal lamina regulates Sertoli cell tight junction dynamics in the rat testis. Endocrinology 2003; 144:371-387.
35. Walsh SV, Hopkins AM, Nusrat A. Modulation of tight junction structure and function by cytokines. Adv Drug Deliv Rev 2000; 41:303-313.
36. Tartaglia LA, Goeddel DV. Two TNF receptors. Immunol Today 1992; 13:151-153.
37. De Cesaris P, Starace D, Starace G et al. Activation of Jun N-terminal kinase/stress-activated protein kinase pathway by tumor necrosis factor α leads to intercellular adhesion molecule-1 expression. J Biol Chem 1999; 274:28978-28982.
38. Pentikainen V, Erkkila K, Suomalainen L et al. TNFα downregulates the Fas ligand and inhibits germ cell apoptosis in the human testis. J Clin Endocrinol Metab 2001; 86:4480-4488.
39. Hong CY, Park JH, Ahn RS et al. Molecular mechanism of suppression of testicular steroidogenesis by proinflammatory cytokine tumor necrosis factor α. Mol Cell Biol 2004; 24:2593-2604.
40. Orth JM. Proliferation of Sertoli cells in fetal and postnatal rats: A quantitative autoradiographic study. Anat Rec 1982; 203:485-492.
41. Wang ZX, Wreford NG, de Kretser DM. Determination of Sertoli cell numbers in the developing rat testis by stereological methods. Int J Androl 1989; 12:58-64.
42. Weber JE, Russell LD, Wong V et al. Three-dimensional reconstruction of a rat stave V Sertoli cell. II. Morphometry of Sertoli-Sertoli and Sertoli-germ-cell relationships. Am J Anaet 1983; 167:163-179.
43. Bartke A. Apoptosis of male germ cells, a generalized or a cell type-specific phenomenon? Endocrinology 1995; 136:3-4.
44. Clermont Y. The cycle of the seminiferous epithelium in man. Am J Anat 1963; 112:35-51.
45. Sinha Hikim AP, Swerdloff RS. Hormonal and genetic control of germ cell apoptosis in the testis. Rev Reprod 1999; 4:38-47.
46. Suominen JS, Wang Y, Kaipia A et al. Tumor necrosis factor-α (TNFα) promotes cell survival during spermatogenesis, and this effect can be blocked by infliximab, a TNF-α antagonist. Eur J Endocrinol 2004; 151:629-640.
47. Ren HP, Russell LD. Clonal development of interconnected germ cells in the rat and its relationship to the segmental and subsegmental organization of spermatogenesis. Am J Anat 1991; 192:121-128.
48. Fawcett DW. Intercellular bridges. Exp Cell Res 1961; 8:174-187.
49. Sternlicht MD, Werb Z. How matrix metalloproteinases regulate cell behavior. Annu Rev Cell Dev Biol 2001; 17:463-516.
50. Tsilibary EC, Charonis AS, Reger LA et al. The effect of nonenzymatic glucosylation on the binding of the main noncollagenous NC1 domain to type IV collagen. J Biol Chem 1988; 263:4302-4308.
51. Vogel W, Gish GD, Alves F et al. The discoidin domain receptor tyrosine kinases are activated by collagen. Mol Cell 1997; 1:13-23.
52. Russell L. Observations on rat Sertoli ectoplasmic ('junctional') specializations in their association with germ cells of the rat testis. Tissue Cell 1977; 9:475-498.
53. Vogl AW, Pfeiffer DC, Mulholland D et al. Unique and multifunctional adhesion junctions in the testis: Ectoplasmic specializations. Arch Histol Cytol 2000; 63:1-15.
54. Lee NP, Mruk D, Lee WM et al. Is the cadherin/catenin complex a functional unit of cell-cell actin-based adherens junctions in the rat testis? Biol Reprod 2003; 68:489-508.
55. Ozaki-Kuroda K, Nakanishi H, Ohta H et al. Nectin couples cell-cell adhesion and the actin scaffold at heterotypic testicular junctions. Curr Biol 2002; 12:1145-1150.
56. Yan HH, Cheng CY. Blood-testis barrier dynamics are regulated by an engagement/disengagement mechanism between tight and adherens junctions via peripheral adaptors. Proc Natl Acad Sci USA 2005; 102:11722-11727.

57. Yan HH, Cheng CY. Laminin α3 forms a complex with β3 and γ3 chains that serves as the ligand for α6β1-integrin at the apical ectoplasmic specialization in adult rat testes. J Biol Chem 2006; 281:17286-17303.
58. Sasaki T, Fassler R, Hohenester E. Laminin: The crux of basement membrane assembly. J Cell Biol 2004; 164:959-963.
59. Lee NP, Cheng CY. Protein kinases and adherens junction dynamics in the seminiferous epithelium of the rat testis. J Cell Physiol 2005; 202:344-360.
60. Wong CH, Xia W, Lee NP et al. Regulation of ectoplasmic specialization dynamics in the seminiferous epithelium by focal adhesion-associated proteins in testosterone-suppressed rat testes. Endocrinology 2005; 146:1192-1204.
61. Palombi F, Salanova M, Tarone G et al. Distribution of β1 integrin subunit in rat seminiferous epithelium. Biol Reprod 1992; 47:1173-1182.
62. Giebel J, Loster K, Rune GM. Localization of integrin β1, α1, α5 and α9 subunits in the rat testis. Int J Androl 1997; 20:3-9.
63. Salanova M, Stefanini M, De Curtis I et al. Integrin receptor α6β1 is localized at specific sites of cell-to-cell contact in rat seminiferous epithelium. Biol Reprod 1995; 52:79-87.
64. Mulholland DJ, Dedhar S, Vogl AW. Rat seminiferous epithelium contains a unique junction (ectoplasmic specialization) with signaling properties both of cell/cell and cell/matrix junctions. Biol Reprod 2001; 64:396-407.
65. Frojdman K, Pelliniemi LJ. Differential distribution of the α6 subunit of integrins in the development and sexual differentiation of the mouse testis. Differentiation 1994; 57:21-29.
66. Juliano RL. Signal transduction by cell adhesion receptors and the cytoskeleton: Functions of integrins, cadherins, selectins, and immunoglobulin-superfamily members. Annu Rev Pharmacol Toxicol 2002; 42:283-323.
67. Mecham RP. Receptors for laminin on mammalian cells. FASEB J 1991; 5:2538-2546.
68. Hallmann R, Horn N, Selg M et al. Expression and function of laminins in the embryonic and mature vasculature. Physiol Rev 2005; 85:979-1000.
69. Aumailley M, Bruckner-Tuderman L, Carter WG et al. A simplified laminin nomenclature. Matrix Biol 2005; 24:326-332.
70. Kuphal S, Bauer R, Bosserhoff AK. Integrin signaling in malignant melanoma. Cancer Metastasis Rev 2005; 24:195-222.
71. Carragher NO, Frame MC. Focal adhesion and actin dynamics: A place where kinases and proteases meet to promote invasion. Trends Cell Biol 2004; 14:241-249.
72. Caswell PT, Norman JC. Integrin trafficking and the control of cell migration. Traffic 2006; 7:14-21.
73. Koch M, Olson PF, Albus A et al. Characterization and expression of the laminin γ3 chain: A novel, nonbasement membrane-associated, laminin chain. J Cell Biol 1999; 145:605-618.
74. Longin J, Guillaumot P, Chauvin MA et al. MT1-MMP in rat testicular development and the control of Sertoli cell proMMP-2 activation. J Cell Sci 2001; 114:2125-2134.
75. Cheng CY, Silvestrini B, Grima J et al. Two new male contraceptives exert their effects by depleting germ cells prematurely from the testis. Biol Reprod 2001; 65:449-461.
76. Grima J, Silvestrini B, Cheng CY. Reversible inhibition of spermatogenesis in rats using a new male contraceptive, 1-(2,4-dichlorobenzyl)-indazole-3-carbohydrazide. Biol Reprod 2001; 64:1500-1508.
77. Mruk DD, Wong CH, Silvestrini B et al. A male contraceptive targeting germ cell adhesion. Nat Med 2006; 12:1323-1328.
78. Koshikawa N, Giannelli G, Cirulli V et al. Role of cell surface metalloprotease MT1-MMP in epithelial cell migration over laminin-5. J Cell Biol 2000; 148:615-624.
79. Udayakumar TS, Chen ML, Bair EL et al. Membrane type-1-matrix metalloproteinase expressed by prostate carcinoma cells cleaves human laminin-5 beta3 chain and induces cell migration. Cancer Res 2003; 63:2292-2299.
80. Giannelli G, Falk-Marzillier J, Schiraldi O et al. Induction of cell migration by matrix metalloprotease-2 cleavage of laminin-5. Science 1997; 277:225-228.
81. Gilles C, Polette M, Coraux C et al. Contribution of MT1-MMP and of human laminin-5 γ2 chain degradation to mammary epithelial cell migration. J Cell Sci 2001; 114:2967-2976.
82. Siu MK, Cheng CY. Interactions of proteases, protease inhibitors, and the β1 integrin/laminin γ3 protein complex in the regulation of ectoplasmic specialization dynamics in the rat testis. Biol Reprod 2004; 70:945-964.
83. Wine RN, Chapin RE. Adhesion and signaling proteins spatiotemporally associated with spermiation in the rat. J Androl 1999; 20:198-213.
84. Velichkova M, Guttman J, Warren C et al. A human homologue of Drosophila kelch associates with myosin-VIIa in specialized adhesion junctions. Cell Motil Cytoskeleton 2002; 51:147-164.

85. Guttman JA, Janmey P, Vogl AW. Gelsolin—evidence for a role in turnover of junction-related actin filaments in Sertoli cells. J Cell Sci 2002; 115:499-505.
86. Maekawa M, Toyama Y, Yasuda M et al. Fyn tyrosine kinase in Sertoli cells is involved in mouse spermatogenesis. Biol Reprod 2002; 66:211-221.
87. Cohen LA, Guan JL. Mechanisms of focal adhesion kinase regulation. Curr Cancer Drug Targets 2005; 5:629-643.
88. McLean GW, Carragher NO, Avizienyte E et al. The role of focal-adhesion kinase in cancer - A new therapeutic opportunity. Nat Rev Cancer 2005; 5:505-515.
89. Parsons JT. Focal adhesion kinase: The first ten years. J Cell Sci 2003; 116:1409-1416.
90. Iwahara T, Akagi T, Fujitsuka Y et al. CrkII regulates focal adhesion kinase activation by making a complex with Crk-associated substrate, p130Cas. Proc Natl Acad Sci USA 2004; 101:17693-17698.
91. Tsuda M, Tanaka S, Sawa H et al. Signaling adaptor protein v-Crk activates Rho and regulates cell motility in 3Y1 rat fibroblast cell line. Cell Growth Differ 2002; 13:131-139.
92. Goldberg GS, Alexander DB, Pellicena P et al. Src phosphorylates Cas on tyrosine 253 to promote migration of transformed cells. J Biol Chem 2003; 278:46533-46540.
93. Shin NY, Dise RS, Schneider-Mergener J et al. Subsets of the major tyrosine phosphorylation sites in Crk-associated substrate (CAS) are sufficient to promote cell migration. J Biol Chem 2004; 279:38331-38337.
94. Gu J, Sumida Y, Sanzen N et al. Laminin-10/11 and fibronectin differentially regulated integrin-dependent Rho and Rac activation via $p130^{Cas}$-CrkII-DOCK180 pathway. J Biol Chem 2001; 276:27090-27097.
95. Grimsley CM, Kinchen JM, Tosello-Trampont AC et al. Dock180 and ELMO1 proteins cooperate to promote evolutionarily conserved Rac-dependent cell migration. J Biol Chem 2004; 279:6087-6097.
96. Xia W, Cheng CY. TGF-β3 regulates anchoring junction dynamics in the seminiferous epithelium of the rat testis via the Ras/ERK signaling pathway: An in vivo study. Dev Biol 2005; 280:321-343.
97. Wang CQ, Mruk DD, Lee WM et al. Coxsackie and adenovirus receptor (CAR) is a product of Sertoli and germ cells in rat testes which is localized at the Sertoli-Sertoli and Sertoli-germ cell interface. Exp Cell Res 2007; 313:1373-1392.
98. Raschperger E, Thyberg J, Pettersson S et al. The coxsackie- and adenovirus receptor (CAR) is an in vivo marker for epithelial tight junctions, with a potential role in regulating permeability and tissue homeostasis. Exp Cell Res 2006; 312:1566-1580.
99. Mirza M, Hreinsson J, Strand ML et al. Coxsackievirus and adenovirus receptor (CAR) is expressed in male germ cells and forms a complex with the differentiation factor JAM-C in mouse testis. Exp Cell Res 2006; 312:817-830.
100. Gliki G, Ebnet K, Aurrand-Lions M et al. Spermatid differentiation requires the assembly of a cell polarity complex downstream of junctional adhesion molecule-C. Nature 2004; 320-324.
57. Yan HH, Cheng CY. Laminin α3 forms a complex with β3 and γ3 chains that serves as the ligand for α6β1-integrin at the apical ectoplasmic specialization in adult rat testes. J Biol Chem 2006; 281:17286-17303.
58. Sasaki T, Fassler R, Hohenester E. Laminin: The crux of basement membrane assembly. J Cell Biol 2004; 164:959-963.
59. Lee NP, Cheng CY. Protein kinases and adherens junction dynamics in the seminiferous epithelium of the rat testis. J Cell Physiol 2005; 202:344-360.
60. Wong CH, Xia W, Lee NP et al. Regulation of ectoplasmic specialization dynamics in the seminiferous epithelium by focal adhesion-associated proteins in testosterone-suppressed rat testes. Endocrinology 2005; 146:1192-1204.
61. Palombi F, Salanova M, Tarone G et al. Distribution of β1 integrin subunit in rat seminiferous epithelium. Biol Reprod 1992; 47:1173-1182.
62. Giebel J, Loster K, Rune GM. Localization of integrin β1, α1, α5 and α9 subunits in the rat testis. Int J Androl 1997; 20:3-9.
63. Salanova M, Stefanini M, De Curtis I et al. Integrin receptor α6β1 is localized at specific sites of cell-to-cell contact in rat seminiferous epithelium. Biol Reprod 1995; 52:79-87.
64. Mulholland DJ, Dedhar S, Vogl AW. Rat seminiferous epithelium contains a unique junction (ectoplasmic specialization) with signaling properties both of cell/cell and cell/matrix junctions. Biol Reprod 2001; 64:396-407.
65. Frojdman K, Pelliniemi LJ. Differential distribution of the α6 subunit of integrins in the development and sexual differentiation of the mouse testis. Differentiation 1994; 57:21-29.
66. Juliano RL. Signal transduction by cell adhesion receptors and the cytoskeleton: Functions of integrins, cadherins, selectins, and immunoglobulin-superfamily members. Annu Rev Pharmacol Toxicol 2002; 42:283-323.

67. Mecham RP. Receptors for laminin on mammalian cells. FASEB J 1991; 5:2538-2546.
68. Hallmann R, Horn N, Selg M et al. Expression and function of laminins in the embryonic and mature vasculature. Physiol Rev 2005; 85:979-1000.
69. Aumailley M, Bruckner-Tuderman L, Carter WG et al. A simplified laminin nomenclature. Matrix Biol 2005; 24:326-332.
70. Kuphal S, Bauer R, Bosserhoff AK. Integrin signaling in malignant melanoma. Cancer Metastasis Rev 2005; 24:195-222.
71. Carragher NO, Frame MC. Focal adhesion and actin dynamics: A place where kinases and proteases meet to promote invasion. Trends Cell Biol 2004; 14:241-249.
72. Caswell PT, Norman JC. Integrin trafficking and the control of cell migration. Traffic 2006; 7:14-21.
73. Koch M, Olson PF, Albus A et al. Characterization and expression of the laminin γ3 chain: A novel, nonbasement membrane-associated, laminin chain. J Cell Biol 1999; 145:605-618.
74. Longin J, Guillaumot P, Chauvin MA et al. MT1-MMP in rat testicular development and the control of Sertoli cell proMMP-2 activation. J Cell Sci 2001; 114:2125-2134.
75. Cheng CY, Silvestrini B, Grima J et al. Two new male contraceptives exert their effects by depleting germ cells prematurely from the testis. Biol Reprod 2001; 65:449-461.
76. Grima J, Silvestrini B, Cheng CY. Reversible inhibition of spermatogenesis in rats using a new male contraceptive, 1-(2,4-dichlorobenzyl)-indazole-3-carbohydrazide. Biol Reprod 2001; 64:1500-1508.
77. Mruk DD, Wong CH, Silvestrini B et al. A male contraceptive targeting germ cell adhesion. Nat Med 2006; 12:1323-1328.
78. Koshikawa N, Giannelli G, Cirulli V et al. Role of cell surface metalloprotease MT1-MMP in epithelial cell migration over laminin-5. J Cell Biol 2000; 148:615-624.
79. Udayakumar TS, Chen ML, Bair EL et al. Membrane type-1-matrix metalloproteinase expressed by prostate carcinoma cells cleaves human laminin-5 beta3 chain and induces cell migration. Cancer Res 2003; 63:2292-2299.
80. Giannelli G, Falk-Marzillier J, Schiraldi O et al. Induction of cell migration by matrix metalloprotease-2 cleavage of laminin-5. Science 1997; 277:225-228.
81. Gilles C, Polette M, Coraux C et al. Contribution of MT1-MMP and of human laminin-5 γ2 chain degradation to mammary epithelial cell migration. J Cell Sci 2001; 114:2967-2976.
82. Siu MK, Cheng CY. Interactions of proteases, protease inhibitors, and the β1 integrin/laminin γ3 protein complex in the regulation of ectoplasmic specialization dynamics in the rat testis. Biol Reprod 2004; 70:945-964.
83. Wine RN, Chapin RE. Adhesion and signaling proteins spatiotemporally associated with spermiation in the rat. J Androl 1999; 20:198-213.
84. Velichkova M, Guttman J, Warren C et al. A human homologue of Drosophila kelch associates with myosin-VIIa in specialized adhesion junctions. Cell Motil Cytoskeleton 2002; 51:147-164.
85. Guttman JA, Janmey P, Vogl AW. Gelsolin—Evidence for a role in turnover of junction-related actin filaments in Sertoli cells. J Cell Sci 2002; 115:499-505.
86. Maekawa M, Toyama Y, Yasuda M et al. Fyn tyrosine kinase in Sertoli cells is involved in mouse spermatogenesis. Biol Reprod 2002; 66:211-221.
87. Cohen LA, Guan JL. Mechanisms of focal adhesion kinase regulation. Curr Cancer Drug Targets 2005; 5:629-643.
88. McLean GW, Carragher NO, Avizienyte E et al. The role of focal-adhesion kinase in cancer—A new therapeutic opportunity. Nat Rev Cancer 2005; 5:505-515.
89. Parsons JT. Focal adhesion kinase: The first ten years. J Cell Sci 2003; 116:1409-1416.
90. Iwahara T, Akagi T, Fujitsuka Y et al. CrkII regulates focal adhesion kinase activation by making a complex with Crk-associated substrate, p130Cas. Proc Natl Acad Sci USA 2004; 101:17693-17698.
91. Tsuda M, Tanaka S, Sawa H et al. Signaling adaptor protein v-Crk activates Rho and regulates cell motility in 3Y1 rat fibroblast cell line. Cell Growth Differ 2002; 13:131-139.
92. Goldberg GS, Alexander DB, Pellicena P et al. Src phosphorylates Cas on tyrosine 253 to promote migration of transformed cells. J Biol Chem 2003; 278:46533-46540.
93. Shin NY, Dise RS, Schneider-Mergener J et al. Subsets of the major tyrosine phosphorylation sites in Crk-associated substrate (CAS) are sufficient to promote cell migration. J Biol Chem 2004; 279:38331-38337.
94. Gu J, Sumida Y, Sanzen N et al. Laminin-10/11 and fibronectin differentially regulated integrin-dependent Rho and Rac activation via $p130^{Cas}$-CrkII-DOCK180 pathway. J Biol Chem 2001; 276:27090-27097.
95. Grimsley CM, Kinchen JM, Tosello-Trampont AC et al. Dock180 and ELMO1 proteins cooperate to promote evolutionarily conserved Rac-dependent cell migration. J Biol Chem 2004; 279:6087-6097.

96. Xia W, Cheng CY. TGF-β3 regulates anchoring junction dynamics in the seminiferous epithelium of the rat testis via the Ras/ERK signaling pathway: An in vivo study. Dev Biol 2005; 280:321-343.
97. Wang CQ, Mruk DD, Lee WM et al. Coxsackie and adenovirus receptor (CAR) is a product of Sertoli and germ cells in rat testes which is localized at the Sertoli-Sertoli and Sertoli-germ cell interface. Exp Cell Res 2007; 313:1373-1392.
98. Raschperger E, Thyberg J, Pettersson S et al. The coxsackie- and adenovirus receptor (CAR) is an in vivo marker for epithelial tight junctions, with a potential role in regulating permeability and tissue homeostasis. Exp Cell Res 2006; 312:1566-1580.
99. Mirza M, Hreinsson J, Strand ML et al. Coxsackievirus and adenovirus receptor (CAR) is expressed in male germ cells and forms a complex with the differentiation factor JAM-C in mouse testis. Exp Cell Res 2006; 312:817-830.
100. Gliki G, Ebnet K, Aurrand-Lions M et al. Spermatid differentiation requires the assembly of a cell polarity complex downstream of junctional adhesion molecule-C. Nature 2004; 320-324.

Chapter 6

Inflammatory Networks in the Control of Spermatogenesis

Chronic Inflammation in an Immunologically Privileged Tissue?

Moira K. O'Bryan* and Mark P. Hedger

Abstract

Spermatogenesis is a complex, organized process involving intimate interactions between the developing germ cells and supporting Sertoli cells. The process is also highly regulated. Studies suggest that regulation in the seminiferous epithelium involves molecules normally associated with either immune or inflammatory processes; in particular, interleukin 1a (IL1a), IL6, tumor necrosis factor (TNFa), activin A and nitric oxide (NO). While there is considerable evidence that these inflammatory mediators have effects on spermatogonial and spermatocyte development as well as critical supportive functions of the Sertoli cells, which are undoubtedly of considerable importance during testicular inflammation, there remains some skepticism regarding the significance of these molecules with respect to normal testicular function. Nonetheless, it is evident that expression of these regulators varies across the cycle of the seminiferous epithelium in a consistent manner, with major changes in production coinciding with key events within the cycle. This review summarizes the evidence supporting the hypothesis that inflammatory cytokines play a role in normal testicular spermatogenesis, as well as in the etiology of inflammation induced sub-fertility. The balance of data leads to the striking conclusion that the cycle of the seminiferous epithelium resembles a chronic inflammatory event. This appears to be a somewhat paradoxical assertion, since the testis is an immunologically privileged tissue based on its well-established ability to support grafts with minimal rejection responses. However, it may be argued that local immunoregulatory mechanisms, which confer protection from immunity on both transplanted tissues and the developing spermatogenic cells, are equally necessary to prevent local inflammation responses associated with the spermatogenic process from activating the adaptive immune response.

Background

Spermatogenesis and the resulting cycle of the seminiferous epithelium are complex and highly organized processes that involve intimate and dynamic interactions between the developing germ cells and their supporting Sertoli cells. The repeating cell associations of the seminiferous epithelium are a consequence of spermatogonia entering the process of spermatogenesis at regularly spaced intervals, which are considerably shorter than the time required for the

*Corresponding Author: Moira K. O'Bryan—Monash Institute of Medical Research and the ARC Centre of Excellence in Biotechnology and Development, Monash University 27-31 Wright St., Clayton 3168, Australia. Email: moira.obryan@med.monash.edu.au

Molecular Mechanisms in Spermatogenesis, edited by C. Yan Cheng.

entire spermatogenic process, and proceeding through the process at a tightly controlled and predictable rate. In the human, for example, it takes approximately 64 days for a spermatogonium to mature into a structurally complete sperm and to be released from the seminiferous epithelium. During this period, 4 rounds of differentiation of the spermatogonial stem cell population, or waves of spermatogenic initiation, occur. Collectively, this leads to the establishment of a complex stratified epithelium comprising 4 separate generations of spermatogenic cells each at different levels of maturation.[1] Spermatogenesis takes about 35 days in the mouse and 48-50 days in the rat,[2,3] but in all mammalian species several rounds of spermatogonial differentiation during this time period produce multiple germ cell generations within each seminiferous tubule cross-section.[4] The regular timing of these events means that the generations form distinct and recurring cellular associations, referred to as stages of the cycle of the seminiferous epithelium. In the human, 6 such stages have been described, while in the mouse the number is 12 and in the rat, 14. How this high degree of coordination is maintained remains largely unknown. In particular, what triggers the stems cells to divide and produce the next generation of developing cells at regular intervals? Conversely, what prevents the spermatogonial stem cells and their offspring from differentiating randomly and continuously? Overall, what is the mechanism that coordinates the process across and along the seminiferous epithelium to ensure that the orderly progression of cellular associations, or stages, is maintained?

Mounting evidence suggests that inflammatory regulators play a key role in the initiation of the spermatogenic wave and in many other aspects of germ cell development. These regulators include the well-characterized cytokines interleukin-1 (IL1) and IL6, but also non-proteinaceous mediators of inflammation and immunity, such as nitric oxide (NO).[5-9] Furthermore, the evidence suggests that such mediators are produced in the testis under normal conditions by somatic cells, including the Sertoli, peritubular and Leydig cells, and the germ cells, rather than by immune cell types.

On the other hand, it is well established that the testis is an immunologically privileged tissue. This is demonstrated by the prolonged survival of grafts into the testicular interstitial tissue,[10,11] and the ability of cotransplanted testicular cells to confer protection from immunological rejection in non-testicular sites.[12,13] The mechanisms responsible for immune privilege of the testis remain incompletely understood, but most evidence suggests that the somatic cells of the testis, and the Sertoli cell in particular, play a key role in the regulation of this property.[12] Moreover, it is evident that the most numerous immune cell type within the testis, the resident macrophages of the testicular interstitium, produces extremely low levels of pro-inflammatory cytokines and mediators when challenged with the potent inflammatory mediator lipopolysaccharide (LPS).[14-17] The fact that these cells also display anti-inflammatory properties and produce cytokines, such as IL10 and transforming growth factor β (TGFβ), when stimulated, suggest that they possess an immunosuppressive phenotype.[15,18-20] Such 'alternatively activated' macrophages are generally associated with sites of reduced immune responses.[21] While lymphocytes and inflammatory monocyte-like macrophages also circulate through the testicular interstitium,[22-24] the unique immune status of the resident macrophages almost certainly serves to reduce the onset and severity of inflammatory and subsequent immunological responses within the testis. Although still a matter for conjecture, these controlled immune/rejection and inflammatory responses are assumed to be in place to benefit the developing spermatogenic cells, which might otherwise be recognized by the host immune system as foreign and come under immunological attack, due to their highly immunogenic properties.[25,26]

It would appear, therefore, that the testis has something of a split immunological personality. On the one hand, there is clear evidence that inflammatory mediators are produced constitutively within the seminiferous epithelium, yet the testis exhibits considerable resistance to the activation of adaptive immune responses. In other words, it appears that testicular immunological privilege coexists with a seminiferous epithelium that otherwise exhibits characteristics of a chronically inflamed tissue! It will be argued in this review that this arrangement is essential for successful spermatogenesis and that disturbances in the balance between these two immunological 'compartments' of the testis result in either immune-mediated damage or spermatogenic failure, leading to germ cell death. Since dysregulation of the networks involved in these processes during systemic or reproductive tract inflammation almost certainly contributes to infertility, a better understanding of this aspect of testicular function is essential.

Production, Regulation and Actions of Inflammatory Mediators in the Seminiferous Epithelium

In general, inflammation occurs when cells of the mononuclear phagocyte lineage (monocytes and macrophages) become activated. This may be triggered by specific pathogenic molecules (e.g., endotoxins such as LPS), phagocytosis of opsonized (antibody- or complement-coated) particles or immune complexes, and/or various intracellular components released by tissue damage.[27] Activation induces the production of cytokines, acute-phase proteins, proteases and complement components, reactive oxygen and nitrogen species, and lipid mediators, such as prostaglandins and platelet activating factor. Non-myeloid cells are less effective than monocytes/macrophages, but also may initiate a response if they share some of the essential receptors and signaling pathways. In this regard, the Sertoli cell is particularly interesting because of several features it shares with cells of the monocyte/macrophage linage, not least its ability to respond to LPS, cyclical phagocytic activity during spermatogenesis, and ability to produce a range of inflammatory mediators.[8,28-32]

The most intensively studied of the inflammatory mediators produced in the seminiferous epithelium are the cytokines IL1α, IL6, tumor necrosis factor (TNFα) and activin A, and the highly reactive nitrogen molecule, nitric oxide (NO). It is on these molecules that this review will focus. While there is evidence that other inflammatory molecules also are involved (e.g., IL2, IL18, interferons and eicosinoids),[33-36] they have been excluded because the evidence for their role in regulating spermatogenesis in the adult remains incomplete or speculative. This is not meant to imply that future studies will not bring such roles to light. Moreover, it should be recognized that some of the mediators discussed here, as well as other immunoregulatory cytokines not discussed (e.g., the TGFβs), have effects on fetal and postnatal testicular development,[37,38] an aspect of testicular biology that also has been excluded from the scope of this review.

Interleukin 1

Interleukin 1 is the most comprehensively studied of all of the cytokines normally expressed in the testis. IL1 is produced in two forms, α and β, which share approximately 25% sequence homology and are encoded by separate genes.[39,40] Both forms act through the same receptor complex (IL1R), and exert essentially the same effects across a broad range of immunological and inflammatory processes. Signaling occurs principally (although not exclusively) through activation of the MyD88/TRAF and MAP kinase/Jnk pathways, regulating many pro-inflammatory genes through stimulation of the transcription factors, NFκB and AP-1 (Fig. 1).[41,42] The IL1s are synthesized as 31 to 33 kDa precursor proteins, which are enzymatically cleaved to produce active 17 kDa forms. In the case of IL1α, both the long and short forms are biologically active, but for IL1β the precursor protein is inactive.[43-45] The precursor of IL1β is cleaved by IL1 converting enzyme (ICE or caspase 1) during the process of secretion into the extracellular space, whereas IL1α is cleaved either by the calcium dependent membrane associated cysteine protease (calpain) or by extracellular proteases.[45,46] As both IL1α and β lack a signal sequence, however, their mechanisms of secretion remain poorly defined.[47] Nonetheless, IL1β is copiously secreted by activated monocyte/macrophages and is the main secreted form during inflammation. IL1α is also found in secretions,[45] but is more commonly found in association with the cell membrane and is thought to act as an autocrine or paracrine growth factor involved in direct cell-to-cell communication.[40] In general, the majority of IL1α usually remains within the cell, from whence it may be released following cell damage.

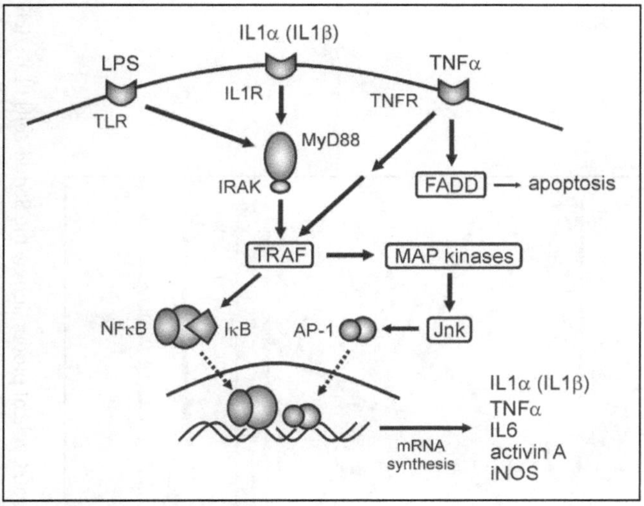

Figure 1. Inflammatory signaling pathways. During inflammation, binding of ligands to their receptors leads to activation of parallel and convergent pathways in responsive cells. IL1α and IL1β act through the IL1 receptor (ILR) via the adaptor protein MyD88, signaling through ILR associated kinases (IRAK) and tumor necrosis factor receptor (TNFR)-associated factors (TRAF), leading to degradation of the nuclear factor (NF)-κB repressor protein IκB and activation of mitogen activated protein (MAP) kinases. MAP kinases activate multiple downstream events, including production of the transcription factor AP1 via the c-jun N-terminal kinase (Jnk). These transcription factors enter the nucleus and activate transcription of a number of inflammation-related genes, including IL1α, IL1β, TNFα, IL6, activin A and inducible NO synthase (iNOS). Depending upon which adaptor molecules are engaged, binding of TNFα to its receptor can lead to activation of TRAF, or to the caspase activation cascade and apoptosis through the Fas-associated death domain protein (FADD). Lipopolysaccharides (LPS) bind to the toll-like receptor (TLR) 4 and also act through the MyD88/TRAF pathway. Note that while the central pathways are depicted, they are by no means the only signaling pathways involved in this complex regulation.

There is a third member of the IL1 cytokine group that is homologous with IL1α and IL1β and binds to IL1R, but lacks the ability to transduce a signal. This molecule acts as an antagonist of IL1 action and is called, naturally enough, IL1 receptor antagonist (IL1ra).[48]

Within the normal testis, the balance of experimental data suggests that IL1α is expressed by the Sertoli cells, where it first appears around day 15-20 in the developing rat testis, and is differentially expressed throughout the cycle of the seminiferous epithelium in the adult (Fig. 2).[5,28,31,49] Specifically, IL1 mRNA and protein production occurs at a more or less constant level throughout the cycle, with the exception of stage VII in the rat, when production is low or non-detectable. Both in vitro, and in vivo data suggest that the Sertoli cell production of IL1α is driven by the presence of spermatogenic cells, but it is most effectively simulated by the phagocytosis of residual bodies produced during spermiation at stage VIII of the cycle.[31] In contrast to studies clearly showing that inflammation stimulates IL1α production by the Sertoli cells in vitro,[28-30] the production of IL1α in the intact rat testis is not stimulated during inflammation in vivo,[15,50] indicating that its production is constitutively and possibly maximally up-regulated under normal conditions.

Within the seminiferous epithelium, the IL1R has been localized to both Sertoli and spermatogenic cells.[51] In vivo and in vitro data suggest that IL1 stimulates DNA synthesis in intermediate and type B spermatogonia as well as preleptotene spermatocytes,[52-55] and acts as

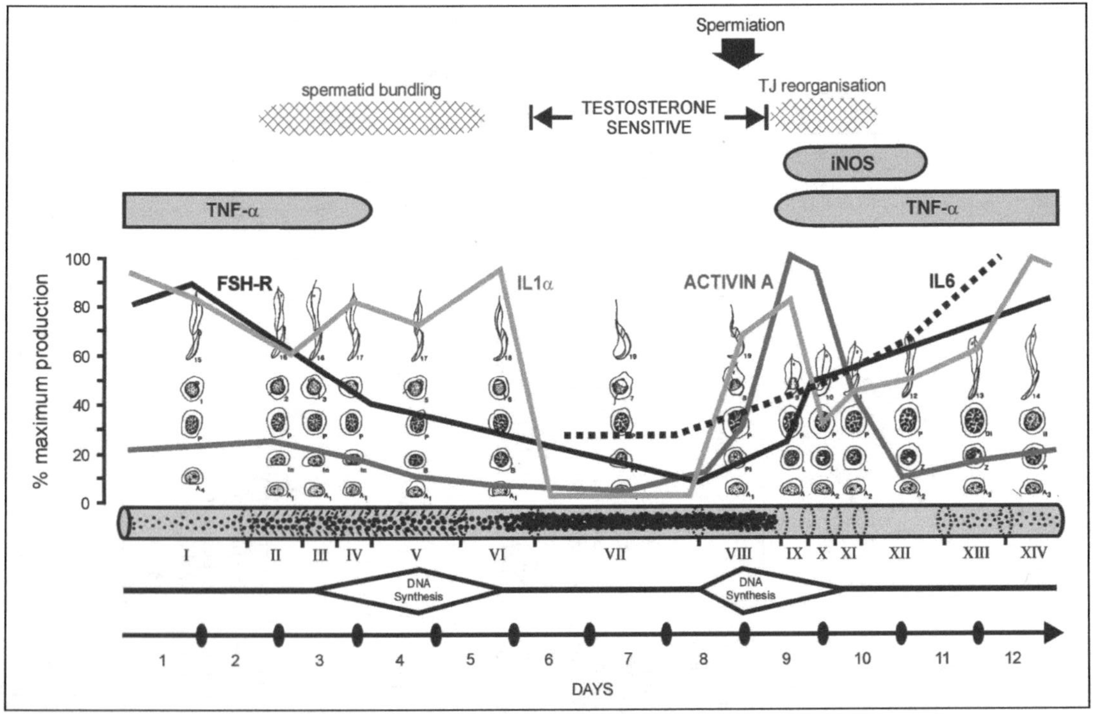

Figure 2. Inflammatory mediator expression during the cycle of the seminiferous epithelium in the rat. Cyclical production by the Sertoli cells (IL1α, IL6 and activin A) and germ cells (TNFα and iNOS) and expression of the FSH receptor (FSHR) are superimposed on critical events during the cycle, such as spermiation, bundling of the spermatids by the Sertoli cells and tight junction (TJ) reorganization to allow meiotic germ cells to pass through the blood-testis barrier. While DNA synthesis occurs throughout the cycle, there are two major peaks of DNA synthesis, at stages IV-VI and at stages VIII-X. The transillumination appearance of the tubules is also shown—the length of each stage of the cycle is presented in proportion to the time taken for each stage to occur. The figure is based on integrated mRNA and protein data from several studies,[9,28,32,49,53,84,123,163,191] and is intended to show relative changes only—some details are approximations based on the available data. Figure modified from original.[32]

an autocrine regulator of several Sertoli cell functions involved in the support of spermatogenesis, including the production of lactate and transferrin.[56,57] It should be noted that Sertoli cells also secrete a 24 kDa testis-specific form of IL1α, which is the product of an alternative mRNA transcript.[58] The 24 kDa variant lacks the calpain cleavage site and consequently is not post-translationally cleaved. The physiological significance of this variant is not entirely clear, although it does possess biological activity.[58,59] It is worth noting here that expression of IL1α also has been reported in isolated late pachytene spermatocytes and round spermatids germ cells,[60,61] although these data are in conflict with other studies.

Although immunohistochemistry has localized IL1β to both the seminiferous epithelium and interstitial tissue of normal mice,[60] quantitative studies in the rat suggest that IL1β expression is comparatively very low in the normal testis.[6,15,49] During inflammation induced by LPS in intact rats, IL1β expression is up-regulated in the testis, but to a much lesser extent than normally occurs in other tissues, such as the liver.[15] In vitro and in vivo studies suggest that production arises from the Leydig cells and a subset of monocyte-like macrophages in the testis, rather than from cells of the seminiferous epithelium.[15,50,62,63] Testicular interstitial fluid IL1β concentrations, as measured by ELISA, also increased following injection of LPS in adult rats, but surprisingly, there was no increase in the overall IL1 bioactivity of testicular interstitial fluid. This was assumed to be due to the constitutively high production of IL1α by the Sertoli cells.[8] A similar observation had been reported previously,[50] wherein the authors suggested that the lack of change in IL1 bioactivity may have been due to a compensatory increase in IL1ra produced by the Sertoli cell.[64] Testicular interstitial fluid fractionation studies, however, established that very little of the IL1β entering the interstitial fluid following LPS stimulation had been cleaved to its active form, suggesting a possible deficiency in the activity of ICE/caspase 1.[15] It appears that pro-inflammatory cytokine activity may be regulated at both the transcriptional and post-translational level in the testis.

Outside the seminiferous tubules, both IL1α and IL1β have direct inhibitory effects on gonadotropin-stimulated androgen production by the Leydig cells.[59,65,66] In the mouse, evidence suggests that the major site of inhibition occurs at the level of 17α-hydroxylase/C17-20 lyase (P450c17) expression, with affects of higher doses on the cholesterol side chain cleavage enzyme (P450scc) and 3β-hydroxysteroid dehydrogenase (3β-HSD).[66,67] In the rat, inhibition appears to involve P450scc, specifically.[68]

Interleukin 6

Interleukin 6 is a member of an important family of mediators involved in the regulation of the acute-phase response to injury and infection, which exert their action via binding to specific receptors that associate with a common membrane signal transducer gp130, leading to the activation of the Jak/Stat and MAP kinase cascades.[69,70] Although evidence suggests that the Leydig cells actually may be the major source of this cytokine in the testis,[7,71] IL6 is produced by isolated rat Sertoli cells in response to stimulation by follicle-stimulating hormone (FSH) and testosterone, or by phagocytosis and other inflammatory stimuli, including IL1α, IL1β, TNFα and LPS (Fig. 1).[7,8,28,29,71,72] Within the seminiferous epithelium, IL6 is produced in a coordinated manner (Fig. 2), and FSH differentially stimulates IL6 secretion during the cycle of the seminiferous epithelium.[28,73] Both gp130 and IL6R mRNA are expressed in rat Sertoli cells, and are stimulated by IL1 and IL6, but only the IL6R subunit is stimulated by FSH.[74]

The data from many studies indicate that that IL1 and IL6 are integrated in a complex network of endocrine and local regulatory mechanisms within the seminiferous epithelium. Stimulation of Sertoli cell IL1α mRNA production, in turn, stimulates IL6 secretion through activation of leukotriene production via the lipoxygenase pathway.[28,29] This results in an endogenous cyclical pattern of secretion that corresponds with the changes in the stages of the spermatogenic cycle, similar to that of IL1α (Fig. 2). IL6 has been found to act as an inhibitor of meiotic DNA synthesis in preleptotene spermatocytes[73] and increases basal and FSH-induced transferrin and cyclic GMP secretion by Sertoli cell.[75,76] On the other hand, IL6 reduces κ opioid receptor mRNA levels in the Sertoli cell.[77] In models of experimental autoimmune orchitis (EAO), IL6 has been implicated as playing an ameliorative or protective role within the seminiferous epithelium.[78,79]

Tumor Necrosis Factor α

Tumor necrosis factor α is a 17 kDa glycosylated polypeptide, principally produced by activated monocytes and macrophages, which binds as a trimer to either of the two TNF receptors (TNFR1 and TNFR2), and plays a central role in the initiation of the inflammatory response by stimulating the production of IL1 and IL6 (Fig. 1).[80,81] As its name suggests, TNFα can also exert a cell-death signal via TNFR1, through interaction with the TNFR-associated death domain protein (TRADD) or the Fas-associated death domain protein (FADD), and activation of the caspase-dependent apoptotic pathway (Fig. 1).[82,83] Whether TNFα has a stimulatory, pro-inflammatory effect, or a destructive effect depends on the receptor subtype engaged and the expression of specific adaptor proteins within the target cell.

In situ hybridization studies in mice have confirmed the presence of TNFα mRNA in round spermatids and pachytene spermatocytes, as well as in testicular interstitial macrophages.[84] Moreover, bioactive TNFα was produced by the round spermatids in vitro and mRNA for the corresponding receptor was located on both Sertoli and Leydig cells. FSH stimulates TNFα receptor subunit protein expression in the Sertoli cell.[85] Expression of TNFα by germ cells within the seminiferous epithelium, like that of IL1α and IL6 in the Sertoli cell, is cyclical (Fig. 2). There is no evidence that TNFα is produced by the Sertoli cell, but treatment of isolated testicular macrophages with LPS induces its secretion.[86,87]

Within the seminiferous epithelium, TNFα appears to play a complex role the regulation of Sertoli cell function and spermatogenesis. TNFα reduces spontaneous germ cell degeneration in cultured human and rat seminiferous tubules, suggesting a germ cell survival effect mediated via the Sertoli cell.[88,89] On the other hand, in vitro studies indicate that TNFα disrupts Sertoli cell tight-junction assembly by inhibiting production of the junction protein, occludin and inducing the expression of matrix metalloprotease-9 and its inhibitor tissue inhibitor of metalloproteases-1.[90] Likewise, TNFα has been reported to increase plasminogen activator inhibitor-1 (PAI1) expression in rat testicular peritubular cells, indicating that it plays a key role in controlling testicular protease activity.[91] Similar to IL1, TNFα stimulates basal lactate production by cultured Sertoli cells,[92,93] but TNFα generally antagonizes the actions of FSH on Sertoli cell function, including the stimulation of aromatase activity and lactate production.[94] Conversely, Delfino and colleagues have shown that TNFα stimulates androgen receptor expression in Sertoli cells via up-regulation of NFκB, which binds to several enhancer motifs in the androgen receptor promoter.[95] These many studies suggest that TNFα produced by the germ cells exerts a complicated paracrine effect on the adjacent Sertoli cell to alter its function at various stages during the cycle of the seminiferous epithelium.

In testicular pathology, TNFα has been implicated as a major causative agent in the development of EAO.[96] In rats with EAO, there is a significant increase in the number of TNFα-positive testicular macrophages and the number of TNFR1-positive germ cells.[97] The majority of TNFR1-positive germ cells were apoptotic, suggesting that TNFα could act to trigger germ cell apoptosis in this model, acting together with other local cell death regulatory systems such as the Fas-Fas ligand system.[98] TNFα also stimulates IL6 and leukocyte adhesion molecule expression in Sertoli cells.[99]

Outside the seminiferous epithelium, TNFα is an effective inhibitor of Leydig cell steroidogenesis acting through the NFκB signaling pathway.[100] Inhibition of LH/hCG binding by TNFα has been reported,[101] but the majority of studies in the mouse suggest that inhibition occurs primarily at the level of steroidogenic gene expression, particularly P450scc, P450c17 and 3β-HSD.[65,102,103] In studies on porcine Leydig cells, the inhibitory affect of TNFα also was reported to involve a decrease in steroidogenic acute regulatory protein (StAR) mRNA and protein levels.[104] In non-stimulated or hCG-treated intact or hypophysectomized rats, intratesticular delivery of TNFα induced a rapid and sustained reduction in StAR protein expression and testosterone biosynthesis.[105]

Activin A

The activins are homodimers or heterodimers of several homologous subunits (designated β_A-β_E), and are members of the much larger TGFβ family of dimeric cytokines. Homodimers of β_A form activin A, which is widely expressed and has been extensively studied.[106] Relatively little is known about the distribution and actions of the other activin forms, which appear to be both less abundant and less widely distributed. Heterodimers of either the β_A or β_B subunits with an homologous α subunit are feedback inhibitors of FSH secretion from the pituitary, which are produced by the testis and are called inhibin A and inhibin B, respectively.[107] Conversely, activin A and B act as stimulators of pituitary FSH secretion. Increasing data, however, illustrate the fact that activin A in particular is also a paracrine growth factor and inflammatory regulator.[108,109] Unlike the other mediators discussed in this review, which have predominantly or exclusively pro-inflammatory actions, the functions of activin A tend towards immunoregulation or immunosuppression, although activin A does appear to play a key role in early inflammation.[106,109-111]

The regulation of activin A production is still poorly characterized, but its synthesis and secretion is stimulated by IL1 in several cell types, including the Sertoli cells and peritubular cells of the testis.[112] This regulation probably involves signaling via the p38 MAP kinase/Jnk pathway through the transcription factor AP1, since the promoter of the β_A subunit includes AP1 sites, but no NFκB sites,[113-115] although this assumption is yet to be formally proven (Fig. 1). In the Sertoli cell, β_A production is negatively regulated by FSH through the protein kinase A pathway, and is stimulated by LPS.[30,112] Binding of activin A to target cells causes dimerization of membrane type II and type I signal-transducing receptors and activation of the Smad family of transcription factors.[116-118]

Activin A bioactivity can be regulated at the transcriptional and translational level, as well as at a post-translational level through the binding of β_A subunit to apparently functionally inactive β subunits (such as the β_C subunit)[119] or to the α subunit of inhibin.[106] Activity is also controlled post-secretion by the activin-binding protein, follistatin.[120,121] Follistatin binds activins, as well as a small number of related TGFβ family members, with very high affinity, competing with their ability to interact with their receptors and essentially neutralizing biological activity.

Under control conditions in the adult testis, immunohistochemical and in situ hybridization studies indicate that the β_A subunit of activin is largely associated with the Sertoli cell, but it appears to have a more widespread distribution within germ cells, extending into spermatogonia, spermatocytes and spermatids.[32,122,123] It is also found in macrophages and mast cells within the interstitial tissue of adult rats.[32] Peritubular cells from immature rats in culture produce activin A,[112,124] but the protein was not detectable by immunohistochemistry in peritubular profiles of adult rat testis,[32] suggesting that activin A production by these cells may decline with age. This possibility is given extra weight by the observation that, in prepubertal rat testes, peritubular cells rather than Sertoli cells appear to be the main source of activin A.[122] Given the ability for activin subunits to form dimers with differential activity, it is critical to measure the whole protein, rather than just the assess the presence of a particular subunit in isolation. This has been facilitated in the case of activin A by the availability of a specific sandwich-type ELISA that detects the dimeric protein.[125,126] A combination of whole protein and mRNA studies on activin A/β_A subunit expression in several species have established that activin A protein is present at all stages of the seminiferous cycle, but undergoes a distinct cyclical pattern of production (Fig. 2).[32,123]

Experiments with adult rat seminiferous tubule cultures indicate that IL1α may be driving activin A production at all stages of the cycle where IL1α is produced, but that the ability of Sertoli cells to respond to IL1α changes throughout the cycle.[32] This may involve changes in

IL1R levels,[51] production of endogenous IL1ra by the Sertoli cells,[60,64] and/or a cycle-specific switch in the inhibitory regulation of activin A by FSH.[32] Regardless of the fine detail of this control, activin A secretion by the seminiferous epithelium displays a very large surge at stages VIII-XII in the rat, immediately following spermiation and the resumption of IL1α production that follows stage VII (Fig. 2). By the end of stage XII, however, activin A production has returned to basal levels. It is likely that the bioavailability of activin A is also regulated at this time by the production of follistatin, which reaches maximal levels of expression within the cycle at stages X-XIV.[123,127]

The surge of activin A at stages VIII-XII coincides with and then extends beyond a burst of DNA synthesis associated with meiotic division in preleptotene spermatocytes and a round of type A spermatogonial division.[4,55] The ability of activin A to stimulate spermatogonial and preleptotene spermatocyte DNA synthesis has been established by several in vitro experiments, using tubule fragment cultures[128] or Sertoli-spermatogonial cell cocultures.[129] However, other studies have shown that activin A inhibits and follistatin stimulates FSH-induced spermatogonial proliferation in testis fragment cultures from younger rats.[130,131] Moreover, activin A delays meiosis in cultures of rat primary spermatocytes,[132] and in many other cell types activin A has been shown to inhibit cell growth and induce apoptosis.[133] To complicate the matter further, activin A can block production and down-stream effects of IL1 and IL6 during inflammatory responses,[109,134] and may have similar effects on endogenous IL1α and IL6 within the seminiferous epithelium. At present, it is difficult to predict exactly what role the surge of activin A might play in the control of germ cell mitosis and meiosis during stages VIII-XII, and studies to address this issue are warranted.

As with activin A, inhibin B is produced in a stage regulated manner in the rat seminiferous epithelium (Fig. 2). Further, the production of inhibin B is regulated by the presence of developing germ cells[135,136] and by FSH and IL1α in a reciprocal pattern with activin A.[30,32,112] For example, the incubation of cultured stage VIII tubules with IL1ra resulted in a reduction in activin A secretion and a corresponding increase in inhibin B production. In rat Sertoli cell cultures, IL1α and IL1β stimulated β_A mRNA production and activin A protein secretion, while concurrently reducing inhibin B protein secretion and transcription of both β_B and inhibin α mRNA.[112] Conversely, FSH inhibits activin A secretion by the Sertoli cell, but stimulates inhibin B secretion. While still only partially revealed, these data highlight the complex and dynamic cytokine and regulatory hormone network that operates within the seminiferous epithelium.

Nitric Oxide

The nitric oxide synthases (NOS) are a group of three related enzymes, neuronal NOS (nNOS or NOS1), inducible NOS (iNOS or NOS2) and endothelial NOS (eNOS or NOS3), which catalyze the conversion of L-arginine to L-citrulline and NO.[137,138] At low levels (<1 μM), NO acts as a regulatory molecule, but at high levels NO causes damage to DNA, proteins and lipids through free radical generation.[139,140] The NOS enzymes are homodimeric proteins composed of identical monomers of ~130-160 kDa and are encoded by three separate genes. Both nNOS and eNOS are constitutively expressed enzymes whose activity is regulated through a calcium-calmodulin mediated mechanism.[141,142] In contrast, iNOS is a constitutively activated form of NOS that is regulated at the transcriptional level by a range of inflammatory mediators, including LPS, IL1 and TNFα (Fig. 1). Consequently, iNOS has both physiological and pathophysiological actions.

All three NOS forms have been identified in testicular tissue from several species.[143] They appear to be involved in the regulation of normal male fertility at multiple levels and are pathogenic under some circumstances. At the cellular level, NOS has been found in Sertoli (nNOS, eNOS, iNOS), Leydig (nNOS, eNOS, iNOS) and peritubular cells (iNOS), spermatogenic cells (eNOS, iNOS) and testicular macrophages (iNOS).[143] It is important to note that macrophage expression of iNOS is confined to the minority of monocyte-like macrophages of the rat testis, and it is not expressed by the majority resident macrophages.[9,14] In the normal rat seminiferous epithelium, iNOS is particularly expressed by elongating spermatids at stage IX of the cycle, and in pachytene spermatocytes at stages IX-XII, with relative lower levels of expression in the Sertoli cells and peritubular cells across all stages.[9] The *nNOS* gene also produces a testis-specific isoform, TnNOS, which has been localized specifically to Leydig cells and is implicated in the control of steroidogenesis through its ability to regulate steroidogenic enzyme levels.[144-147] Regardless of its source, NO has been shown to inhibit Leydig cell steroidogenesis directly, and treatment with NOS inhibitors counteracts the decrease in testosterone associated with sepsis or stress.[148-151] The mechanism of action probably involves oxidative damage through generation of reactive nitrogen species, such as the peroxynitrite anion.[141,142] In addition to the regulation of androgen production and germ cell number, NO production has been implicated in the control of the formation and disassembly of the Sertoli cell junctions that constitute the blood-testis barrier, as well as the junctional complexes involved in Sertoli-germ cell adhesion.[152]

Surprisingly, male mice with deletions of each *NOS* form are fertile, although only the fertility of *iNOS* null mice has been studied in great depth. Potentially, considerable redundancy exists in all of these processes whereby the substitution of another NOS enzymes, as well as reactive species other than NO, may occur in the genetic absence of each individual NOS form. Significantly, *iNOS* null mice have increased testis weights (131% of control) as a result of decreased pachytene and round spermatid apoptosis, which leads to a 65% increase in daily sperm output.[153] The susceptibility of pachytene spermatocytes to iNOS is entirely consistent with the expression of iNOS in normal wildtype rat testes, and is strongly indicative of a key role for iNOS in determining the germ cell carrying capacity of Sertoli cells.[9,153]

Not surprisingly, given the response of the NOS forms to stress in other tissues, iNOS expression and NO production in the testis is greatly up-regulated during inflammatory events induced by the injection of LPS,[9] testicular torsion[154] or testicular heating.[153] NO over-production leads to stage-specific germ cell damage and loss by both apoptosis and necrosis, as well as changes in testicular blood flow and interstitial fluid content.[9,155]

Cytokines in the Regulation of Normal Spermatogenesis—What Should We Believe?

On the face of it, the large body of data outlined in the preceding section would seem to indicate that pro-inflammatory mediators must play an important role in the functions of the seminiferous epithelium. However, because these molecules are associated with inflammation and can be artefactually induced in many cell types by inflammation, stress or even the very act of cell isolation, doubts have been expressed regarding their actual contribution to normal testicular function. This attitude is not entirely unjustified. The sensitivity of many cells to stimulation by LPS and other endotoxic agents and the failure of many earlier studies in particular to eliminate the complication of endogenous endotoxin contamination has led some researchers to question the validity of the observations that these mediators are expressed by testicular cells under normal conditions. In other words, it is suspected that the production of inflammatory mediators by testicular cells in the absence of an apparent inflammatory stimulus may be due to stressing of the cells during their isolation, endotoxin contamination of in vitro preparations, or even an underlying pathology in the animals used as a source of tissue. For example, conflicting results concerning IL1α localization in spermatogenic cells may be attributable to such uncontrolled experimental variables.[6,61] The problem is compounded by the use of RT-PCR to detect these mediators because of the sensitivity of such methods. Indeed, using RT-PCR alone, one can "demonstrate" the presence or absence of an mRNA species by simply increasing or decreasing the number of cycles, respectively. Fortunately, the development of quantitative RT-PCR methods in recent years has gone a long way towards reducing this problem. Nonetheless, a reliance on mRNA data alone ignores well documented variations in cytokine translational efficiency and the requirement for post-translational processing to produce a bioactive protein (Fig. 3). Finally, a number of immunohistochemical studies using antibodies of poorly defined specificity, often with inadequate controls or using poorly-fixed testicular tissue, may have contributed to confusion in the literature as well.

Skepticism has been compounded by the fact that, with the exception of activin A, which is fetal lethal,[156] breeding studies show that male mice with deletions of IL1, IL6, TNFα and iNOS, or of the relevant receptors, are all fertile.[153,157-159] Accordingly, in spite of considerable evidence that IL1α is produced by the Sertoli cell and has regulatory effects on spermatogonial proliferation and development, mice lacking the IL1R, and hence unresponsive to IL1, display relatively normal fertility.[157] Yet it cannot be ignored that numerous studies have shown by quantitative mRNA and protein methods using both in vivo and in vitro approaches that the mediators discussed in this review are produced by testicular cells and that they have effects on spermatogenesis. Moreover, most of the findings have been consistent and reproducible in different research laboratories over many years, and it seems unlikely that endotoxin contamination or sick animals can account for all the observations. In fact, some studies have gone to considerable lengths to completely eliminate these possibilities.[160,161] While there is still much room for debate concerning the details, there are sufficient data to declare that IL1α, TNFα, IL6, activin A and iNOS/NO have a case to answer with regards to their role in normal testicular function.

As outlined above, the expression of IL1α, TNFα, IL6, activin A and iNOS occurs in a regulated manner across the cycle of the seminiferous epithelium (Fig. 2). These proteins show distinct patterns of cyclical production and their patterns of production coincide with key events in Sertoli cells and spermatogenic cells. A critical series of events occurs at, and immediately after, stage VIII in the rat: the release of sperm from the epithelium (spermiation), a peak

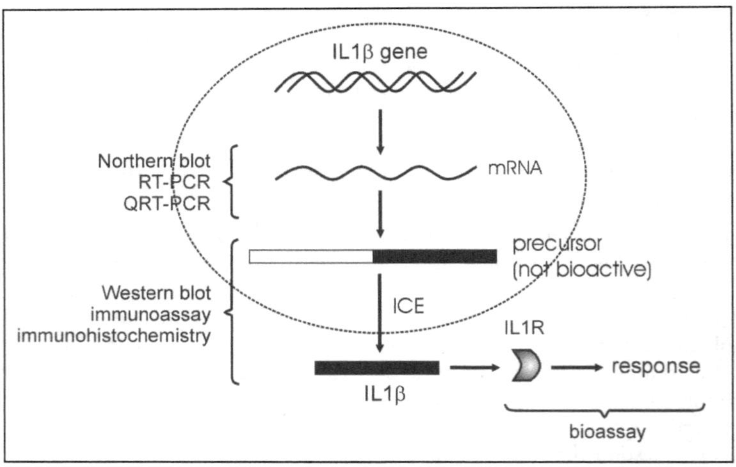

Figure 3. Measurement of IL1β. This cytokine displays a particularly complex regulation, involving a biologically inactive precursor which is activated by the enzyme IL1 cleaving enzyme, ICE or caspase 1, at the time of its secretion from the cell. The mechanisms of production, processing and secretion are poorly understood, but appear to be relatively inefficient, and there can be large discrepancies between the levels of mRNA expression and the amount of bioactive protein secreted by the cell.[47,192,193] Moreover, significant secretion of the inactive precursor without processing may occur, as has been observed in the testis and other systems.[15,47,194] As a result, what is measured can make very big differences to the conclusions reached. Even quantitative methods which detect mRNA may tell us relatively little about the actual levels of protein produced. Methods which detect the protein may also detect the precursor, leading to an overestimation of the bioactive protein. Bioassays provide the most informative measure of the physiological levels of IL1, although even this measurement may be compromised by the presence of anti-inflammatory cytokines that inhibit its activity in various assays.

of DNA synthesis by preleptotene primary spermatocytes cells and type A spermatogonia prior to meiotic and mitotic division, respectively, and the reorganization of tight junctions of the blood-testis barrier to allow the meiotic cells to enter the adluminal compartment. These events also coincide with a recovery of the responsiveness of the Sertoli cell to FSH.[162,163] At the same time, there is a resumption in production of IL1α by the Sertoli cells and of TNFα and iNOS by the germ cells, a rise in Sertoli cell IL6 production, and a transient peak of activin A production. These responses are highly reminiscent of an inflammatory event. Could the epithelium be experiencing a cyclical inflammatory burst, associated with sperm release and phagocytosis of the residual bodies?

Significantly, nuclear localization of the key pro-inflammatory transcription factor, NFκB in the Sertoli cell and the germ cells also shows a cyclical pattern within the seminiferous epithelium.[164] There is a good relationship between nuclear NFκB levels in spermatocytes and both TNFα and iNOS expression by these cells. Curiously, however, there does not appear to be a close concordance between the content of NFκB in the Sertoli cell nucleus, which is elevated at most stages of the cycle but appears to decline during stages VIII and IX, and the production of IL1α or IL6 by this cell. This is, perhaps, less surprising in the case of activin A and inhibin B, since NFκB almost certainly does not regulate their expression. However, it should be borne in mind that the overlying regulatory influence of the developing germ cells, as well as FSH and testosterone in the control of several of these mediators may distort the cyclical expression patterns observed. For example, production of IL6 by the Sertoli cell is stimulated by FSH and, although it is regulated by IL1α and nuclear NFκB, its production appears to be most closely aligned with changes in the expression of the FSH receptor (Fig. 2). More detailed studies on the regulation of these and other transcriptional regulators and signaling pathways involved in inflammatory cytokine production throughout the cycle of the seminiferous epithelium will be required to resolve these issues.

Additional questions remain regarding the precise biological effects exerted by some of these mediators within the seminiferous epithelium. It appears that different in vitro models can lead to very different conclusions. This is best exemplified by the fact that TNFα reduces germ cell apoptosis in seminiferous tubule cultures and, hence, could be considered a germ cell survival factor.[88,89] However, TNFα is also implicated in the breakdown of Sertoli cell tight junctions,[90,152] stimulation of apoptosis by Fas-Fas ligand activity in spermatogenic cells,[98] and the onset of orchitis.[97] It would appear that the role of TNFα in regulation of spermatogenesis may depend upon its context, i.e., when and for how long it is produced, how much of it is produced and which receptors are available to respond to it. In a similar manner, activin A has been identified as both a stimulator and inhibitor of spermatogonial development by different experiments.[73,129-131]

Nonetheless, even though there are many questions still to be answered, it is possible to propose a model of cytokine network signaling in the Sertoli cell based on the available data (Fig. 4). It can be postulated that release of sperm and resorption of residual bodies at stage VIII-IX of the cycle triggers an inflammatory response in the Sertoli cell as evidenced by an up-regulation of IL1α. IL1α in turn stimulates a surge of spermatogonial proliferation and a new generation of germ cells entering the spermatogenic cycle. IL1α also induces the production of IL6, which acts to regulate the number of spermatocytes progressing through meiosis. The role of activin A in this model is not entirely clear, but this cytokine may cooperate with IL1α to stimulate spermatogonial proliferation, or with IL6 to control meiotic progression, or it may even act to block the activity of IL1α and IL6. As a result of this network, the entry of spermatogonia into spermatogenesis occurs in short bursts that are timed to coincide with the release of sperm into the lumen, while at the same time the entry into meiosis is being modulated. A parallel network involving the spermatocytes and spermatids is also triggered at this time, possibly involving IL1α from the Sertoli cells, stimulating the production of TNFα and iNOS/NO, which induce the disassembly of the intercellular tight junctions to allow the meiotic cells to transit the blood-testis barrier. Variants of these regulatory networks may also

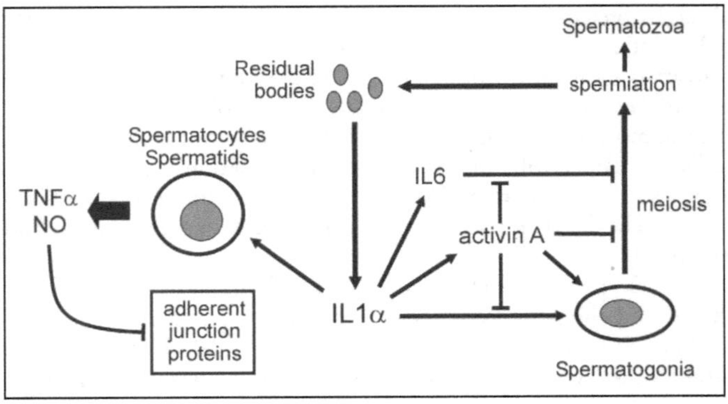

Figure 4. A model of cytokine networks in control of Sertoli-germ cell interactions. Residual bodies produced during spermiation stimulate production of IL1α by the Sertoli cell, which in turn stimulates IL6 and activin A. All three cytokines have been shown to have stimulatory and/or inhibitory actions on spermatogonial proliferation and meiotic progression of the spermatocytes in vitro. Activin A also modulates the activity of IL1α and IL6. Spermatocytes and spermatids produce TNFα and NO, most likely in response to stimulation by IL1α from the Sertoli cell, which are regulators of Sertoli cell tight junction formation and degradation. It is hypothesized that these interactions coordinate germ cell initiated events, such as spermiation and release of the residual bodies with spermatogonial proliferation, meiosis and intercellular junction reorganization throughout the cycle of the seminiferous epithelium. This process appears to be most relevant at stages VIII-XI, but variants may also operate elsewhere during the cycle.

operate at other times and in different ways throughout the remainder of the cycle, for example, in controlling the proliferation of intermediate and B type spermatogonia during stage V.[4,55]

Given the considerable evidence for a direct role for cytokine networks in the control of spermatogenesis under normal conditions, therefore, how can we explain the fact that the relevant 'knockout' mice are fertile? Three main issues need to be considered here:

Redundancy of Action

Most cytokines and enzymes involved in inflammatory pathways share overlapping functions and signaling pathways, as in the case of IL1 and TNFα (Fig. 1), or belong to families with similar properties and range of actions (e.g., the NOS forms). Absence of a critical gene, particularly during development, may even stimulate appropriation of other genes with similar function. It is common knowledge that deletions of even fundamental regulators like IL1, TNFα or IL6 results in relatively subtle immunity phenotypes.[165] Rather than focusing on the individual players, the inflammatory response itself should be considered as being responsible for spermatogenic regulation. Consequently, the retention of fertility in mice lacking the IL1R, and presumably insensitive to either IL1α or IL1β,[157] may be due to the fact that IL1 is just one of several inflammatory mediators with overlapping functions induced by phagocytosis in the Sertoli cells. Moreover, the possibility for alternative or non-classical actions of IL1α in the seminiferous epithelium, which bypass the classical ILR must also be considered.[166,167]

Superficial Assessments of Fertility

Few of the knockouts relevant to the present discussion have been carefully examined for subtle testicular phenotypes, which may occur: the *iNOS* null mouse is a notable exception.[153] Null mice may be considered to be fertile, because they are capable of breeding in an animal house environment, but further examination may expose testicular or germ cell anomalies.[168] The genetic background of the animal also should be considered, since phenotypes observed in one strain of knockout mice can disappear when backcrossed onto another background.

"Hidden" Phenotypes

Fertility or other physiological phenotypes may not manifest under normal animal house conditions, or in the absence of some stressor or other intervention, such as ageing or infection. A good example of this is the *IL6* null mouse,[159] which has apparently normal testicular function, but actually possesses an aromatase deficiency that can lead to anomalous steroidogenic responses (Fig. 5).

In summary, we have outlined a complex model of spermatogenic regulation involving inflammatory networks that leads to the hypothesis that the cycle of the seminiferous epithelium is actually a cyclical inflammatory event. As such, spermatogenesis may be viewed as a localized inflammatory process wherein the Sertoli cell functions in the role of the monocyte/macrophage. With this concept is mind, it is particularly important that the testis maintains a tight immunoregulatory environment to suppress local antigen-specific immune responses. Although outside the scope of this review, it is clear that the testicular resident macrophages, in concert with the Sertoli and Leydig cells, conspire to inhibit immune responses, which might otherwise be triggered by the ongoing inflammatory process within the seminiferous tubules (reviewed in detail by Hedger and Hales, ref. 169).

Inflammation and Testis Function—Role of Inflammatory Mediators and Implications for Fertility

While the role of inflammatory mediators in normal spermatogenesis may be disputed, there is no doubt that they play a critical role in the suppression of spermatogenesis by inflammation. Normal testicular function can be directly inhibited by local or systemic illness, infection and chronic inflammatory disease in men,[170-172] and similar decreases in gonadal function occur in experimental animal models of chronic inflammation and systemic immune activation.[149,173-178] In spite of a common assumption that such reproductive failure is related to the negative effects of a raised body temperature on spermatogenesis, there is very little evidence to support this contention in febrile

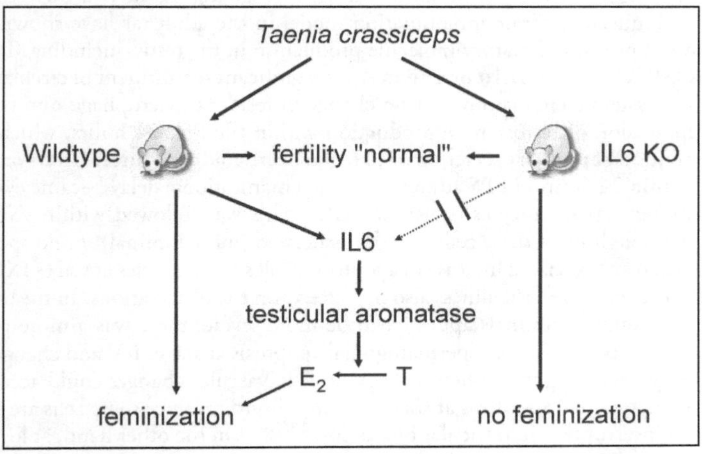

Figure 5. The "hidden" phenotype of the *IL6* null mouse model. Infection of mice with *Taenia crassiceps* leads to a testicular feminization syndrome, as a result of up-regulation of aromatase activity. While testicular function and fertility in *IL6* null mice is virtually indistinguishable from that of the wild-type mouse, these mice show no feminization following infection directly implicating IL6 in the control of aromatase activity in the testis of both normal and infected animals. Thus, a role for IL6 in testicular function and pathology is only evident if the appropriate experiment is carried out. This model provides an excellent example of a significant phenotype that appears only under conditions of modified function.

patients, or in experimental animals.[173,174] In fact, it is much more likely that specific inflammatory events are directly involved. As a logical extension of the key role of inflammatory mediators in normal male spermatogenesis and steroidogenesis, it is not surprising that inflammatory events, either within the testis itself or in the rest of the body, compromise testis function. Indeed, based on the normal expression pattern of such mediators, one would expect certain aspects of spermatogenesis to be particularly sensitive to shifts in their expression.

Another general perception is that reduced fertility following an illness is due to decreased androgen production. Serum androgen levels are generally decreased with illness, and certainly contribute to a lack of libido and well-being.[179] The experimental models that have helped to elucidate this aspect of immune-testis interactions have involved administration of the inflammatory mediator LPS or studies on the effects of agents and treatments that alter the vasculature of the testis. These models involve an increase in both systemic levels and testicular expression of inflammatory mediators in addition to effects on androgens and spermatogenesis.[15,154,173,175,180-182] There is no doubt that IL1, TNFα and NO, in particular, have largely negative effects on Leydig cell steroidogenesis, and that this inhibition involves both central and direct effects on the Leydig cell itself.[65,66,68,101,103,150,151] Consequently, inflammation leads to suppression of the hypothalamic-pituitary-Leydig cell axis, and a corresponding decline in androgen levels, and all the subsequent clinical implications. However, it is not certain that this is the main cause of damage to spermatogenesis during inflammation. For one thing, there are distinct species differences in the dynamics and severity of the inhibition of the endocrine axis in the LPS-induced inflammation models. While the mouse displays a rapid onset and prolonged suppression of steroidogenesis after treatment with LPS,[181,183] in the rat model, even very high doses of LPS do not reduce intratesticular levels of testosterone in the rat much below 30% of control,[173,184] well above the threshold necessary to sustain spermatogenesis in this species.[185,186] Moreover, serum testosterone levels actually appear to rise in the boar following LPS treatment due to an increase in pulsatile LH secretion.[178]

In contrast to the many studies on endocrine parameters, there have been few detailed studies of the direct effects of inflammation on spermatogenesis itself. Our own studies, using an acute LPS induced systemic inflammation model in the adult rat have shown a selective up-regulation of pro-inflammatory molecule production in the testis, including IL1β, TNFα, IL6 and iNOS/NO, but not IL1α or activin A,[9,15] significant recruitment of circulating monocytes from the systemic circulation, but no change in resident macrophage numbers,[14] and a transient suppression of testosterone production within the first 24 hours, which involves a complex inhibition of pituitary secretion of LH, glucocorticoids and direct effects on the Leydig cell.[173,184] Within 24 hours of LPS administration, a maturational delay became evident in the leptotene/zygotene spermatocytes (stages IX-XIII). This was followed within six days by an increase in the sloughing of these cells and the associated (more luminal) round spermatids (at stages I-VIII) and an associated increase in apoptosis of all spermatocytes at stages IX-XIII.[173,187] Significantly, the severity of the illness also had effects on the observations. In the earlier study, where illness among the animals appeared to be more severe, there was a more pronounced spermatocyte and spermatid loss, spermatogonial apoptosis at stages I-V and changes in vascular permeability, including micro-hemorrhage. In fact, vascular changes could account for the increased spermatogonial apoptosis at stages I-V in this group, since these cells are particularly sensitive to an interruption in testicular blood flow.[182,188] On the other hand, at lower doses of LPS, even those that caused maximal inhibition of intratesticular testosterone, little or no germ cell loss was observed.[173] Remarkably, even following a high dose of LPS, spermatogenesis had returned to qualitatively normal levels by 28 days post-injection.[187] This recovery suggests that a compensatory reduction in normal germ cell attrition and possibly an increase in proliferation may occur following an acute inflammatory event, restoring the spermatogenic capacity of the testis to its pre-inflammation levels. It should be noted, however, that this model involves an acute inflammatory episode only. Very little quantitative data exists concerning the effects of on-going systemic or testicular inflammation similar to that occurring in a significant proportion of the human male population suffering chronic inflammatory conditions such as arthritis.

Altogether, the data point towards a direct effect of inflammation on the seminiferous epithelium, and that the effects of acute inflammation are most pronounced and earliest on the seminiferous epithelium at stages IX-XIII, i.e., immediately following spermiation. Importantly, the effects of LPS-induced inflammation on spermatogenesis in the rat were not consistent with withdrawal of either testosterone, which initially affects the release of mature spermatids into the tubule lumen and the integrity of the junctions between the Sertoli cells and mid-phase round spermatids at stages VII-VIII, or of FSH, which particularly affects spermatogonia at stages XIV-III.[189,190] While there is no doubt that loss of hormonal support may contribute to spermatogenic damage in some models, the observations suggest that alternative explanations must be sought to explain spermatogenic failure in the acute inflammatory model. A potential cause of damage in this model is the action of LPS and pro-inflammatory mediators on the seminiferous epithelium itself. This could involve increased levels of circulating mediators as well as local production by leukocytes and somatic cells in the testis. In addition to systemic increase in these mediators, LPS causes the up-regulation of testicular IL1β, TNFα, IL6 and iNOS expression.[9,15,50,86,184] Although the absolute levels of expression of IL1α and activin A do not appear to change, their distribution and timing may be affected. As discussed in the previous section, these inflammatory mediators are produced in a regulated fashion during the normal cycle of the seminiferous epithelium and have direct and complex effects on both Sertoli cell and spermatogenic cell function. Changes in IL1, activin A and IL6 would disrupt the signaling processes involved in controlling meiotic progression and spermatogonial proliferation. Similarly, local increases in TNFα and NO would disrupt Sertoli tight junction integrity and germ cell attachment. All of these factors, as well as direct effects of LPS on the Sertoli cell itself may affect critical supportive functions of the Sertoli cells. Consequently, it is particularly significant that the region of the seminiferous epithelium that is first affected by LPS induced inflammation is the stages immediately following spermiation (IX-XIII), where these cytokine networks appear to play their most complex roles (Fig. 2). Overall, these data suggest that inflammation directly affects spermatogenesis through interfering with these critical inflammatory networks of the seminiferous epithelium.

Acknowledgements

This research has been supported by grants from the National Health and Medical Research Council (NHMRC) and the Australian Research Council (ARC).

References

1. Clermont Y, Leblond CP. Spermiogenesis of man, monkey, ram and other mammals as shown by the periodic acid-Schiff technique. Am J Anat 1955; 96:229-253.
2. Clermont Y, Harvey SC. Duration of the cycle of the seminiferous epithelium of normal, hypophysectomized and hypophysectomized-hormone treated albino rats. Endocrinology 1965; 76:80-89.
3. Oakberg EF. Duration of spermatogenesis in the mouse and timing of stages of the cycle of the seminiferous epithelium. Am J Anat 1956; 99:507-516.
4. Clermont Y. Kinetics of spermatogenesis in mammals: Seminiferous epithelium cycle and spermatogonial renewal. Physiol Rev 1972; 52:198-236.
5. Syed V, Söder O, Arver S et al. Ontogeny and cellular origin of an interleukin-1-like factor in the reproductive tract of the male rat. Int J Androl 1988; 11:437-447.
6. Gérard N, Syed V, Bardin W et al. Sertoli cells are the site of interleukin-1α synthesis in rat testis. Mol Cell Endocrinol 1991; 82:R13-16.
7. Okuda Y, Sun XR, Morris PL. Interleukin-6 (IL-6) mRNAs expressed in Leydig and Sertoli cells are regulated by cytokines, gonadotropins and neuropeptides. Endocrine 1994; 2:617-624.
8. Cudicini C, Kercret H, Touzalin AM et al. Vectorial production of interleukin 1 and interleukin 6 by rat Sertoli cells cultured in a dual culture compartment system. Endocrinology 1997; 138:2863-2870.
9. O'Bryan MK, Schlatt S, Gerdprasert O et al. Inducible nitric oxide synthase in the rat testis: Evidence for potential roles in both normal function and inflammation-mediated infertility. Biol Reprod 2000; 63:1285-1293.
10. Head JR, Billingham RE. Immune privilege in the testis. II. Evaluation of potential local factors. Transplantation 1985; 40:269-275.

11. Ferguson J, Scothorne RJ. Extended survival of pancreatic islet allografts in the testis of guinea-pigs. J Anat 1977; 124:1-8.
12. Sanberg PR, Borlongan CV, Saporta S et al. Testis-derived Sertoli cells survive and provide localized immunoprotection for xenografts in rat brain. Nat Biotechnol 1996; 14:1692-1695.
13. Korbutt GS, Elliott JF, Rajotte RV. Cotransplantation of allogeneic islets with allogeneic testicular cell aggregates allows long-term graft survival without systemic immunosuppression. Diabetes 1997; 46:317-322.
14. Gerdprasert O, O'Bryan MK, Muir JA et al. The response of testicular leukocytes to lipopolysaccharide-induced inflammation: Further evidence for heterogeneity of the testicular macrophage population. Cell Tiss Res 2002; 308:277-285.
15. O'Bryan MK, Gerdprasert O, Nikolic-Paterson DJ et al. Cytokine profiles in the testes of rats treated with lipopolysaccharide reveal localized suppression of inflammatory responses. Am J Physiol—Reg Int Comp Physiol 2005; 288:R1744-1755.
16. Hayes R, Chalmers SA, Nikolic-Paterson DJ et al. Secretion of bioactive interleukin 1 by rat testicular macrophages in vitro. J Androl 1996; 17:41-49.
17. Kern S, Robertson SA, Mau VJ et al. Cytokine secretion by macrophages in the rat testis. Biol Reprod 1995; 53:1407-1416.
18. Kern S, Maddocks S. Indomethacin blocks the immunosuppressive activity of rat testicular macrophages cultured in vitro. J Reprod Immunol 1995; 28:189-201.
19. Bryniarski K, Szczepanik M, Maresz K et al. Subpopulations of mouse testicular macrophages and their immunoregulatory function. Am J Reprod Immunol 2004; 52:27-35.
20. Hedger MP. Macrophages and the immune responsiveness of the testis. J Reprod Immunol 2002; 57:19-34.
21. Mantovani A, Sica A, Locati M. Macrophage polarization comes of age. Immunity 2005; 23:344-346.
22. Wang J, Wreford NG, Lan HY et al. Leukocyte populations of the adult rat testis following removal of the Leydig cells by treatment with ethane dimethane sulfonate and subcutaneous testosterone implants. Biol Reprod 1994; 51:551-561.
23. Pöllänen P, Maddocks S. Macrophages, lymphocytes and MHC II antigen in the ram and the rat testis. J Reprod Fertil 1988; 82:437-445.
24. Pöllänen P, Niemi M. Immunohistochemical identification of macrophages, lymphoid cells and HLA antigens in the human testis. Int J Androl 1987; 10:37-42.
25. Hendry WF, Morgan H, Stedronska J. The clinical significance of antisperm antibodies in male subfertility. Br J Urol 1977; 49:757-762.
26. Pattinson HA, Mortimer D. Prevalence of sperm surface antibodies in the male partners of infertile couples as determined by immunobead screening. Fertil Steril 1987; 48:466-469.
27. Rosenberg HF, Gallin JI. Inflammation. In: Paul WE, ed. Fundamental Immunology. 5th ed. Philadelphia: Lippincott, Williams and Wilkins, 2003:1151-1169.
28. Syed V, Stéphan JP, Gérard N et al. Residual bodies activate Sertoli cell interleukin-1α (IL-1α) release, which triggers IL-6 production by an autocrine mechanism, through the lipoxygenase pathway. Endocrinology 1995; 136:3070-3078.
29. Stéphan JP, Syed V, Jégou B. Regulation of Sertoli cell IL-1 and IL-6 production in vitro. Mol Cell Endocrinol 1997; 134:109-118.
30. Okuma Y, O'Connor AE, Muir JA et al. Regulation of activin A and inhibin B secretion by inflammatory mediators in adult rat Sertoli cell cultures. J Endocrinol 2005; 187:125-134.
31. Gérard N, Syed V, Jégou B. Lipopolysaccharide, latex beads and residual bodies are potent activators of Sertoli cell interleukin-1a production. Biochem Biophys Res Commun 1992; 185:154-161.
32. Okuma Y, O'Connor AE, Hayashi T et al. Regulated production of activin A and inhibin B throughout the cycle of the seminiferous epithelium in the rat. J Endocrinol 2006; 190:331-340.
33. Dejucq N, Lienard MO, Guillaume E et al. Expression of interferons-α and -γ in testicular interstitial tissue and spermatogonia of the rat. Endocrinology 1998; 139:3081-3087.
34. Guo H, Calkins JH, Sigel MM et al. Interleukin-2 is a potent inhibitor of Leydig cell steroidogenesis. Endocrinology 1990; 127:1234-1239.
35. Strand ML, Wahlgren A, Svechnikov K et al. Interleukin-18 is expressed in rat testis and may promote germ cell growth. Mol Cell Endocrinol 2005; 240:64-73.
36. Ishikawa T, Morris PL. A multistep kinase-based sertoli cell autocrine-amplifying loop regulates prostaglandins, their receptors, and cytokines. Endocrinology 2006; 147:1706-1716.
37. Teerds KJ, Dorrington JH. Localization of transforming growth factor β_1 and β_2 during testicular development in the rat. Biol Reprod 1993; 48:40-45.
38. Mullaney BP, Skinner MK. Transforming growth factor-β (β1, β2, and β3) gene expression and action during pubertal development of the seminiferous tubule: Potential role at the onset of spermatogenesis. Mol Endocrinol 1993; 7:67-76.

39. Dinarello CA. Proinflammatory cytokines. Chest 2000; 118:503-508.
40. Dinarello CA. Biologic basis for interleukin-1 in disease. Blood 1996; 87:2095-2147.
41. Medzhitov R, Preston-Hurlburt P, Kopp E et al. MyD88 is an adaptor protein in the hToll/IL-1 receptor family signaling pathways. Mol Cell 1998; 2:253-258.
42. Wesche H, Henzel WJ, Shillinglaw W et al. MyD88: An adapter that recruits IRAK to the IL-1 receptor complex. Immunity 1997; 7:837-847.
43. Hazuda DJ, Lee JC, Young PR. The kinetics of interleukin 1 secretion from activated monocytes: Differences between interleukin 1a and interleukin 1b. J Biol Chem 1988; 263:8473-8479.
44. Black RA, Kronheim SR, Cantrell M et al. Generation of biologically active interleukin-1β by proteolytic cleavage of the inactive precursor. J Biol Chem 1988; 263:9437-9442.
45. Watanabe N, Kobayashi Y. Selective release of a processed form of interleukin 1α. Cytokine 1994; 6:597-601.
46. Thornberry NA, Molineaux SM. Interleukin-1β converting enzyme: A novel cysteine protease required for IL-1β production and implicated in programmed cell death. Prot Sci 1995; 4:3-12.
47. Rubartelli A, Bajetto A, Allavena G et al. Post-translational regulation of interleukin 1β secretion. Cytokine 1993; 5:117-124.
48. Arend WP. Interleukin-1 receptor antagonist. Adv Immunol 1993; 54:167-227.
49. Jonsson CK, Zetterström RH, Holst M et al. Constitutive expression of interleukin-1α messenger ribonucleic acid in rat Sertoli cells is dependent upon interaction with germ cells. Endocrinology 1999; 140:3755-3761.
50. Jonsson CK, Setchell BP, Martinelle N et al. Endotoxin-induced interleukin 1 expression in testicular macrophages is accompanied by downregulation of the constitutive expression in Sertoli cells. Cytokine 2001; 14:283-288.
51. Gomez E, Morel G, Cavalier A et al. Type I and type II interleukin-1 receptor expression in rat, mouse, and human testes. Biol Reprod 1997; 56:1513-1526.
52. Pöllänen P, Söder O, Parvinen M. Interleukin-1α stimulation of spermatogonial proliferation in vivo. Reprod Fertil Dev 1989; 1:85-87.
53. Söder O, Syed V, Callard GV et al. Production and secretion of an interleukin-1-like factor is stage-dependent and correlates with spermatogonial DNA synthesis in the rat seminiferous epithelium. Int J Androl 1991; 14:223-231.
54. Hakovirta H, Pentitilä TL, Pöllänen P et al. Interleukin-1 bioactivity and DNA synthesis in X-irradiated rat testes. Int J Androl 1993; 16:159-164.
55. Parvinen M, Söder O, Mali P et al. In vitro stimulation of stage-specific deoxyribonucleic acid synthesis in rat seminiferous tubule segments by interleukin-1α. Endocrinology 1991; 129:1614-1620.
56. Hoeben E, Van Damme J, Put W et al. Cytokines derived from activated human mononuclear cells markedly stimulate transferrin secretion by cultured Sertoli cells. Endocrinology 1996; 137:514-521.
57. Nehar D, Mauduit C, Boussouar F et al. Interleukin 1α stimulates lactate dehydrogenase A expression and lactate production in cultured porcine Sertoli cells. Biol Reprod 1998; 59:1425-1432.
58. Sultana T, Svechnikov K, Weber G et al. Molecular cloning and expression of a functionally different alternative splice variant of prointerleukin-1α from the rat testis. Endocrinology 2000; 141:4413-4418.
59. Svechnikov KV, Sultana T, Söder O. Age-dependent stimulation of Leydig cell steroidogenesis by interleukin-1 isoforms. Mol Cell Endocrinol 2001; 182:193-201.
60. Huleihel M, Lunenfeld E, Blindman A et al. Over expression of interleukin-1α, interleukin-1β and interleukin-1 receptor antagonist in testicular tissues from sexually immature mice as compared to adult mice. Eur Cyto Netw 2003; 14:27-33.
61. Haugen TB, Landmark BF, Josefsen GM et al. The mature form of interleukin-1 α is constitutively expressed in immature male germ cells from rat. Mol Cell Endocrinol 1994; 105:R19-23.
62. Lin T, Wang D, Nagpal ML. Human chorionic gonadotropin induces interleukin-1 gene expression in rat Leydig cells in vivo. Mol Cell Endocrinol 1993; 95:139-145.
63. Rozwadowska N, Fiszer D, Kurpisz M. Interleukin-1 system in testis—Quantitative analysis. Expression of immunomodulatory genes in male gonad. Adv Exp Biol Med 2001; 495:177-180.
64. Zeyse D, Lunenfeld E, Beck M et al. Interleukin-1 receptor antagonist is produced by Sertoli cells in vitro. Endocrinology 2000; 141:1521-1527.
65. Xiong Y, Hales DB. Immune-endocrine interactions in the mouse testis: Cytokine-mediated inhibition of Leydig cell steroidogenesis. Endocrine 1994; 2:223-228.
66. Hales DB. Interleukin-1 inhibits Leydig cell steroidogenesis primarily by decreasing 17α-hydroxylase/C17-20 lyase cytochrome P450 expression. Endocrinology 1992; 131:2165-2172.

67. Xiong Y, Hales DB. Differential effects of tumor necrosis factor-α and interleukin-1 on 3β-hydroxysteroid dehydrogenase/D5 —> D4 isomerase expression in mouse Leydig cells. Endocrine 1997; 7:295-301.
68. Lin T, Wang D, Stocco DM. Interleukin-1 inhibits Leydig cell steroidogenesis without affecting steroidogenic acute regulatory protein messenger ribonucleic acid or protein levels. J Endocrinol 1998; 156:461-467.
69. Heinrich PC, Behrmann I, Haan S et al. Principles of interleukin (IL)-6-type cytokine signalling and its regulation. Biochem J 2003; 374:1-20.
70. Tilg H, Dinarello CA, Mier JW. IL-6 and APPs: Anti-inflammatory and immunosuppressive mediators. Immunol Today 1997; 18:428-432.
71. Cudicini C, Lejeune H, Gomez E et al. Human Leydig cells and Sertoli cells are producers of interleukins-1 and -6. J Clin Endocrinol Metab 1997; 82:1426-1433.
72. Okuda Y, Bardin CW, Hodgskin LR et al. Interleukins-1α and -1β regulate interleukin-6 expression in Leydig and Sertoli cells. Recent Prog Horm Res 1995; 50:367-372.
73. Hakovirta H, Syed V, Jégou B et al. Function of interleukin-6 as an inhibitor of meiotic DNA synthesis in the rat seminiferous epithelium. Mol Cell Endocrinol 1995; 108:193-198.
74. Fujisawa M, Okuda Y, Fujioka H et al. Expression and regulation of gp130 messenger ribonucleic acid in cultured immature rat Sertoli cells. Endocr Res 2002; 28:1-8.
75. Boockfor FR, Schwarz LK. Effects of interleukin-6, interleukin-2, and tumor necrosis factor alpha on transferrin release from Sertoli cells in culture. Endocrinology 1991; 129:256-262.
76. Hoeben E, Wuyts A, Proost P et al. Identification of IL-6 as one of the important cytokines responsible for the ability of mononuclear cells to stimulate Sertoli cell functions. Mol Cell Endocrinol 1997; 132:149-160.
77. Jenab S, Morris PL. Interleukin-6 regulation of κ opioid receptor gene expression in primary Sertoli cells. Endocrine 2000; 13:11-15.
78. Rival C, Theas MS, Guazzone VA et al. Interleukin-6 and IL-6 receptor cell expression in testis of rats with autoimmune orchitis. J Reprod Immunol 2006; 70:43-58.
79. Li L, Itoh M, Ablake M et al. Prevention of murine experimental autoimmune orchitis by recombinant human interleukin-6. Clin Immunol 2002; 102:135-137.
80. Spooner CE, Markowitz NP, Sarvolatz LD. The role of tumor necrosis factor in sepsis. Clin Immunol Immunopath 1992; 62:S11-S17.
81. Cerami A. Inflammatory cytokines. Clin Immunol Immunopath 1992; 62:S3-S10.
82. Hsu H, Shu HB, Pan MG et al. TRADD-TRAF2 and TRADD-FADD interactions define two distinct TNF receptor 1 signal transduction pathways. Cell 1996; 84:299-308.
83. Mak T, Yeh WC. Signaling for survival and apoptosis in the immune system. Arthritis Res 2002; 4:S243-S252.
84. De SK, Chen HL, Pace JL et al. Expression of tumor necrosis factor-α in mouse spermatogenic cells. Endocrinology 1993; 133:389-396.
85. Mauduit C, Besset V, Caussanel V et al. Tumor necrosis factor a receptor p55 is under hormonal (follicle-stimulating hormone) control in testicular Sertoli cells. Biochem Biophys Res Commun 1996; 224:631-637.
86. Moore C, Hutson JC. Physiological relevance of tumor necrosis factor in mediating macrophage-Leydig cell interactions. Endocrinology 1994; 134:63-69.
87. Xiong Y, Hales DB. Expression, regulation, and production of tumor necrosis factor-α in mouse testicular interstitial macrophages in vitro. Endocrinology 1993; 133:2568-2573.
88. Pentikäinen V, Erkkilä K, Suomalainen L et al. TNFα down-regulates the Fas ligand and inhibits germ cell apoptosis in the human testis. J Clin Endocrinol Metab 2001; 86:4480-4488.
89. Suominen JS, Wang Y, Kaipia A et al. Tumor necrosis factor-alpha (TNF-α) promotes cell survival during spermatogenesis, and this effect can be blocked by infliximab, a TNF-α antagonist. Eur J Endocrinol 2004; 151:629-640.
90. Siu MK, Lee WM, Cheng CY. The interplay of collagen IV, tumor necrosis factor-α, gelatinase B (matrix metalloprotease-9), and tissue inhibitor of metalloproteases-1 in the basal lamina regulates Sertoli cell-tight junction dynamics in the rat testis. Endocrinology 2003; 144:371-387.
91. Le Magueresse-Battistoni B, Pernod G, Kolodié L et al. Tumor necrosis factor-α regulates plasminogen activator inhibitor-1 in rat testicular peritubular cells. Endocrinology 1997; 138:1097-1105.
92. Nehar D, Mauduit C, Boussouar F et al. Tumor necrosis factor-α-stimulated lactate production is linked to lactate dehydrogenase A expression and activity increase in porcine cultured Sertoli cells. Endocrinology 1997; 138:1964-1971.
93. Riera MF, Meroni SB, Gómez GE et al. Regulation of lactate production by FSH, IL1β, and TNFα in rat Sertoli cells. Gen Comp Endocrinol 2001; 122:88-97.

94. Mauduit C, Jaspar JM, Poncelet E et al. Tumor necrosis factor-α antagonizes follicle-stimulating hormone action in cultured Sertoli cells. Endocrinology 1993; 133:69-76.
95. Delfino FJ, Boustead JN, Fix C et al. NF-κB and TNF-α stimulate androgen receptor expression in Sertoli cells. Mol Cell Endocrinol 2003; 201:1-12.
96. Yule TD, Tung KS. Experimental autoimmune orchitis induced by testis and sperm antigen-specific T cell clones: An important pathogenic cytokine is tumor necrosis factor. Endocrinology 1993; 133:1098-1107.
97. Suescun MO, Rival C, Theas MS et al. Involvement of tumor necrosis factor-α in the pathogenesis of autoimmune orchitis in rats. Biol Reprod 2003; 68:2114-2121.
98. Riccioli A, Starace D, D'Alessio A et al. TNF-α and IFN-γ regulate expression and function of the Fas system in the seminiferous epithelium. J Immunol 2000; 165:743-749.
99. Riccioli A, Filippini A, De Cesaris P et al. Inflammatory mediators increase surface expression of integrin ligands, adhesion to lymphocytes, and secretion of interleukin 6 in mouse Sertoli cells. Proc Natl Acad Sci USA 1995; 92:5808-5812.
100. Hong CY, Park JH, Ahn RS et al. Molecular mechanism of suppression of testicular steroidogenesis by proinflammatory cytokine tumor necrosis factor α. Mol Cell Biol 2004; 24:2593-2604.
101. Mauduit C, Hartmann DJ, Chauvin MA et al. Tumor necrosis factor α inhibits gonadotropin action in cultured porcine Leydig cells: Site(s) of action. Endocrinology 1991; 129:2933-2940.
102. Li X, Youngblood GL, Payne AH et al. Tumor necrosis factor-α inhibition of 17α-hydroxylase/C17-20 lyase gene (Cyp17) expression. Endocrinology 1995; 136:3519-3526.
103. Xiong Y, Hales DB. The role of tumor necrosis factor-α in the regulation of mouse Leydig cell steroidogenesis. Endocrinology 1993; 132:2438-2444.
104. Mauduit C, Gasnier F, Rey C et al. Tumor necrosis factor-α inhibits leydig cell steroidogenesis through a decrease in steroidogenic acute regulatory protein expression. Endocrinology 1998; 139:2863-2868.
105. Morales V, Santana P, Diaz R et al. Intratesticular delivery of tumor necrosis factor-α and ceramide directly abrogates steroidogenic acute regulatory protein expression and Leydig cell steroidogenesis in adult rats. Endocrinology 2003; 144:4763-4772.
106. Phillips DJ. The activin/inhibin family. In: Thomson AW, Lotze MT, eds. The Cytokine Handbook, Vol 2. 4th ed. Amsterdam: Academic Press, 2003:1153-1177.
107. de Kretser DM, Hedger MP, Loveland KL et al. Inhibins, activins and follistatin in reproduction. Human Reprod Update 2002; 8:529-541.
108. Yu J, Dolter KE. Production of activin A and its roles in inflammation and hematopoiesis. Cytokines Cell Mol Ther 1997; 3:169-177.
109. Phillips DJ, Jones KL, Scheerlinck JY et al. Evidence for activin A and follistatin involvement in the systemic inflammatory response. Mol Cell Endocrinol 2001; 180:155-162.
110. Hedger MP, Phillips DJ, de Kretser DM. Divergent cell-specific effects of activin-A on thymocyte proliferation stimulated by phytohemagglutinin, and interleukin 1β or interleukin 6 in vitro. Cytokine 2000; 12:595-602.
111. Hedger MP, Drummond AE, Robertson DM et al. Inhibin and activin regulate [^{3}H]thymidine uptake by rat thymocytes and 3T3 cells in vitro. Mol Cell Endocrinol 1989; 61:133-138.
112. Okuma Y, Saito K, O'Connor AE et al. Reciprocal regulation of activin A and inhibin B by interleukin-1 (IL-1) and follicle-stimulating hormone (FSH) in rat Sertoli cells in vitro. J Endocrinol 2005; 185:99-110.
113. Yoshida E, Tanimoto K, Murakami K et al. Isolation and characterization of 5'-regulatory region of mouse activin βA subunit gene. Biochem Mol Biol Int 1998; 44:325-332.
114. Tanimoto K, Yoshida E, Mita S et al. Human activin βA gene: Identification of novel 5' exon, functional promoter, and enhancers. J Biol Chem 1996; 271:32760-32769.
115. Ardekani AM, Romanelli JC, Mayo KE. Structure of the rat inhibin and activin β_A-subunit gene and regulation in an ovarian granulosa cell line. Endocrinology 1998; 139:3271-3279.
116. Bilezikjian LM, Corrigan AZ, Blount AL et al. Regulation and actions of Smad7 in the modulation of activin, inhibin, and transforming growth factor-β signaling in anterior pituitary cells. Endocrinology 2001; 142:1065-1072.
117. Chen X, Weisberg E, Fridmacher V et al. Smad4 and FAST-1 in the assembly of activin-responsive factor. Nature 1997; 389:85-89.
118. Ethier JF, Findlay JK. Roles of activin and its signal transduction mechanisms in reproductive tissues. Reproduction 2001; 121:667-675.
119. Mellor SL, Ball EM, O'Connor AE et al. Activin βC-subunit heterodimers provide a new mechanism of regulating activin levels in the prostate. Endocrinology 2003; 144:4410-4419.
120. Mather JP, Roberts PE, Krummen LA. Follistatin modulates activin activity in a cell- and tissue-specific manner. Endocrinology 1993; 132:2732-2734.

121. Nakamura T, Takio K, Eto Y et al. Activin-binding protein from rat ovary is follistatin. Science 1990; 247:836-838.
122. Buzzard JJ, Loveland KL, O'Bryan MK et al. Changes in circulating and testicular levels of inhibin A and B and activin A during postnatal development in the rat. Endocrinology 2004; 145:3532-3541.
123. Kaipia A, Penttila TL, Shimasaki S et al. Expression of inhibin β_A and β_B, follistatin and activin-A receptor messenger ribonucleic acids in the rat seminiferous epithelium. Endocrinology 1992; 131:2703-2710.
124. de Winter JP, Vanderstichele HM, Verhoeven G et al. Peritubular myoid cells from immature rat testes secrete activin-A and express activin receptor type II in vitro. Endocrinology 1994; 135:759-767.
125. Knight PG, Muttukrishna S, Groome NP. Development and application of a two-site enzyme immunoassay for the determination of 'total' activin-A concentrations in serum and follicular fluid. J Endocrinol 1996; 148:267-279.
126. Groome NP, Tsigou A, Cranfield M et al. Enzyme immunoassays for inhibins, activins and follistatins. Mol Cell Endocrinol 2001; 180:73-77.
127. Meinhardt A, O'Bryan MK, McFarlane JR et al. Localization of follistatin in the rat testis. J Reprod Fertil 1998; 112:233-241.
128. Hakovirta H, Kaipia A, Söder O et al. Effects of activin-A, inhibin-A, and transforming growth factor-β1 on stage-specific deoxyribonucleic acid synthesis during rat seminiferous epithelial cycle. Endocrinology 1993; 133:1664-1668.
129. Mather JP, Attie KM, Woodruff TK et al. Activin stimulates spermatogonial proliferation in germ-Sertoli cell cocultures from immature rat testis. Endocrinology 1990; 127:3206-3214.
130. Meehan T, Schlatt S, O'Bryan MK et al. Regulation of germ cell and Sertoli cell development by activin, follistatin, and FSH. Dev Biol 2000; 220:225-237.
131. Boitani C, Stefanini M, Fragale A et al. Activin stimulates Sertoli cell proliferation in a defined period of rat testis development. Endocrinology 1995; 136:5438-5444.
132. Meinhardt A, McFarlane JR, Seitz J et al. Activin maintains the condensed type of mitochondria in germ cells. Mol Cell Endocrinol 2000; 168:111-117.
133. Chen YG, Lui HM, Lin SL et al. Regulation of cell proliferation, apoptosis, and carcinogenesis by activin. Exp Biol Med 2002; 227:75-87.
134. de Kretser DM, Hedger MP, Phillips DJ. Activin A and follistatin: Their role in the acute phase reaction and inflammation. J Endocrinol 1999; 161:195-198.
135. Illingworth PJ, Groome NP, Byrd W et al. Inhibin-B: A likely candidate for the physiologically important form of inhibin in men. J Clin Endocrinol Metab 1996; 81:1321-1325.
136. Clifton RJ, O'Donnell L, Robertson DM. Pachytene spermatocytes in coculture inhibit rat Sertoli cell synthesis of inhibin βB-subunit and inhibin B but not the inhibin α-subunit. J Endocrinol 2002; 172:565-574.
137. Stuehr DJ. Structure-function aspects in the nitric oxide synthases. Ann Rev Pharmacol Toxicol 1997; 37:339-359.
138. Alderton WK, Cooper CE, Knowles RG. Nitric oxide synthases: Structure, function and inhibition. Biochem J 2001; 357:593-615.
139. Davis KL, Martin E, Turko IV et al. Novel effects of nitric oxide. Ann Rev Pharmacol Toxicol 2001; 41:203-236.
140. Droge W. Free radicals in the physiological control of cell function. Physiol Rev 2002; 82:47-95.
141. Schmidt HH, Walter U. NO at work. Cell 1994; 78:919-925.
142. Nathan C, Xie QW. Nitric oxide synthases: Roles, tolls, and controls. Cell 1994; 78:915-918.
143. Lee NP, Cheng CY. Nitric oxide/nitric oxide synthase, spermatogenesis, and tight junction dynamics. Biol Reprod 2004; 70:267-276.
144. Brenman JE, Xia H, Chao DS et al. Regulation of neuronal nitric oxide synthase through alternative transcripts. Dev Neurosci 1997; 19:224-231.
145. Wang Y, Goligorsky MS, Lin M et al. A novel, testis-specific mRNA transcript encoding an NH_2-terminal truncated nitric-oxide synthase. J Biol Chem 1997; 272:11392-11401.
146. Wang Y, Newton DC, Miller TL et al. An alternative promoter of the human neuronal nitric oxide synthase gene is expressed specifically in Leydig cells. Am J Pathol 2002; 160:369-380.
147. Herman M, Rivier C. Activation of a neural brain-testicular pathway rapidly lowers Leydig cell levels of the steroidogenic acute regulatory protein and the peripheral-type benzodiazepine receptor while increasing levels of neuronal nitric oxide synthase. Endocrinology 2006; 147:624-633.
148. Kostic TS, Andric SA, Maric D et al. Inhibitory effects of stress-activated nitric oxide on antioxidant enzymes and testicular steroidogenesis. J Steroid Biochem Molec Biol 2000; 75:299-306.
149. Sharma AC, Sam IInd AD, Lee LY et al. Effect of N^G-nitro-L-arginine methyl ester on testicular blood flow and serum steroid hormones during sepsis. Shock 1998; 9:416-421.

150. Welch C, Watson ME, Poth M et al. Evidence to suggest nitric oxide is an interstitial regulator of Leydig cell steroidogenesis. Metabolism 1995; 44:234-238.
151. Del Punta K, Charreau EH, Pignataro OP. Nitric oxide inhibits Leydig cell steroidogenesis. Endocrinology 1996; 137:5337-5343.
152. Lee NP, Cheng CY. Regulation of Sertoli cell tight junction dynamics in the rat testis via the nitric oxide synthase/soluble guanylate cyclase/3',5'-cyclic guanosine monophosphate/protein kinase G signaling pathway: An in vitro study. Endocrinology 2003; 144:3114-3129.
153. Lue Y, Sinha Hikim AP, Wang C et al. Functional role of inducible nitric oxide synthase in the induction of male germ cell apoptosis, regulation of sperm number, and determination of testes size: Evidence from null mutant mice. Endocrinology 2003; 144:3092-3100.
154. Shiraishi K, Naito K, Yoshida K. Nitric oxide promotes germ cell necrosis in the delayed phase after experimental testicular torsion of rat. Biol Reprod 2001; 65:514-521.
155. Lissbrant E, Löfmark U, Collin O et al. Is nitric oxide involved in the regulation of the rat testicular vasculature? Biol Reprod 1997; 56:1221-1227.
156. Chang H, Lau AL, Matzuk MM. Studying TGF-β superfamily signaling by knockouts and knockins. Mol Cell Endocrinol 2001; 180:39-46.
157. Cohen PE, Pollard JW. Normal sexual function in male mice lacking a functional type I interleukin-1 (IL-1) receptor. Endocrinology 1998; 139:815-818.
158. Pasparakis M, Alexopoulou L, Episkopou V et al. Immune and inflammatory responses in TNFα-deficient mice: A critical requirement for TNFα in the formation of primary B cell follicles, follicular dendritic cell networks and germinal centers, and in the maturation of the humoral immune response. J Exp Med 1996; 184:1397-1411.
159. Morales-Montor J, Baig S, Mitchell R et al. Immunoendocrine interactions during chronic cysticercosis determine male mouse feminization: Role of IL-6. J Immunol 2001; 167:4527-4533.
160. Granholm T, Fröysa B, Lundström C et al. Cytokine responsiveness in germfree and conventional NMRI mice. Cytokine 1992; 4:545-550.
161. Granholm T, Fröysa B, Midtvedt T et al. Ontogeny of lymphocyte activating factors in conventional and germfree rats. Reg Immunol 1992; 4:209-215.
162. Kangasniemi M, Kaipia A, Mali P et al. Modulation of basal and FSH-dependent cyclic AMP production in rat seminiferous tubules staged by an improved transillumination technique. Anat Rec 1990; 227:62-76.
163. Kangasniemi M, Kaipia A, Toppari J et al. Cellular regulation of follicle-stimulating hormone (FSH) binding in rat seminiferous tubules. J Androl 1990; 11:336-343.
164. Delfino F, Walker WH. Stage-specific nuclear expression of NF-κB in mammalian testis. Mol Endocrinol 1998; 12:1696-1707.
165. Kluger MJ, Kozak W, Leon LR et al. The use of knockout mice to understand the role of cytokines in fever. Clin Exp Pharmacol Physiol 1998; 25:141-144.
166. Born TL, Smith DE, Garka KE et al. Identification and characterization of two members of a novel class of the interleukin-1 receptor (IL-1R) family: Delineation of a new class of IL-1R-related proteins based on signaling. J Biol Chem 2000; 275:29946-29954.
167. Andre R, Moggs JG, Kimber I et al. Gene regulation by IL-1β independent of IL-1R1 in the mouse brain. Glia 2006; 53:477-483.
168. Cohen PE, Chisholm O, Arceci RJ et al. Absence of colony-stimulating factor-1 in osteopetrotic ($csfm^{op}/csfm^{op}$) mice results in male fertility defects. Biol Reprod 1996; 55:310-317.
169. Hedger MP, Hales DB. Immunophysiology of the male reproductive tract. In: Neill JD, ed. Knobil and Neill's Physiology of Reproduction, Vol 1. 3rd ed. Amsterdam: Elsevier, 2006:1195-1286.
170. Cutolo M, Balleari E, Giusti M et al. Sex hormone status of male patients with rheumatoid arthritis: Evidence of low serum concentrations of testosterone at baseline and after human chorionic gonadotropin stimulation. Arthritis Rheum 1988; 31:1314-1317.
171. Buch JP, Havlovec SK. Variation in sperm penetration assay related to viral illness. Fertil Steril 1991; 55:844-846.
172. Adamopoulos DA, Lawrence DM, Vassilopoulos P et al. Pituitary-testicular interrelationships in mumps orchitis and other viral infections. Br Med J 1978; 1:1177-1180.
173. O'Bryan MK, Schlatt S, Phillips DJ et al. Bacterial lipopolysaccharide-induced inflammation compromises testicular function at multiple levels in vivo. Endocrinology 2000; 141:238-246.
174. Tulassay Z, Viczián M, Böjthe L et al. Quantitative histological studies on the injury of spermatogenesis induced by endotoxin in rats. J Reprod Fertil 1970; 22:161-164.
175. Bosmann HB, Hales KH, Li X et al. Acute in vivo inhibition of testosterone by endotoxin parallels loss of steroidogenic acute regulatory (StAR) protein in Leydig cells. Endocrinology 1996; 137:4522-4525.
176. Clemens JW, Bruot BC. Testicular dysfunction in the adjuvant-induced arthritic rat. J Androl 1989; 10:419-424.

177. Wallgren M, Kindahl H, Larsson K. Clinical, endocrinological and spermatological studies after endotoxin in the ram. Zentralbl Veterinarmed [A] 1989; 36:90-103.
178. Wallgren M, Kindahl H, Rodriguez-Martinez H. Alterations in testicular function after endotoxin injection in the boar. Int J Androl 1993; 16:235-243.
179. Baker HW. Reproductive effects of nontesticular illness. Endocrinol Metab Clin North Am 1998; 27:831-850.
180. Hedger M, Klug J, Fröhlich S et al. Regulatory cytokine expression and interstitial fluid formation in the normal and inflamed rat testis are under Leydig cell control. J Androl 2005; 26:379-386.
181. Hales KH, Diemer T, Ginde S et al. Diametric effects of bacterial endotoxin lipopolysaccharide on adrenal and Leydig cell steroidogenic acute regulatory protein. Endocrinology 2000; 141:4000-4012.
182. Turner TT, Tung KS, Tomomasa H et al. Acute testicular ischemia results in germ cell-specific apoptosis in the rat. Biol Reprod 1997; 57:1267-1274.
183. Hales DB, Diemer T, Hales KH. Role of cytokines in testicular function. Endocrine 1999; 10:201-217.
184. Gow RM, O'Bryan MK, Canny BJ et al. Differential effects of dexamethasone treatment on lipopolysaccharide-induced testicular inflammation and reproductive hormone inhibition in adult rats. J Endocrinol 2001; 168:193-201.
185. Sharpe RM, Donachie K, Cooper I. Re-evaluation of the intratesticular level of testosterone required for quantitative maintenance of spermatogenesis in the rat. J Endocrinol 1988; 117:19-26.
186. Cunningham GR, Huckins C. Persistence of complete spermatogenesis in the presence of low intratesticular concentrations of testosterone. Endocrinology 1979; 105:177-186.
187. Liew SH, Meachem SJ, Hedger MP. A stereological analysis of the response of spermatogenesis to an acute inflammatory episode in adult rats. J Androl 2007; 28, (in press).
188. Tjioe DY, Steinberger E. A quantitative study of the effect of ischaemia on the germinal epithelium of rat testes. J Reprod Fertil 1970; 21:489-494.
189. Meachem SJ, McLachlan RI, Stanton PG et al. FSH immunoneutralization acutely impairs spermatogonial development in normal adult rats. J Androl 1999; 20:756-762, (discussion 755).
190. O'Donnell L, McLachlan RI, Wreford NG et al. Testosterone promotes the conversion of round spermatids between stages VII and VIII of the rat spermatogenic cycle. Endocrinology 1994; 135:2608-2614.
191. Heckert LL, Griswold MD. Expression of follicle-stimulating hormone receptor mRNA in rat testes and Sertoli cells. Mol Endocrinol 1991; 5:670-677.
192. Schindler R, Clark BD, Dinarello CA. Dissociation between interleukin-1b mRNA and protein synthesis in human peripheral blood mononuclear cells. J Biol Chem 1990; 265:10232-10237.
193. Lord PC, Wilmoth LM, Mizel SB et al. Expression of interleukin-1a and b genes by human blood polymorphonuclear leukocytes. J Clin Invest 1991; 87:1312-1321.
194. Herzyk DJ, Allen JN, Marsh CB et al. Macrophage and monocyte IL-1β regulation differs at multiple sites: Messenger RNA expression, translation, and post-translational processing. J Immunol 1992; 149:3052-3058.

CHAPTER 7

Transcription Regulation in Spermatogenesis

Wing-Yee Lui* and C. Yan Cheng

Introduction

Spermatogenesis is a highly coordinated process in which diploid spermatogonia (2n) differentiate into mature haploid (1n) spermatozoa in the seminiferous epithelium. In this process, spermatogonia undergo several mitotic divisions and either enter a stem cell renewal pathway, or commit themsevles for further development. Diploid spermatocytes subsequently undergo two meiotic divisions and result in the production of haploid round spermatids. They then enter the process of spermiogenesis in which profound morphological and biochemical restructuring, such as the formation of acrosome and flagellum occur, and give rise to mature spermatozoa.

The cyclic and synchronous nature of spermatogenesis leads to specific pattern of cellular associations at a given segment in the tubules in which germ cells at particular stages of differentiation will associate with one another. Such cellular associations have been classified into the stages of the seminiferous epithelium. There are twelve (stages I-XII) and fourteen stages (stages I-XIV) of the seminiferous epithelium in mouse and rat, respectively[1,2] according to their cellular associations. Such differentiation pattern apparently requires precise regulation of specific genes at a given stage. In order to have a better understanding how transcription factors exerts their regulatory function to modulate cellular and stage-specific gene expression during spermatogenesis, we summarize herein some of the recent findings in the study of transcription regulation during spermatogenesis into five categories: (i) general transcription factors, (ii) nuclear receptor superfamily of transcription factors, (iii) other transcription factors involved in testicular functions, (iv) testis-specific gene transcription, and (v) transcriptional regulation of cell junction dynamics. The chapter is not intended to be exhaustive, rather, it serves as a guide for future studies based on latest findings in the field.

Transcription Regulation in Spermatogenesis

General Transcription Factors

Regulation of stringent stage-specific gene expression in testicular cells and the massive wave of transcriptional activity in germ cells following meiosis are governed by a highly specialized transcriptional mechanism.[3] Such temporal and restricted pattern of gene transcription is achieved by the presence of germ cell-specific transcription factors (Table 1). In addition, various general transcription factors, in term of their expression levels and their testis-specific isoforms, are differentially regulated in germ cells and in testes. It is believed that the differential expression of general transcription factors also play a crucial role to ensure proper and efficient transcription in germ cells throughout spermatogenesis.[4] For instance, TFIIB (a transcription factor that serves as a positioning factor for polymerase), TATA-binding protein (TBP)

*Corresponding Author: Wing-Yee Lui—School of Biological Sciences, The University of Hong Kong, Pokfulam Road, Hong Kong, China. Email: wylui@hku.hk

Molecular Mechanisms in Spermatogenesis, edited by C. Yan Cheng. ©2008 Landes Bioscience and Springer Science+Business Media.

Table 1. List of the genes encoding the transcription factors whose deletion in the mice generate defects in males

Gene Disrupted	Male Phenotype	Female Phenotype	References
AR	Complete arrest at pachytene spermatocyte stage Female-like appearance Small testis with a decrease in serum testosterone concentration	Fertile	Yeh, 2002[23]
RARα	Complete arrest and severe degeneration of the seminiferous epithelium	Fertile	Lufkin, 1993[34]
RXRβ	All survivers are sterile Partial arrest at primary spermatocyte stage Structural abnormalities in spermatozoa	Fertile	Kastner, 1996[35]
GCNF	Embryonic lethality	Embryonic lethality	Chung, 2001[156]
TR2	Functional testis having normal sperm number and motility	Fertile	Shyr, 2002[73]
TR4	Delay in the first wave of spermatogenesis Prolonged stages XI to XII of spermatogenesis Reduced fertility	Fertile	Mu, 2004[72]
CREM	Complete arrest at pachytene spermatocyte stage	Fertile	Nantel, 1996;[81] Blendy, 1996[157]
CREB (α and δ isoforms)	Fertile	Fertile	Hummler, 1994[158]
CREB (α, β and δ)	Die shortly after birth	Die shortly after birth	Rudolph, 1998[159]
Rhox5	Subfertile Increased frequency of apoptotic meiotic spermatocytes	Fertile	Pitman, 1998;[95] MacLean, 2005[26]
Sperm-1	Subfertile	Fertile	Pearse, 1997[97]
Plzf	Exhibit progressive loss of spermatogonia and increase in apoptosis with age	Fertile	Costoya, 2004[102] Buaas, 2004[103]
WT1	Conditional knockout mice show impaired spermatogenesis and predicted to be fertile	—	Gao, 2006[106]
GATA-1	Embryonic lethality	Embryonic lethality	Pevny, 1991[160]
GATA-4	Embryonic lethality	Embryonic lethality	Narita, 1997[161]
GATA-6	Embryonic lethality	Embryonic lethality	Koutsourakis, 1999[162]
MSY2	Infertile	Infertile	Yang, 2005[139]
CAF1	Infertile	Fertile	Nakamura, 2004[143]; Berthet, 2004[144]

and RNA polymerase II were found to be accumulated in early haploid germ cells. Their levels in haploid germ cells are much higher than in somatic cells.[5] Adult rodent testes contain 80-200 molecules of TBP mRNA per haploid genome-equivalent, whereas adult spleen and liver contains 0.7 and 2.3 molecules of TBP mRNA per haploid genome-equivalent, respectively.[5] Such organization of transcription factors enable early spermatids accumulate enough mRNA for their development until the final stages of spermiogenesis.

In addition to the unique expression pattern of various general transcription factors in germ cells, the presence of their testis-specific isoforms may play a specialized function in spermatogenesis. ALF or TFIIA-τ is a testis-specific isoform of TFIIA which may have specificity for a subset of transcriptional activators.[6,7]

Nuclear Receptor Superfamily

Lipophilic Hormone Nuclear Receptors

Androgen Receptor

Androgens are crucial steroid hormones in male reproduction and their actions ranging from regulating sexual differentiation, sexual maturation, spermatogenesis to production of gonadotropins.[8-12] Androgens exert their effects through the androgen receptor (AR). AR is a ligand-inducible transcription factor (110 kDa) that regulates the expression of target genes in response to its cognate ligand (androgen) through binding to an androgen response element (ARE).[12,13]

Similar to other members of the nuclear receptor superfamily, AR can be divided into four functional domains. They are: NH_2-terminal transactivation domain, DNA-binding domain (DBD), hinge region, and ligand-binding domain (LBD). AR has two separate NH_2-terminal transactivation domains which possibly interact with different coregulators or transcription factors in a promoter content-dependent manner.[14] The DBD contains two zinc fingers that recognize specific DNA consensus sequences. AR homodimer binds to the inverted repeat ARE, GGTACAnnnTGTTCT.[15-18] Apart from the formation of homodimer, it was reported that AR is capable of forming the heterodimers with TR4 (human testicular receptor 4, TR4, is an orphan member of the nuclear receptor superfamily) or ERα (estrogen receptor α), which results in a decrease in AR transcriptional activity.[19,20] The LBD is responsible for the formation of the ligand-binding pocket, facilitating the interaction between AR and heat shock protein, and also interacting with AR NH_2 terminus to stabilize the bound androgen.[21,22]

AR is of particular interest because of the observation that knockout of AR produced male mice displaying female-like appearance with arrested spermatogenesis.[23] Although AR plays an indispensable role in spermatogenesis, only a few number of genes have been identified so far that are directly regulated by AR in the testis. The expression of X-linked Rhox5/PEM homeobox gene is a typical example of AR-mediated gene regulation in the testis.[24-26] Barbulescu et al. have identified two functional AREs within 300-bp upstream of the Rhox5 transcription start site.[27,28] The promoter region containing the regulatory sequences that directs AR-dependent expression specifically in Sertoli cells and confers AR stage-specific expression in adult testis.[29,30] Recent studies from MacLean et al. have shown that another four Rhox genes (namely Rhox2, 3, 10 and 11) are dramatically upregulated in response to incubation with testosterone and cotransfection with an AR expression plasmid. Although the promoter sequences of the four Rhox genes have not yet been characterized, it is apparent that they all are androgen-dependent.[26]

Apart from AR knockout mice, a tissue-specific knockout mouse with the AR gene deleted in Sertoli cells [SC AR knockout mice] was generated to investigate how androgen/AR in Sertoli cells influence spermatogenesis.[31,32] It was found that the SC AR knockout male exhibit similar phenotypes as that of $AR^{-/-}$ mice with more severe testis atrophy. SC AR knockout mice showed alterations in the expression of anti-Mullerian hormone (AMH), cyclin A1, Pem and sperm-1.[31,32] The increase in the expression of AMH in mice leads to the reduction of testosterone production in Leydig cells. Significant reduction in germ cell number in SC AR knockout is associated with increased germ cell apoptosis and reduced expression of cyclin A1, Pem and sperm-1 genes that are important for late stage of germ cell development.[31,32] Sertoli cell-specific AR knockout mice clearly demonstrated the functional significance of AR in Sertoli cells in maintaining spermatogenesis and steroidogenesis.

Using another SC AR knock-out model,[32a] it was shown that the loss of androgen receptors in Sertoli cells led to a disruption of the blood-testis barrier (BTB) integrity since biotin could diffuse through the BTB.[32b] Using techniques of gene profiling, it was shown that the gene responsible for the "leaky" BTB in SC AR knock-out mice is likely to be claudin 3, which displays transient expression in newly formed tight junctions.[32b] However, it is noted that the SC AR knock-out mice used in this study were made with a floxed exon 1, yet the floxed animals had already displayed marked hypomorphic phenotype and the ultimate AR knockout was neither complete nor Sertoli cell selective,[32a] which may explain why did the SC AR knock-out mice had a serum testosterone level almost 40-fold of that of the wild type.[32a] Furthermore, the testicular claudin 3 level in adult rat testes was extremely low,[32b] and it is virtually undetectable beyond 45 days of age (Yan and Cheng, unpublished observations), making claudin 3 hardly an important structural component of the BTB in adult rats. Nonetheless, it is likely that testosterone and its receptor are important components that regulate BTB dynamics, much work is needed in the field to define the precise molecular target(s) of testosterone and AR at the BTB.

Retinoid Receptors

Retinoic acid receptors (RARs) and retinoid X receptors (RXRs) are two members of this family found in the testis. Ligand-dependent activation of RAR and RXR are essential to spermatogenesis based on the fact that infertility was observed in vitamin A-deficient rats and in RARα and RXRβ transgenic mice.[33-36] In vitro binding studies have demonstrated that the natural metabolites all-trans-RA and 9-cis-RA are high-affinity ligands for RARs, whereas only 9-cis-RA has been shown to bind RXRs. Each family consists of three genes, namely α, β, and γ, and each of them exists as multiple isoforms. RXR is capable of forming homodimers (RXR/RXR), heterodimers with RAR (RXR/RAR) and with other types of nuclear receptors such as thyroid hormone receptor (RXR/TR),[37] such characteristic enables this receptor family exerts combinatorial regulatory properties.

The homodimer and heterodimer function as RA-inducible transcriptional regulatory proteins through binding to DNA sequences called retinoic acid response element (RARE) or retinoid X response element (RXRE) located within the promoter of target genes. The consensus sequence of RARE is AGGTCAnnnnnAGGTCA, whilst RXRE is direct repeats of AGGTCA with one nucleotide spacing (AGGTCAnAGGTCA). The RAR/RXR heterodimer binds to the RARE, with RXR occupying the 5' upstream half-site and RAR occupying the 3' downstream half-site.[38]

Extensive studies using RARα and RXRβ transgenic mice have clearly demonstrated that retinoic acid-mediated gene regulation via RAR, and RXR play a crucial role in spermatogenesis. For instance, detailed morphological analysis in RARα knockout mouse testes showed that the typical characteristic of stage VIII tubule, where mature step 16 spermatids aligning along the tubular lumen, was not observed.[39] Instead, a mixed population of germ cells was found in stage VIII tubule in RARα knockout male.[39] For RXRβ knockout mice, failure of spermatid release occurred within the germinal epithelium and the epididymis contained very few spermatozoa. Although knockout of RARα and RXRβ resulted in male infertility, they displayed different seminiferous tubule morphology. These observations suggest that the downstream targets of RARα and RXRβ are not the same. Genes expressed in different testicular cells, namely Stra8 and bone morphogenetic protein 4 (BMP4) in germ cells, prostaglandin D2 synthetase in Sertoli cells, and fibronectin and laminin in myoid cells, were shown to be regulated by retinoic acid or retinol.[40-44] However, the precise mechanisms of vitamin A-mediated gene regulations have yet to be elucidated. Whether the regulation of those genes are direct effects mediated through the interaction of retinoid receptors and their corresponding promoters, or whether other retinoid-regulated proteins mediate indirect regulatory effects remain to be determined. Identification of the regulatory mechanism on RA-RAR-mediated BMP4 expression in other cell lines has provided a blueprint to study the transcription regulation of BMP4 gene in germ cells.[45]

Orphan Receptors

Germ Cell Nuclear Factor

Germ cell nuclear factor (GCNF), which is also known as retinoid receptor-related testis-associated receptor (RTR), is a novel member of the nuclear receptor superfamily of ligand-activated transcription factors.[46,47] Since the natural ligand for GCNF has not been identified, GCNF is classified as an orphan receptor. GCNF binds as a homodimer either to direct repeat response elements (AGGTCA) without additional nucleotide or to extended half-site such as TCAAGGTCA (XRE).[46,48-51] It does not form heterodimer with other nuclear receptors such as RXR.[48] In vitro studies have revealed that GCNF is a sequence-specific repressor of transcription and it folds into a β-sheet that contributes to dimerization and the recruitment of corepressors.[51-54] It can interact with other nuclear corepressors and with the repressor, RAP80, that is highly expressed in the testis.[54-56]

GCNF expression is restricted to the developing nervous system during embryogenesis, whereas the receptor is expressed during specific stages in maturing germ cells. Two transcripts of GCNF gene with sizes of 7.4 kb and 2.3 kb have been identified in spermatogenic cells. The 7.4 kb transcript is expressed during testicular development and is the predominant form in pachytene spermatocytes, whereas the 2.3 kb transcript is expressed predominantly in round spermatids.[47,57,58] In situ hybridization studies have shown that the GCNF transcript levels remain low during the meiotic prophase in rats and mice, and increase substantially and reach maximal level in round spermatids at stages VI-VIII.[58]

Up to now, several genes expressed in the testis were found to be regulated by GCNF. The temporal expression of protamine genes, prm-1 and prm-2, at stage I round spermatid is regulated reciprocally by GCNF and cAMP-response element modulator, CREMτ.[59-61] Binding of GCNF to GCNF response elements of prm-1 and prm-2 promoters represses both basal and CREMτ-activated transcription, thus GCNF may play a role to shut down protamine gene expression in elongating spermatids.[61] Apart from prm-1 and prm-2 genes, mitochondrial glycerol-3-phosphate dehydrogenase (mGPDH) and endozepine-like peptide (ELP) are two other testis-specific genes that are regulated by GCNF.[62,63] Both promoters of mGPDH and ELP genes contain CRE/GCNF elements that can effectively bind to GCNF. The binding of GCNF to these motifs can interfere with CREMτ-transactivation. Apparently, GCNF is a crucial transcription regulator that regulates the temporal and spatial expression of several testicular genes during meiosis and the early haploid phase of spermatogenesis.

Testicular Orphan Receptors 2 and 4

Testicular orphan receptor 2 (TR2) and testicular orphan receptor 4 (TR4) constitute a subfamily of nuclear receptors.[64,65] The TR2 and TR4 can modulate its target gene expression by forming homodimers and binding to the AGGTCA direct repeat (DR) sequences in its target genes.[66,67] TR4 can modulate transactivation mediated by other steroid nuclear receptors through interaction with these steroid receptors. For instance, TR4 could interact with the androgen receptor (AR) and the estrogen receptor (ER) that suppress AR- and ER-mediated transactivation.[19,68]

TR2 and TR4 have been shown to be expressed in mouse testes. TR2 is confined to meiotic and postmeiotic germ cells,[69,70] whereas TR4 is predominantly expressed in primary spermatocytes, especially in late-stage pachytene spermatocytes.[71,72] The expression of TR4 in round spermatid is stage-dependent and is confined to stage VII.[72] Although the male knockout mice of TR2 and TR4 are fertile, the disruption of TR4 gene does affect spermatogenesis at the end of late meiotic prophase and subsequent meiotic divisions, thus delays the first wave of spermatogenesis in the $TR4^{-/-}$ mice.[72,73] Gene disruption analyses indicated that TR4, but not TR2, is essential for normal spermatogenesis in mice.

Recent studies has demonstrated that TR4 can suppress the expression of 25-hydroxyvitamin D3 24-hydroxylase, Cyp24a1, through direct binding of TR4 to the vitamin D3 receptor response element (VDRE) in Chinese hamster ovary (CHO) cells. The VDRE shares similarity with the hormone response element for the TR4, which contains two repeated half sites of AGGTCA; however, it is separated by a 3-nucleotide space. Using the $TR4^{-/-}$ knockout mice model, Mu et al. showed that the expression level of Cyp24a1 increased in adult mice testes when TR4 gene was knocked out. Such observation indicates that testicular Cyp24a1 expression is also under the precise control of TR4.[72] Cyp24a1 is the only gene identified so far that is regulated by TR in the testis, identification of the molecular targets, such as putative ligands of TR2 and TR4, and the mechanisms that affect meiosis may help in a better understanding of the role of TR in spermatogenesis.

Transcription Factors Involved in Testicular Functions

Basic-Domain-Leucine-Zipper (b-zip) Family

Members of the b-zip family that are known to be expressed in the testis include cAMP response element modulator (CREM), cAMP response element binding protein (CREB), and activating transcription factor 1 (ATF1).[74,75] These proteins contain a basic DNA-binding domain with an adjacent leucine zipper that is required for dimerization and binding to a specific cis-acting element.[76,77] CREM, CREB and ATF-1 are capable of forming homodimers and heterodimers in response to cAMP signaling pathway and bind to a regulatory DNA sequence, known as cAMP responsive element (CRE). A CRE is constituted by the palindromic consensus sequence, TGACGTCA.[76-78]

CREM

Many isoforms of CREM are generated by alternative splicing. Among them, CREMτ is the isoform which has been extensively studied as its expression is restricted to the testis and is highly regulated during spermatogenesis.[79] CREMτ mRNA transcript is found at high levels in pachytene spermatocytes and more advanced germ cells, while its protein is present only in post-meiotic spermatids, suggesting that CREMτ plays a role in late stages of spermatogenesis.[80] The importance of CREMτ in spermatogenesis could be reflected in the gene knockout studies since spermatogenic arrest was observed at pachytene spermatocyte stage.[81] A list of postmeiotic genes encoding structural proteins required for spermatid differentiation, including the transition proteins (TP1 and TP2), protamines (prm1 and prm2), RT7, testis angiotensin-converting enzyme (ACE), proacrosin and calspermin, were found to be the direct targets of CREMτ.[82-85] All of these genes contain the putative CREs for the binding of CREMτ. It is apparent that CREMτ is a key transcription factor that controls postmeiotic germ cell differentiation.

Different from other CREM isoforms, the activation of CREMτ requires the association of a coactivator known as activator of CREM in testes (ACT).[86] ACT is exclusively expressed in testes.[86] ACT shows similar developmental expression pattern as CREMτ in testes and they are colocalized in spermatids.[86-88] ACT displays intrinsic transactivation potential capable of converting CREMτ into a potent transcriptional activator, leading to the activation of CREMτ in a phosphorylation-independent manner.[87,88] The presence of ACT in post-meiotic germ cells enables stage-specific activation of CREMτ-mediated gene transcription.

To elucidate the significance of ACT in CREMτ-mediated gene transcription in testes, gene targeting disruption in mice has been performed. It is surprising that male mice lacking ACT are fertile, which is different from the CREM knockout counterpart. Mice lacking ACT show some male reproductive defects including abnormalities in sperm heads and tails and reduced sperm motility.[89] However, the expressions of CREMτ-dependent genes, such as TP1 and prm1, were not affected in ACT knockout mice. These results seemingly suggest that other yet-to-be identified coactivators exist in testes could compensate for the loss of ACT to modulate CREMτ-dependent gene transcription.

CREB

Similar to CREM, many CREB isoforms are generated by alternative splicing in the testis. Although the gene knockout analyses of CREB isoforms have been performed, the role of CREB in spermatogenesis has not been fully elucidated. Since mice carrying mutations in all CREB isoforms exhibited severe developmental disorders and died shortly after birth. In situ hybridization analysis has shown that CREB mRNA is present in Sertoli cells in stages I-VIII tubules and the amount decreases to an undetectable level at stages IX-XIV.[90] The cellular localization of CREB in the testis is quite different from CREM, whose protein is present only in post-meiotic spermatids. Several genes involved in spermatogenesis such as murine spermatogenesis-associated protein, claudin-II and nectin-2 have been found to be regulated directly by CREB via the CRE motif in the corresponding promoters.[91,92,153] Interaction of CREB with other transcription factors, such as c-Jun, was found to be involved in regulating the nectin-2 gene transcription in Sertoli cells.[92] In addition, overexpression of dominant-negative CREB in primary Sertoli cells could completely inhibit the FSH-induced c-Fos expression. Taken collectively, these data illustrate that CREB seems to play an intriguing role in regulating gene transcription in Sertoli cells.

Homeobox Family

Transcription factors belonging to this family contain the homeobox motif that is a highly conserved DNA-binding domain constituted by 61 amino acids. Transcription factors belonging to this family are grouped in subfamilies based on the homeodomain sequence as well as the gene structure.[93] Our chapter does not attempt to cover all members of this family but highlights two subfamilies that show intimate relationships with spermatogenesis. They are the reproductive homeobox X-linked (Rhox) gene cluster and the POU-domain gene family.

Reproductive Homeobox X-Linked (Rhox) Gene Cluster

Rhox gene cluster presents a newly homeobox subfamily that contains 12 related homeobox genes.[24,26] All 12 Rhox genes are organized into three subclusters, namely α (Rhox 1-4), β (Rhox 5-9) and γ (Rhox 10-12) on the X chromosome and are expressed in male and female reproductive tissues. All of them exhibit cell type-specific expression.[26] In testes, all Rhox genes are restricted to Sertoli cells except Rhox4 which is predominantly expressed in Leydig cells.[26] Apart from cell-type specificity, these 12 Rhox genes exhibit a colinear expression pattern in which an expression gradient is achieved spatially, temporally, or quantitatively, pertinent to their relative position within subclusters. For instance, the genes in subcluster α display both temporal and quantitative colinearity.[26] Rhox1, the gene located at the distal 5' end of subcluster α express first (days 7-12 postpartum) followed by Rhox2 (day 12 postpartum), Rhox3 and Rhox4 (days 20-22 postpartum).[26] Among them, Rhox1 is expressed at the highest level during testis development than other gene members in same subcluster and each subsequent gene in the same subcluster exhibits a stepwise decline in its expression level.[26] It is believed that such colinear expression pattern observed in the Rhox cluster might provide Sertoli cells with a precise regulatory system to transduce temporally variable signals to germ cells at all stages of development.[94] Clearly, future studies such as targeted disruption or knockdown approaches will be required to reveal the individual and overlapping function of these Rhox genes in spermatogenesis.

The importance of the Rhox gene cluster in spermatogenesis could be demonstrated at least by target disruption of Rhox5 gene in male mice.[26,95] Ablation of Rhox5 gene by homologous recombination was subsequently found that mutant male are subfertile.[26] Reduced sperm count and sperm motility along with increased germ cell apoptosis were observed in Rhox5$^{-/-}$ mice. Since the expression of Rhox5 is restricted to Sertoli cells,[24,26,95] it is likely that Rhox5 plays a role in regulating the expression of Sertoli-cell genes that can modulate germ cell survival. Efforts should be made to elucidate the functional significance of each Rhox member in spermatogenesis and identify target genes that are regulated by the Rhox gene cluster.

POU Homedomain Proteins

Sperm-1

Sperm-1, belonging to the family of the POU (Pit, Oct, Unc) homeodomain proteins, is selectively expressed in male germ cells immediately preceding the first meiotic division and in the haploid spermatids.[96,97] Sperm-1 preferentially binds to an octamer DNA-response element with sequence of 5'-GCATATGTTATT-3' in which the optimal sequence differs from that preferred by other POU protein members.[96]

Knockout studies of Sperm-1 in mice have been performed, null mice develop normal testis, apparently with normal spermatogenesis and produce normal number of motile sperms as those of normal mice, except that the Sperm-1 null male mice are subfertile.[97] However, the molecular basis for this subfertile phenotype has not yet been elucidated. Thus, identification of the molecular targets and mechanism of action of sperm-1 may help in a better understanding its role in spermatogenesis.

Oct-4

Oct-4 is expressed in the postproliferative prospermatogonia until after birth in male embryos. Oct-4 expression continues in undifferentiated type A spermatogonia as spermatogenesis starts, and is downregulated when germ cells enter their differentiation pathway. There is no reexpression of Oct-4 in germ cells at any developemental stages of spermatogenesis.[98,99] The downregulation of Oct-4 seems to be one of the molecular triggers in the commitment of meiosis in male germ cells, although the target gene(s) involved in such event has not been identified.

C_2H_2 Zinc Finger Family

Transcription factors belong to this family must contain C_2H_2 zinc finger motif (also known as Krüppel zinc finger motif), which is generally present in tandem arrays with the sequence of Y/F-X-C-$X_{2\text{-}4}$-C-X_3-F-X_5-L-X_2-H-$X_{3\text{-}5}$-H, where X can be variable amino acids.[100] These conserved cysteine and histidine residues are able to bond tetrahedrally to a zinc ion. Plzf and WT1 are two transcription factors that are known to possess a C_2H_2 zinc finger and have been reported to have significant impact on spermatogenesis.[101]

Plzf

Plzf is also known as zinc-finger protein 145 (zfp145) that is expressed in the developing male gonad.[102] In postnatal and adult testes, Plzf is restricted to spermatogonia that exhibit stem-cell like properties and is coexpressed with Oct-4, a transcription factor implicated in maintaining stem-cell population.[102,103] The functional importance of Plzf has been revealed by two in vivo studies. Studies of naturally occurring Plzf-mutant (luxoid) mice and Plzf knockout mice have shown that both mutant mice exhibit a progressive loss of spermatogonia with age, associated with an increase in apoptosis, but without apparent defects in Sertoli cells.[102,103] Spermatogonial transplantation experiments demonstrated that Plzf is a spermatogonia-specific transcription factor that is required to regulate self-renewal and maintenance of the stem cell pool as transplantation of spermatogonia isolated from Plzf-null mice failed to repopulate gonads that had been chemically depleted of germ cells.[102] Up to now, no direct target gene of Plzf regulation has been identified. Apparently, it is an area that needs further investigation.

Wilms' Tumor Protein (WT1)

WT1 protein contains four COOH-terminal C_2H_2 zinc fingers for DNA binding and one of each transcriptional repression and activation domains at its NH_2 terminus.[104] WT1 plays a crucial role in the development of the genitourinary system.[105] Conditional knockout of WT1 protein in Sertoli cells by embryonic day 14.5 could result in disruption of developing seminiferous tubules and progressive loss of Sertoli cells and germ cells.[106] Using tissue-specific RNA interference (RNAi) approach that disrupts the expression of WT1 in mouse testis, studies have shown that increased germ cell apoptosis, loss of adherens junctions and impaired spermatogenesis were observed in siRNA-WT1 mice.[107] Microarray analysis on siRNA-WT1 testes has found that a spectrum of genes encoding signaling molecules and structural proteins whose expressions were altered.[107] For instance, integrin cytoplasmic domain associated protein 1α (Icap1-α) and epidermal growth factor receptor pathway substrate 8 (Eps8), which are signaling molecules that regulate actin-mediated cytoskeletal events, are altered in siRNA-WT1 testes.[107] These results suggest that Icap1-α and Eps8 are the target proteins of WT1 and WT1 is a crucial transcription factor in regulating spermatogenesis.

GATA Family

All GATA proteins contain a DNA-binding domain composed of two conserved multifunctional zinc fingers, $C\text{-}X_2\text{-}C\text{-}X_{17}\text{-}C\text{-}X_2\text{-}C$, where X represents variable amino acids.[108,109] GATA proteins recognize and bind to the DNA consensus motif, WGATAR.[109] The N-terminal zinc finger is required for the specificity and stability of the DNA binding, whilst the C-terminal zinc finger is for the recognition and binding to the core GATA motif.[110-113] GATA interacts with cofactors such as Friend of GATA-1 and -2 (FOG-1 and FOG-2) and p300/CBP via the N-terminal or C-terminal zinc fingers, resulting in either activation or repression of gene transcription.[114-119]

GATAs are essential transcription factors in mammalian reproductive development and function. Among six members of this family, GATA-1, -4 and -6 are found in testes. GATA-1 is expressed in mouse Sertoli cells from stages VII to IX of the seminiferous epithelial cycle.[120] GATA-4 is present in mouse testis throughout all developmental stages and localized to Sertoli cells and Leydig cells.[121-123] GATA-6 is expressed in neonatal, prepubertal, and adult testes and localized in Sertoli cells.[116,122] The GATA family members play equally important role in gonadal development, testosterone production and regulation of gene expression in testicular somatic cells such as Sertoli and Leydig cells.[118,119,124] For instance, GATA-4 is capable of activating the promoters of testicular genes including Mullerian-inhibiting substance (MIS), PII aromatase (Cyp19), SF-1, StAR and inhibin α.[124] The examples mentioned herein are not intended to be exhaustive, readers are strongly encouraged to read earlier review to gain a more comprehensive view of this protein family.[118,119]

Nuclear Factor Kappa B (NF-κB) Family

The NF-κB family of transcription factors regulates a wide variety of genes involved in spermatogenesis. The NF-κB family is composed of p50, p52, p65 (RelA), RelB and c-Rel,[125,126] which regulates transcription by binding as homo- or heterodimers to κB enhancer elements in the regulatory region of genes. Among five protein subunits, p50 and p65 have been shown to express in rat testes. Nuclear expression of p50 and p65 are cell-type and stage-specific. Nuclear p50 and p60 are highest at stages XIV-VII in Sertoli cells and stages VII-XI in spermatocytes.[127]

Like another transcription factors, the NF-κB family of transcription factors can activate and repress testicular gene transcription. For example, TNF-α induces NF-κB binding to the cAMP-response element-binding protein (CREB) in AR promoters and elevates their promoter activities in Sertoli cells.[128,129] TNF-α has been reported to downregulate SF-1 transactivation of Mullerian inhibiting substance (MIS) gene in the testis by NF-κB. The SF-1-bound NF-κB could recruit histone deacetylases to inhibit the SF-1-mediated MIS gene activation.[130] Since TNF-α is a major cytokine secreted by germ cells, it is believed that the effect of TNF-α and its downstream regulators, NF-κB, may not be limited to those identified genes. Clearly, there is much remains to be investigated with regard to the function of NF-κB in spermatogenesis.

Y-Box

The family of Y-box proteins contains a conserved cold-shock domain (CSD) for DNA binding, a variable N-terminal domain thought for transactivation and a C-terminal tail for protein-protein interaction.[131,132] YB-1 was the first identified transcription factor that bound to the Y-box and the consensus DNA sequence was determined as CTGATTGGYYUU, a reverse sequence motif of the CCAAT box.[133]

Mammalian germ cell homologues of *Xenopus* FRG Y1 and FRG Y2 have been identified in mouse testis, namely MSY1 and MSY2 respectively.[134,135] Similar to *Xenopus* homologues, MSY1 is ubiquitously expressed in somatic tissues; whereas MSY2 is expressed in meiotic and postmeiotic germ cells.[134,136] Several studies have revealed that Y-box proteins are needed to activate gene transcription in male germ cells, such as protamine 2 and cytochrome c genes.[137,138] Recent knockout studies further confirmed the functional significance of MSY2 in spermatogenesis.

Spermatogenesis is disrupted in postmeiotic null germ cells with many misshapen and multinucleated spermatids.[139]

Apart from MSY2, at least two other Y-box proteins, MSY1 and MSY4, are expressed in meiotic and postmeiotic germ cells.[134,140] However, their roles on gene transcription pertinent to spermatogenesis remain entirely unknown.

CAF1

Chromatin assembly factor-1 (CAF1), also called as Cnot7, is the mammalian homolog of yeast CAF1.[141] It is a component of the CCR4-NOT complex that has multiple roles in regulating transcription.[142] CAF1-deficient male mice are sterile owning to oligo-astheno-teratozoospermia shown in two independent knockout studies.[143,144] Maturation of spermatids is unsynchronized and impaired. Further studies have shown that the proper function of retinoid X receptor β (RXRβ)-mediated transcription in the testis requires the interaction of CAF1 through the AF-1 domain of RXRβ, suggesting CAF1 functions as a coregulator of RXRβ in regulating transcription in testicular somatic cells as RXRβ is expressed in somatic Sertoli cells and Leydig cell.[143]

Testis-Specific Gene Expression

Testis-specific gene expression could be in part achieved through the expression of testis-specific transcription factors, such as CREMτ, and cell type-specific components of the general or core transcription machinery as an increasing number of tissue or cell type-specific components of general transcription factors has been identified, such as TFIIA-τ, a testis-specific isoform of TFIIA.[145-147]

An alternative approach to achieve tissue-specific gene expression is by permanent transcriptional repression of that particular promoter in nonexpressing cells via DNA methylation.[148] A testis-specific expression of histone H1t is one of the examples belonging to this category. The repression of the histone H1t gene in nonexpressing cells is achieved by partial and full methylation of all seven CpG dinucleotides within the H1t proximal promoter, while these CpG dinucleotides are completely unmethylated in primary spermatocytes.[149,150]

Transcriptional Regulation of Cell Junction Dynamics

The translocation of germ cells across the seminiferous epithelium during spermatogenesis requires extensive restructuring of cell junctions at the Sertoli-germ and Sertoli-Sertoli interface.[151] It is believed that the transcriptional, post-transcriptional and post-translational regulations of cell junction proteins play crucial roles in controlling the assembly and disassembly of cell junctions, resulting in the progressive movement of germ cells to the adluminal from the basal compartment for the completion of spermatogenesis.[152] Therefore, studies of the transcriptional regulation of junction proteins found at the ectoplasmic specialization (ES) and the blood-testis barrier (BTB) are crucial for the thorough understanding of spermatogenesis. In our laboratory, the transcriptional regulations of nectin-2 and claudin-11 in Sertoli cells have been studied.[92,153] Nectin-2 is a junction protein localized at Sertoli cells and interacts at nectin-3 that is expressed in germ cells to form the heterotypic interlock between Sertoli and germ cells at the apical ES.[154] Our recent studies have demonstrated that CREB and c-Jun are bound to the cAMP responsive element (CRE) motif of the nectin-2 promoter located between nucleotides -316 and -211 (relative to the translation start site), resulting in the upregulation of nectin-2 gene transcription. Apart from CREB and c-Jun, two members of Sp1 family, Sp1 and Sp3, are also positive regulators of the nectin-2 transcription.[92] Analysis of the staged tubules has confirmed that the cyclic expressions of CREB and nectin-2 coincide with the event of apical ES restructuring between Sertoli cells and germ cells. It is believed that the tight regulation of the basal nectin-2 transcription by CREB, c-Jun and Sp1 are crucial to regulate the disassembly of adherens junctions between Sertoli cells and germ cells during spermiation (Fig. 1).

Apart from adherens junction proteins, we have also studied the transcriptional regulation of tight junction (TJ) proteins in Sertoli cells. Claudin-11 is a TJ integral protein found in testis and

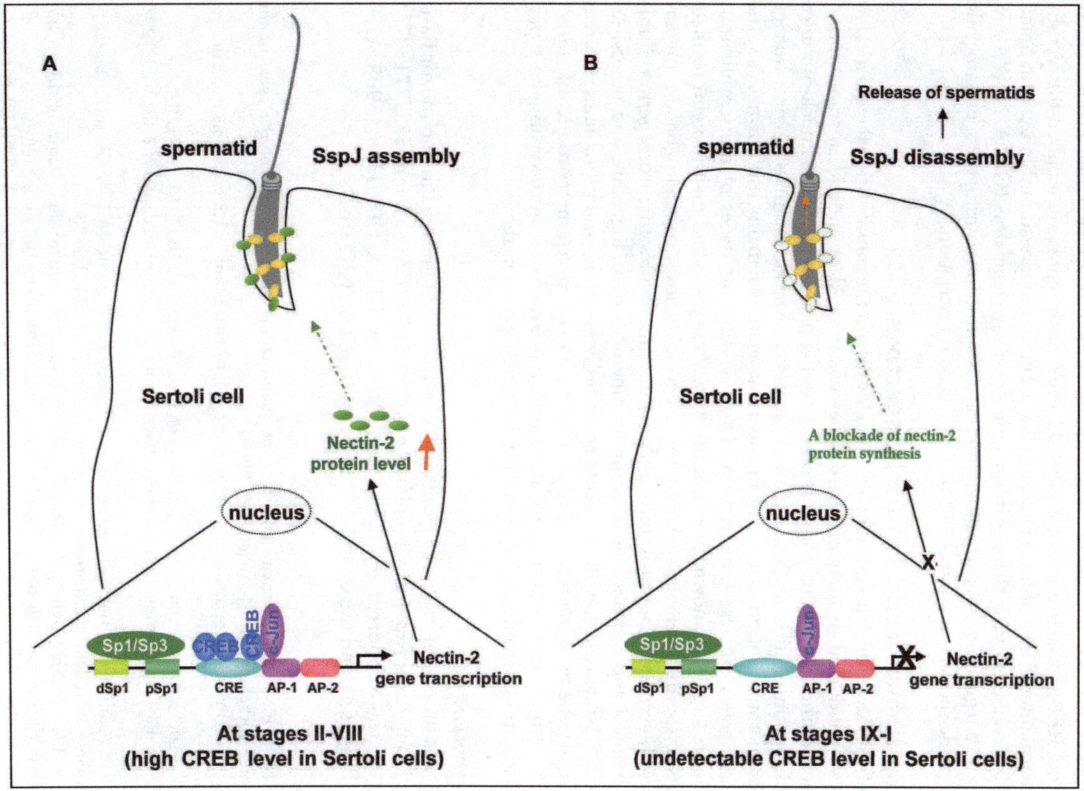

Figure 1. A-B) A proposed model for the regulation of nectin-2 expression in testis. This model accounts for the functional cooperation of multiple transcription factors (Sp1 protein family, CREB and c-Jun) in regulating the basal nectin-2 gene transcription. It also illustrates how the cyclic expression of CREB in a spermatogenic cycle influences the nectin-2 gene transcription, which in turn regulates the assembly of SspJ (A) at stages II-VIII and disassembly at stages IX-I (B), resulting in spermiation.

CNS (central nervous system) myelin.[155] In our study, we demonstrated that the overlapping GATA/NF-Y motif within the core promoter of claudin-11 gene is modulated by differential binding of various transcription factors, resulting in dual transcriptional control.[153] We confirmed that GATA, nuclear factor YA (NF-YA), and cAMP response element-binding protein (CREB) form a complex in vivo and bind to the GATA/NF-Y region to promote claudin-11 gene transcription. GATA and CREB transactivation could be further modulated by the presence of Smad3 and Smad4 proteins. Binding of Smad proteins at the GATA/NF-Y motif could repress the GATA and CREB transactivation of claudin-11 gene. Such repression required the recruitment and physical interactions of histone deacetylase 1 and its corepressor, mSin3A, with Smad proteins. It is believed that cyclic changes in the ratio of positive regulators (GATA, NF-YA and CREB) to negative regulators (Smads) in the seminiferous epithelium during the spermatogenic cycle might provide the precise control in claudin-11 gene transcription.

Concluding Remarks and Future Perspectives

As we briefly reviewed and discussed herein, much work on the transcriptional regulation of spermatogenesis conducted in the past two decades was focused on individual transcription factor, and most of these studies relied solely on changes in phenotypes of the knock-out mice to assess the function of different transcription factors. However, the physiological linkage between different transcription factors during spermatogenesis remains unknown. Also, the molecular target genes of these transcription factors at different stages of the seminiferous epithelial cycle are largely unknown. Furthermore, how these genes and their proteins regulate different facets of spermatogenesis, such as germ cell cycle, meiosis, spermatogonial proliferation and renewal, germ cell apoptosis, cell adhesion and junction restructuring, germ cell migration, biochemical and morphological events pertinent to spermiogenesis, and others, remain unexplored. Nonetheless, with the recent advances in genomics and proteomics research, such as the use of gene profiling techniques coupled with mass spectrometry to identify target genes (proteins) important to transcriptional regulation in knock-out mice versus wild types, this shall provide an unprecedented opportunity for investigators in the field.

Acknowledgement

This work was supported in part by grants from CRCG Seed Funding Programme for Basic Research and Hong Kong Research Grant Council (HKU7609/06M and and HKU771507M to WYL). CYC was supported by grants from NIH (NICHD, U01 HD045908; U54 HD029990, Project 3), and the CONRAD Program (CICCR, CIG 01-72).

References

1. Oakberg EF. Duration of spermatogenesis in the mouse and timing of stages of the cycle of the seminiferous epithelium. Am J Anat 1956; 99:507-516.
2. Russell L. Movement of spermatocytes from the basal to the adluminal compartment of the rat testis. Am J Anat 1977; 148:313-328.
3. Eddy EM. Male germ cell gene expression. Recent Prog Horm Res 2002; 57:103-128.
4. Sassone-Corsi P. Transcriptional checkpoints determining the fate of male germ cells. Cell 1997; 88:163-166.
5. Schmidt EE, Schibler U. High accumulation of components of the RNA polymerase II transcription machinery in rodent spermatids. Development 1995; 121:2373-2383.
6. Upadhyaya AB, Lee SH, DeJong J. Identification of a general transcription factor TFIIAα/β homolog selectively expressed in testis. J Biol Chem 1999; 274:18040-18048.
7. Ozer J, Moore PA, Lieberman PM. A testis-specific transcription factor IIA (TFIIAτ) stimulates TATA-binding protein-DNA binding and transcription activation. J Biol Chem 2000; 275:122-128.
8. McLachlan RI, Wreford NG, O'Donnell L et al. The endocrine regulation of spermatogenesis: Independent roles for testosterone and FSH. J Endocrinol 1996; 148:1-9.
9. Sheckter CB, Matsumoto AM, Bremner WJ. Testosterone administration inhibits gonadotropin secretion by an effect directly on the human pituitary. J Clin Endocrinol Metab 1989; 68:397-401.
10. Keller ET, Ershler WB, Chang C. The androgen receptor: A mediator of diverse responses. Front Biosci 1996; 1:d59-71.

11. Roy AK, Lavrovsky Y, Song CS et al. Regulation of androgen action. Vitam Horm 1999; 55:309-352.
12. Heinlein CA, Chang C. Androgen receptor (AR) coregulators: An overview. Endocr Rev 2002; 23:175-200.
13. Bagchi MK, Tsai MJ, O'Malley BW et al. Analysis of the mechanism of steroid hormone receptor-dependent gene activation in cell-free systems. Endocr Rev 1992; 13:525-535.
14. Jenster G, van der Korput HA, Trapman J et al. Identification of two transcription activation units in the N-terminal domain of the human androgen receptor. J Biol Chem 1995; 270:7341-7346.
15. Kasper S, Rennie PS, Bruchovsky N et al. Cooperative binding of androgen receptors to two DNA sequences is required for androgen induction of the probasin gene. J Biol Chem 1994; 269:31763-31769.
16. Zhou Z, Corden JL, Brown TR. Identification and characterization of a novel androgen response element composed of a direct repeat. J Biol Chem 1997; 272:8227-8235.
17. Verrijdt G, Schoenmakers E, Alen P et al. Androgen specificity of a response unit upstream of the human secretory component gene is mediated by differential receptor binding to an essential androgen response element. Mol Endocrinol 1999; 13:1558-1570.
18. Claessens F, Verrijdt G, Schoenmakers E et al. Selective DNA binding by the androgen receptor as a mechanism for hormone-specific gene regulation. J Steroid Biochem Mol Biol 2001; 76:23-30.
19. Lee YF, Shyr CR, Thin TH et al. Convergence of two repressors through heterodimer formation of androgen receptor and testicular orphan receptor-4: A unique signaling pathway in the steroid receptor superfamily. Proc Natl Acad Sci USA 1999; 96:14724-14729.
20. Panet-Raymond V, Gottlieb B, Beitel LK et al. Interactions between androgen and estrogen receptors and the effects on their transactivational properties. Mol Cell Endocrinol 2000; 167:139-150.
21. He B, Kemppainen JA, Voegel JJ et al. Activation function 2 in the human androgen receptor ligand binding domain mediates interdomain communication with the NH(2)-terminal domain. J Biol Chem 1999; 274:37219-37225.
22. Fang Y, Fliss AE, Robins DM et al. Hsp90 regulates androgen receptor hormone binding affinity in vivo. J Biol Chem 1996; 271:28697-28702.
23. Yeh S, Tsai MY, Xu Q et al. Generation and characterization of androgen receptor knockout (ARKO) mice: An in vivo model for the study of androgen functions in selective tissues. Proc Natl Acad Sci USA 2002; 99:13498-13503.
24. Lindsey JS, Wilkinson MF. Pem: A testosterone- and LH-regulated homeobox gene expressed in mouse Sertoli cells and epididymis. Dev Biol 1996; 179:471-484.
25. Maiti S, Doskow J, Li S et al. The Pem homeobox gene: Androgen-dependent and -independent promoters and tissue-specific alternative RNA splicing. J Biol Chem 1996; 271:17536-17546.
26. MacLean IInd JA, Chen MA, Wayne CM et al. Rhox: A new homeobox gene cluster. Cell 2005; 120:369-382.
27. Barbulescu K, Geserick C, Schuttke I et al. New androgen response elements in the murine pem promoter mediate selective transactivation. Mol Endocrinol 2001; 15:1803-1816.
28. Geserick C, Meyer HA, Barbulescu K et al. Differential modulation of androgen receptor action by deoxyribonucleic acid response elements. Mol Endocrinol 2003; 17:1738-1750.
29. Rao MK, Wayne CM, Wilkinson MF. Pem homeobox gene regulatory sequences that direct androgen-dependent developmentally regulated gene expression in different subregions of the epididymis. J Biol Chem 2002; 277:48771-48778.
30. Rao MK, Wayne CM, Meistrich ML et al. Pem homeobox gene promoter sequences that direct transcription in a Sertoli cell-specific, stage-specific, and androgen-dependent manner in the testis in vivo. Mol Endocrinol 2003; 17:223-233.
31. Chang C, Chen YT, Yeh SD et al. Infertility with defective spermatogenesis and hypotestosteronemia in male mice lacking the androgen receptor in Sertoli cells. Proc Natl Acad Sci USA 2004; 101:6876-6881.
32. De Gendt K, Swinnen JV, Saunders PT et al. A Sertoli cell-selective knockout of the androgen receptor causes spermatogenic arrest in meiosis. Proc Natl Acad Sci USA 2004; 101:1327-1332.

32a. Holdcraft RW, Braun RE. Androgen receptor function is required in Sertoli cells for the terminal differentiation of haploid spermatids. Development 2004; 131:459-467

32b. Meng J, Holdcraft RW, Shima JE et al. Androgens regulate the permeability of the blood-testis barrier. Proc Natl Acad Sci USA 2005; 102:16696-16700.

33. van Pelt AM, van den Brink CE, de Rooij DG et al. Changes in retinoic acid receptor messenger ribonucleic acid levels in the vitamin A-deficient rat testis after administration of retinoids. Endocrinology 1992; 131:344-350.
34. Lufkin T, Lohnes D, Mark M et al. High postnatal lethality and testis degeneration in retinoic acid receptor α mutant mice. Proc Natl Acad Sci USA 1993; 90:7225-7229.

35. Kastner P, Mark M, Leid M et al. Abnormal spermatogenesis in RXRβ mutant mice. Genes Dev 1996; 10:80-92.
36. Akmal KM, Dufour JM, Vo M et al. Ligand-dependent regulation of retinoic acid receptor α in rat testis: In vivo response to depletion and repletion of vitamin A. Endocrinology 1998; 139:1239-1248.
37. Lee S, Privalsky ML. Heterodimers of retinoic acid receptors and thyroid hormone receptors display unique combinatorial regulatory properties. Mol Endocrinol 2005; 19:863-878.
38. Soprano DR, Qin P, Soprano KJ. Retinoic acid receptors and cancers. Annu Rev Nutr 2004; 24:201-221.
39. Chung SS, Sung W, Wang X et al. Retinoic acid receptor α is required for synchronization of spermatogenic cycles and its absence results in progressive breakdown of the spermatogenic process. Dev Dyn 2004; 230:754-766.
40. Ricci G, Catizone A, Scarcella MF et al. Vitamin A modulation of basement membrane production by purified testicular myoid cells. Exp Cell Res 1999; 249:102-108.
41. Samy ET, Li JC, Grima J et al. Sertoli cell prostaglandin D2 synthetase is a multifunctional molecule: Its expression and regulation. Endocrinology 2000; 141:710-721.
42. Oulad-Abdelghani M, Bouillet P, Decimo D et al. Characterization of a premeiotic germ cell-specific cytoplasmic protein encoded by Stra8, a novel retinoic acid-responsive gene. J Cell Biol 1996; 135:469-477.
43. Rogers MB, Hosler BA, Gudas LJ. Specific expression of a retinoic acid-regulated, zinc-finger gene, Rex-1, in preimplantation embryos, trophoblast and spermatocytes. Development 1991; 113:815-824.
44. Baleato RM, Aitken RJ, Roman SD. Vitamin A regulation of BMP4 expression in the male germ line. Dev Biol 2005; 286:78-90.
45. Thompson DL, Gerlach-Bank LM, Barald KF et al. Retinoic acid repression of bone morphogenetic protein 4 in inner ear development. Mol Cell Biol 2003; 23:2277-2286.
46. Chen F, Cooney AJ, Wang Y et al. Cloning of a novel orphan receptor (GCNF) expressed during germ cell development. Mol Endocrinol 1994; 8:1434-1444.
47. Hirose T, O'Brien DA, Jetten AM. RTR: A new member of the nuclear receptor superfamily that is highly expressed in murine testis. Gene 1995; 152:247-251.
48. Borgmeyer U. Dimeric binding of the mouse germ cell nuclear factor. Eur J Biochem 1997; 244:120-127.
49. Yan ZH, Medvedev A, Hirose T et al. Characterization of the response element and DNA binding properties of the nuclear orphan receptor germ cell nuclear factor/retinoid receptor-related testis-associated receptor. J Biol Chem 1997; 272:10565-10572.
50. Greschik H, Schule R. Germ cell nuclear factor: An orphan receptor with unexpected properties. J Mol Med 1998; 76:800-810.
51. Greschik H, Wurtz JM, Hublitz P et al. Characterization of the DNA-binding and dimerization properties of the nuclear orphan receptor germ cell nuclear factor. Mol Cell Biol 1999; 19:690-703.
52. Bauer UM, Schneider-Hirsch S, Reinhardt S et al. Neuronal cell nuclear factor—A nuclear receptor possibly involved in the control of neurogenesis and neuronal differentiation. Eur J Biochem 1997; 249:826-837.
53. Cooney AJ, Hummelke GC, Herman T et al. Germ cell nuclear factor is a response element-specific repressor of transcription. Biochem Biophys Res Commun 1998; 245:94-100.
54. Yan Z, Jetten AM. Characterization of the repressor function of the nuclear orphan receptor retinoid receptor-related testis-associated receptor/germ cell nuclear factor. J Biol Chem 2000; 275:35077-35085.
55. Fuhrmann G, Chung AC, Jackson KJ et al. Mouse germline restriction of Oct4 expression by germ cell nuclear factor. Dev Cell 2001; 1:377-387.
56. Yan Z, Kim YS, Jetten AM. RAP80, a novel nuclear protein that interacts with the retinoid-related testis-associated receptor. J Biol Chem 2002; 277:32379-32388.
57. Katz D, Niederberger C, Slaughter GR et al. Characterization of germ cell-specific expression of the orphan nuclear receptor, germ cell nuclear factor. Endocrinology 1997; 138:4364-4372.
58. Zhang YL, Akmal KM, Tsuruta JK et al. Expression of germ cell nuclear factor (GCNF/RTR) during spermatogenesis. Mol Reprod Dev 1998; 50:93-102.
59. Mali P, Kaipia A, Kangasniemi M et al. Stage-specific expression of nucleoprotein mRNAs during rat and mouse spermiogenesis. Reprod Fertil Dev 1989; 1:369-382.
60. Hummelke GC, Meistrich ML, Cooney AJ. Mouse protamine genes are candidate targets for the novel orphan nuclear receptor, germ cell nuclear factor. Mol Reprod Dev 1998; 50:396-405.
61. Hummelke GC, Cooney AJ. Reciprocal regulation of the mouse protamine genes by the orphan nuclear receptor germ cell nuclear factor and CREMτ. Mol Reprod Dev 2004; 68:394-407.

62. Rajkovic M, Middendorff R, Wetzel MG et al. Germ cell nuclear factor relieves cAMP-response element modulator τ-mediated activation of the testis-specific promoter of human mitochondrial glycerol-3-phosphate dehydrogenase. J Biol Chem 2004; 279:52493-52499.
63. Valentin M, Balvers M, Pusch W et al. Structure and expression of the mouse gene encoding the endozepine-like peptide from haploid male germ cells. Eur J Biochem 2000; 267:5438-5449.
64. Chang C, Kokontis J. Identification of a new member of the steroid receptor super-family by cloning and sequence analysis. Biochem Biophys Res Commun 1988; 155:971-977.
65. Chang C, Da Silva SL, Ideta R et al. Human and rat TR4 orphan receptors specify a subclass of the steroid receptor superfamily. Proc Natl Acad Sci USA 1994; 91:6040-6044.
66. Lee YF, Young WJ, Lin WJ et al. Differential regulation of direct repeat 3 vitamin D3 and direct repeat 4 thyroid hormone signaling pathways by the human TR4 orphan receptor. J Biol Chem 1999; 274:16198-16205.
67. Young WJ, Lee YF, Smith SM et al. A bidirectional regulation between the TR2/TR4 orphan receptors (TR2/TR4) and the ciliary neurotrophic factor (CNTF) signaling pathway. J Biol Chem 1998; 273:20877-20885.
68. Shyr CR, Hu YC, Kim E et al. Modulation of estrogen receptor-mediated transactivation by orphan receptor TR4 in MCF-7 cells. J Biol Chem 2002; 277:14622-14628.
69. Lee CH, Chang L, Wei LN. Molecular cloning and characterization of a mouse nuclear orphan receptor expressed in embryos and testes. Mol Reprod Dev 1996; 44:305-314.
70. Lee CH, Chang L, Wei LN. Distinct expression patterns and biological activities of two isoforms of the mouse orphan receptor TR2. J Endocrinol 1997; 152:245-255.
71. Hirose T, Fujimoto W, Tamaai T et al. TAK1: Molecular cloning and characterization of a new member of the nuclear receptor superfamily. Mol Endocrinol 1994; 8:1667-1680.
72. Mu X, Lee YF, Liu NC et al. Targeted inactivation of testicular nuclear orphan receptor 4 delays and disrupts late meiotic prophase and subsequent meiotic divisions of spermatogenesis. Mol Cell Biol 2004; 24:5887-5899.
73. Shyr CR, Collins LL, Mu XM et al. Spermatogenesis and testis development are normal in mice lacking testicular orphan nuclear receptor 2. Mol Cell Biol 2002; 22:4661-4666.
74. Lalli E, Lee JS, Masquilier D et al. Nuclear response to cyclic AMP: Central role of transcription factor CREM (cyclic-AMP-responsive-element modulator). Biochem Soc Trans 1993; 21:912-917.
75. Lalli E, Sassone-Corsi P. Signal transduction and gene regulation: The nuclear response to cAMP. J Biol Chem 1994; 269:17359-17362.
76. Sassone-Corsi P. Transcription factors responsive to cAMP. Annu Rev Cell Dev Biol 1995; 11:355-377.
77. Montminy M. Transcriptional regulation by cyclic AMP. Annu Rev Biochem 1997; 66:807-822.
78. Montminy MR, Bilezikjian LM. Binding of a nuclear protein to the cyclic-AMP response element of the somatostatin gene. Nature 1987; 328:175-178.
79. Foulkes NS, Mellstrom B, Benusiglio E et al. Developmental switch of CREM function during spermatogenesis: From antagonist to activator. Nature 1992; 355:80-84.
80. Nantel F, Sassone-Corsi P. CREM: A transcriptional master switch during the spermatogenesis differentiation program. Front Biosci 1996; 1:d266-269.
81. Nantel F, Monaco L, Foulkes NS et al. Spermiogenesis deficiency and germ-cell apoptosis in CREM-mutant mice. Nature 1996; 380:159-162.
82. Delmas V, van der Hoorn F, Mellstrom B et al. Induction of CREM activator proteins in spermatids: Down-stream targets and implications for haploid germ cell differentiation. Mol Endocrinol 1993; 7:1502-1514.
83. Zhou Y, Sun Z, Means AR et al. cAMP-response element modulator τ is a positive regulator of testis angiotensin converting enzyme transcription. Proc Natl Acad Sci USA 1996; 93:12262-12266.
84. Sassone-Corsi P. CREM: A master-switch governing male germ cells differentiation and apoptosis. Semin Cell Dev Biol 1998; 9:475-482.
85. Steger K, Klonisch T, Gavenis K et al. Round spermatids show normal testis-specific H1t but reduced cAMP-responsive element modulator and transition protein 1 expression in men with round-spermatid maturation arrest. J Androl 1999; 20:747-754.
86. Fimia GM, De Cesare D, Sassone-Corsi P. A family of LIM-only transcriptional coactivators: Tissue-specific expression and selective activation of CREB and CREM. Mol Cell Biol 2000; 20:8613-8622.
87. De Cesare D, Fimia GM, Sassone-Corsi P. Signaling routes to CREM and CREB: Plasticity in transcriptional activation. Trends Biochem Sci 1999; 24:281-285.
88. Fimia GM, De Cesare D, Sassone-Corsi P. CBP-independent activation of CREM and CREB by the LIM-only protein ACT. Nature 1999; 398:165-169.

89. Kotaja N, De Cesare D, Macho B et al. Abnormal sperm in mice with targeted deletion of the act (activator of cAMP-responsive element modulator in testis) gene. Proc Natl Acad Sci USA 2004; 101:10620-10625.
90. Waeber G, Meyer TE, LeSieur M et al. Developmental stage-specific expression of cyclic adenosine 3',5'-monophosphate response element-binding protein CREB during spermatogenesis involves alternative exon splicing. Mol Endocrinol 1991; 5:1418-14130.
91. Slongo M, Zotti L, Onisto M. Cloning and characterization of the promoter region of human spata2 (spermatogenesis-associated protein 2) gene. Biochim Biophys Acta 2003; 1625:192-196.
92. Lui WY, Sze KL, Lee WM. Nectin-2 expression in testicular cells is controlled via the functional cooperation between transcription factors of the Sp1, CREB, and AP-1 families. J Cell Physiol 2006; 207:144-157.
93. Samuel S, Naora H. Homeobox gene expression in cancer: Insights from developmental regulation and deregulation. Eur J Cancer 2005; 41:2428-2437.
94. Hogeveen KN, Sassone-Corsi P. Homeobox galore: When reproduction goes RHOX and roll. Cell 2005; 120:287-288.
95. Pitman JL, Lin TP, Kleeman JE et al. Normal reproductive and macrophage function in Pem homeobox gene-deficient mice. Dev Biol 1998; 202:196-214.
96. Andersen B, Pearse IInd RV, Schlegel PN et al. Sperm 1: A POU-domain gene transiently expressed immediately before meiosis I in the male germ cell. Proc Natl Acad Sci USA 1993; 90:11084-11088.
97. Pearse II RV, Drolet DW, Kalla KA et al. Reduced fertility in mice deficient for the POU protein sperm-1. Proc Natl Acad Sci USA 1997; 94:7555-7560.
98. Pesce M, Gross MK, Scholer HR. In line with our ancestors: Oct-4 and the mammalian germ. Bioessays 1998; 20:722-732.
99. Pesce M, Wang X, Wolgemuth DJ et al. Differential expression of the Oct-4 transcription factor during mouse germ cell differentiation. Mech Dev 1998; 71:89-98.
100. Pavletich NP, Pabo CO. Crystal structure of a five-finger GLI-DNA complex: New perspectives on zinc fingers. Science 1993; 261:1701-1707.
101. Chen Z, Brand NJ, Chen A et al. Fusion between a novel Kruppel-like zinc finger gene and the retinoic acid receptor-α locus due to a variant t(11;17) translocation associated with acute promyelocytic leukaemia. EMBO J 1993; 12:1161-1167.
102. Costoya JA, Hobbs RM, Barna M et al. Essential role of Plzf in maintenance of spermatogonial stem cells. Nat Genet 2004; 36:653-659.
103. Buaas FW, Kirsh AL, Sharma M et al. Plzf is required in adult male germ cells for stem cell self-renewal. Nat Genet 2004; 36:647-652.
104. Rauscher FJ, Morris JF, Tournay OE et al. Binding of the Wilms' tumor locus zinc finger protein to the EGR-1 consensus sequence. Science 1990; 250:1259-1262.
105. Scholz H, Kirschner KM. A role for the Wilms' tumor protein WT1 in organ development. Physiology (Bethesda) 2005; 20:54-59.
106. Gao F, Maiti S, Alam N et al. The Wilms tumor gene, Wt1, is required for Sox9 expression and maintenance of tubular architecture in the developing testis. Proc Natl Acad Sci USA 2006; 103:11987-11992.
107. Rao MK, Pham J, Imam JS et al. Tissue-specific RNAi reveals that WT1 expression in nurse cells controls germ cell survival and spermatogenesis. Genes Dev 2006; 20:147-152.
108. Tsai SF, Martin DI, Zon LI et al. Cloning of cDNA for the major DNA-binding protein of the erythroid lineage through expression in mammalian cells. Nature 1989; 339:446-451.
109. Lowry JA, Atchley WR. Molecular evolution of the GATA family of transcription factors: Conservation within the DNA-binding domain. J Mol Evol 2000; 50:103-115.
110. Martin DI, Orkin SH. Transcriptional activation and DNA binding by the erythroid factor GF-1/NF-E1/Eryf 1. Genes Dev 1990; 4:1886-1898.
111. Yang HY, Evans T. Distinct roles for the two cGATA-1 finger domains. Mol Cell Biol 1992; 12:4562-4570.
112. Omichinski JG, Trainor C, Evans T et al. A small single-"finger" peptide from the erythroid transcription factor GATA-1 binds specifically to DNA as a zinc or iron complex. Proc Natl Acad Sci USA 1993; 90:1676-1680.
113. Omichinski JG, Clore GM, Schaad O et al. NMR structure of a specific DNA complex of Zn-containing DNA binding domain of GATA-1. Science 1993; 261:438-446.
114. Fox AH, Kowalski K, King GF et al. Key residues characteristic of GATA N-fingers are recognized by FOG. J Biol Chem 1998; 273:33595-33603.

115. Tevosian SG, Deconinck AE, Cantor AB et al. FOG-2: A novel GATA-family cofactor related to multitype zinc-finger proteins Friend of GATA-1 and U-shaped. Proc Natl Acad Sci USA 1999; 96:950-955.
116. Robert NM, Tremblay JJ, Viger RS. Friend of GATA (FOG)-1 and FOG-2 differentially repress the GATA-dependent activity of multiple gonadal promoters. Endocrinology 2002; 143:3963-3973.
117. Dai YS, Cserjesi P, Markham BE et al. The transcription factors GATA4 and dHAND physically interact to synergistically activate cardiac gene expression through a p300-dependent mechanism. J Biol Chem 2002; 277:24390-24398.
118. LaVoie HA. The role of GATA in mammalian reproduction. Exp Biol Med (Maywood) 2003; 228:1282-1290.
119. Viger RS, Taniguchi H, Robert NM et al. Role of the GATA family of transcription factors in andrology. J Androl 2004; 25:441-452.
120. Yomogida K, Ohtani H, Harigae H et al. Developmental stage- and spermatogenic cycle-specific expression of transcription factor GATA-1 in mouse Sertoli cells. Development 1994; 120:1759-1766.
121. Viger RS, Mertineit C, Trasler JM et al. Transcription factor GATA-4 is expressed in a sexually dimorphic pattern during mouse gonadal development and is a potent activator of the Mullerian inhibiting substance promoter. Development 1998; 125:2665-2675.
122. Ketola I, Rahman N, Toppari J et al. Expression and regulation of transcription factors GATA-4 and GATA-6 in developing mouse testis. Endocrinology 1999; 140:1470-1480.
123. Ketola I, Anttonen M, Vaskivuo T et al. Developmental expression and spermatogenic stage specificity of transcription factors GATA-1 and GATA-4 and their cofactors FOG-1 and FOG-2 in the mouse testis. Eur J Endocrinol 2002; 147:397-406.
124. Tremblay JJ, Viger RS. GATA factors differentially activate multiple gonadal promoters through conserved GATA regulatory elements. Endocrinology 2001; 142:977-986.
125. Baldwin Jr AS. The NF-κB and IκB proteins: New discoveries and insights. Annu Rev Immunol 1996; 14:649-683.
126. Ghosh S, May MJ, Kopp EB. NF-κB and Rel proteins: Evolutionarily conserved mediators of immune responses. Annu Rev Immunol 1998; 16:225-260.
127. Delfino F, Walker WH. Stage-specific nuclear expression of NF-κB in mammalian testis. Mol Endocrinol 1998; 12:1696-1707.
128. Delfino FJ, Walker WH. NF-κB induces cAMP-response element-binding protein gene transcription in Sertoli cells. J Biol Chem 1999; 274:35607-35613.
129. Delfino FJ, Boustead JN, Fix C et al. NF-κB and TNF-α stimulate androgen receptor expression in Sertoli cells. Mol Cell Endocrinol 2003; 201:1-12.
130. Hong CY, Park JH, Seo KH et al. Expression of MIS in the testis is downregulated by tumor necrosis factor α through the negative regulation of SF-1 transactivation by NF-κB. Mol Cell Biol 2003; 23:6000-6012.
131. Kohno K, Izumi H, Uchiumi T et al. The pleiotropic functions of the Y-box-binding protein, YB-1. Bioessays 2003; 25:691-698.
132. Ladomery M, Sommerville J. A role for Y-box proteins in cell proliferation. Bioessays 1995; 17:9-11.
133. Didier DK, Schiffenbauer J, Woulfe SL et al. Characterization of the cDNA encoding a protein binding to the major histocompatibility complex class II Y box. Proc Natl Acad Sci USA 1988; 85:7322-7326.
134. Tafuri SR, Familari M, Wolffe AP. A mouse Y box protein, MSY1, is associated with paternal mRNA in spermatocytes. J Biol Chem 1993; 268:12213-12220.
135. Kwon YK, Murray MT, Hecht NB. Proteins homologous to the Xenopus germ cell-specific RNA-binding proteins p54/p56 are temporally expressed in mouse male germ cells. Dev Biol 1993; 158:99-100.
136. Oko R, Korley R, Murray MT et al. Germ cell-specific DNA and RNA binding proteins p48/52 are expressed at specific stages of male germ cell development and are present in the chromatoid body. Mol Reprod Dev 1996; 44:1-13.
137. Yiu GK, Hecht NB. Novel testis-specific protein-DNA interactions activate transcription of the mouse protamine 2 gene during spermatogenesis. J Biol Chem 1997; 272:26926-26933.
138. Yiu GK, Murray MT, Hecht NB. Deoxyribonucleic acid-protein interactions associated with transcriptional initiation of the mouse testis-specific cytochrome c gene. Biol Reprod 1997; 56:1439-1449.
139. Yang J, Medvedev S, Yu J et al. Absence of the DNA-/RNA-binding protein MSY2 results in male and female infertility. Proc Natl Acad Sci USA 2005; 102:5755-5760.
140. Giorgini F, Davies HG, Braun RE. Translational repression by MSY4 inhibits spermatid differentiation in mice. Development 2002; 129:3669-3679.

141. Rouault JP, Prevot D, Berthet C et al. Interaction of BTG1 and p53-regulated BTG2 gene products with mCaf1, the murine homolog of a component of the yeast CCR4 transcriptional regulatory complex. J Biol Chem 1998; 273:22563-22569.
142. Draper MP, Salvadore C, Denis CL. Identification of a mouse protein whose homolog in Saccharomyces cerevisiae is a component of the CCR4 transcriptional regulatory complex. Mol Cell Biol 1995; 15:3487-3495.
143. Nakamura T, Yao R, Ogawa T et al. Oligo-astheno-teratozoospermia in mice lacking Cnot7, a regulator of retinoid X receptor β. Nat Genet 2004; 36:528-533.
144. Berthet C, Morera AM, Asensio MJ et al. CCR4-associated factor CAF1 is an essential factor for spermatogenesis. Mol Cell Biol 2004; 24:5808-5820.
145. Hochheimer A, Tjian R. Diversified transcription initiation complexes expand promoter selectivity and tissue-specific gene expression. Genes Dev 2003; 17:1309-1320.
146. Kimmins S, Kotaja N, Davidson I et al. Testis-specific transcription mechanisms promoting male germ-cell differentiation. Reproduction 2004; 128:5-12.
147. Monaco L, Kotaja N, Fienga G et al. Specialized rules of gene transcription in male germ cells: The CREM paradigm. Int J Androl 2004; 27:322-327.
148. Jaenisch R, Bird A. Epigenetic regulation of gene expression: How the genome integrates intrinsic and environmental signals. Nat Genet 2003; 33:245-254.
149. Singal R, van Wert J, Bashambu M et al. Testis-specific histone H1t gene is hypermethylated in nongerminal cells in the mouse. Biol Reprod 2000; 63:1237-1244.
150. Grimes SR, Wilkerson DC, Noss KR et al. Transcriptional control of the testis-specific histone H1t gene. Gene 2003; 304:13-21.
151. Mruk DD, Cheng CY. Sertoli-Sertoli and Sertoli-germ cell interactions and their significance in germ cell movement in the seminiferous epithelium during spermatogenesis. Endocr Rev 2004; 25:747-806.
152. Lui WY, Lee WM. Regulation of junction dynamics in the testis—Transcriptional and post-translational regulations of cell junction proteins. Mol Cell Endocrinol 2006; 250:25-35.
153. Lui WY, Wong EWP, Guan Y et al. Dual transcriptional control of claudin-11 via an overlapping GATA/NF-Y motif: Positive regulation through the interaction of GATA, NF-YA and CREB and negative regulation through the interaction of Smad, HDAC1 and mSin3A. J Cell Physiol 2007, 211:638-648.
154. Ozaki-Kuroda K, Nakanishi H, Ohta H et al. Nectin couples cell-cell adhesion and the actin scaffold at heterotypic testicular junctions. Curr Biol 2002; 12:1145-1150.
155. Morita K, Sasaki H, Fujimoto K et al. Claudin-11/OSP-based tight junctions of myelin sheaths in brain and Sertoli cells in testis. J Cell Biol 1999; 145:579-588.
156. Chung AC, Katz D, Pereira FA et al. Loss of orphan receptor germ cell nuclear factor function results in ectopic development of the tail bud and novel posterior truncation. Mol Cell Biol 2001; 21:663-677.
157. Blendy JA, Kaestner KH, Weinbauer GF et al. Severe impairment of spermatogenesis in mice lacking the CREM gene. Nature 1996; 380:162-165.
158. Hummler E, Cole TJ, Blendy FA et al. Targeted mutation of the CREB gene: compensation within the CREB/ATF family of transcription factors. Proc Natl Acad Sci USA 1998; 95:4481-4486.
159. Rudolph D, Tafuri A, Gass P et al. Impaired fetal T cell development and perinatal lethality in mice lacking the cAMP response element binding protein. Proc Natl Acad Sci USA 1998; 95:4481-4486.
160. Pevny L, Simon MC, Robertson E et al. Erythoid differentiation in chimaeric mice blocked by a targeted mutation in the gene for transcription factor GATA-1. Nature 1991 349:257-260.
161. Narita N, Bielinska M, Wilson DB. Wild-type endoderm abrogates the ventral developmental defects associated with GATA-4 deficiency in the mouse. Dev Biol 1997; 189:270-274.
162. Koutsourakis M, Langeveld A, Patient R et al. The transcription factor GATA6 is essential for early extraembryonic development. Development 1999; 126:723-732.

Chapter 8

Proteases and Their Cognate Inhibitors of the Serine and Metalloprotease Subclasses, in Testicular Physiology

Brigitte Le Magueresse-Battistoni*

The testis is a highly dynamic organ not only in the fetal stage but also during postnatal development and in adult life. It is composed of two major compartments: the interstitium with the steroidogenic Leydig cells, and the seminiferous tubules. The seminiferous tubules are surrounded by peritubular cells. Tubules are composed of Sertoli cells and germ cells at different developmental stages. Sertoli cells play key roles in spermatogenesis. They are target cells for follicle stimulating hormone (FSH) and testosterone, responsible for the initiation and maintenance of spermatogenesis. They form the tubules and provide structural and nutritional support for the developing germ cells.[1-4]

The gonads emerge as an outgrowth and will develop either as a testis or an ovary, depending on the presence of the *Sry* gene located on the Y chromosome.[5-6] In response to *Sry*, Sertoli cells differentiate. They synthesize the Müllerian Inhibiting substance, and they aggregate to form the cords together with peritubular cells originating from the mesonephros. Subsequently, Leydig cells differentiate in the interstitial milieu and start producing testosterone.[7-10] At puberty, dynamic changes are associated with the transformation of the cords into tubules and the initiation of spermatogenesis. In adult life, germ cells migrate from the base to the apex of the tubule epithelium while differentiating further. Finally spermatids are released from the apex of the seminiferous epithelium into the tubular lumen, becoming spermatozoa. A new wave of spermatogenesis will initiate again.

Previous reports suggested that proteases or their inhibitors of the serine-, cysteine-, or metallo- protease family were involved in this spatiotemporal and highly orchestrated process, either during testis development[11-13] or at specific stages of spermatogenesis.[14-17] This chapter summarizes current knowledge about the occurrence and expression pattern of members of the metallo- and of the serine- family of proteases and inhibitors synthesized within the testis. We also report the various predicted functions for these molecules in the establishment and /or maintenance of the testicular architecture and in the process of spermatogenesis.

General Aspects of Proteases and Protease Inhibitors

A number of important processes that regulate the activity and fate of many proteins are strictly dependent on proteolytic events. For example, proteases are involved in the ectodomain shedding of cell surface proteins, the activation or inactivation of cytokines, hormones and growth factors, the exposure of cryptic neoproteins exhibiting functional roles distinct from

*Corresponding Author: Brigitte Le Magueresse-Battistoni—Inserm U418 and INRA UMR 1245 and Université Lyon 1, Hopital Debrousse, 29 rue soeur Bouvier, 69322 Lyon cedex 05, France. Email: lemagueresse@lyon.inserm.fr

Molecular Mechanisms in Spermatogenesis, edited by C. Yan Cheng. ©2008 Landes Bioscience and Springer Science+Business Media.

the parent molecule, degradation of multiple extracellular matrix components facilitating cell migration and invasion. Accordingly, proteases are fundamental in nearly all complex processes of tissue maintenance, repair, growth and development, and alterations in the structure and expression patterns of proteases underlie many pathological processes including cancer, arthritis, osteoporosis, neurodegenerative disorders and cardiovascular diseases. The completion of the human genome sequence has allowed the determination of more than 2% of all human genes are proteases or protease inhibitors, reflecting the importance of proteolysis in human biology.[18,19] The activity of proteases is regulated at multiple levels including the level of production, the activation of the protease which is generally synthesized in an inactive pro-form, and the production of specific inhibitors.

Proteases catalyse the hydrolysis of peptide bonds in proteins. They are of two types, the exopeptidases and the endopeptidases. The exopeptidases attack only peptide bonds localized at/ or near the amino or carboxy terminal portion of peptide chains. The endopeptidases, also named the proteinases, catalyse the hydrolysis of internal bonds in polypeptides. They are divided into 5 classes. Aspartic and metzincins proteases use an activated water molecule as a nucleophile to attack the peptide bond of the substrate. In the cysteine, serine and threonine classes the nucleophile is a catalytic amino-acid residue (Cys, Ser or Thr, respectively) that is located in the active site from which the class name derives. Analysis of the full repertoire of proteases present in the human, mouse and rat genome indicated that serine, metzincins and cysteine proteases are the most abundant proteolytic enzymes in rat, mouse and human (Table 1).[20]

The Metzincins

Members of the metzincin superfamily are metalloproteinases that require zinc at their catalytic sites. Metzincins are distinguished by a conserved structural topology, a consensus motif containing three histidines that bind zinc at the catalytic site, and a conserved 'Met-turn' motif that sits below the proteinase active site zinc ion. The metzincins can be further subdivided into four distinct families, two of which i.e., the matrixins or matrix metalloproteinases (MMPs) and the adamalysin-related proteinases are abundantly expressed in the testis. The actions of these proteinases are inhibited by the tissue inhibitors of metalloproteinases (TIMPs).

Matrix Metalloproteinases (MMPs)

The MMPs are a family of extracellular matrix (ECM) degrading enzymes that share common functional domains and activation mechanism. These are Ca^{2+} and Zn^{2+}-dependent endopeptidases that are active at neutral pH. They are synthesized as secreted or transmembrane proenzymes and processed to an active form by the removal of an amino-terminal propeptide. MMPs can be activated by chaotropic agents or by cleavage of the propeptide by members of the MMP family or other proteases such as the plasminogen activator of the urokinase-type. To date, more than 30 members of the MMP family have been identified. There are several distinct subgroups based on preferential substrates or similar structural domains: collagenases that are active against fibrillar collagen, gelatinases that have high activity against denatured collagens,

Table 1. Disribution of proteases in human, mouse and rat genomes

	Total	Aspartic	Cysteine	Metzincins	Serine	Threonine
Human	561	21	148	186	178	28
Mouse	641	27	163	198	227	26
Rat	626	24	160	192	221	29

Adapted from references 19,20.

stromelysins that degrade noncollagen components of the ECM, membrane-type MMPs (MT-MMPs) that are transmembrane molecules and other less characterized members. Much of the functions attributed to MMPs to date are the results of the cleavage products of ECM components. These include the release of bioactive ECM fragments which may alter the ECM microenvironment, changing the cell from an adhesive to a migratory phenotype. MMPs may also activate chemokines, cytokines and growth factors synthesized as inactive pro-forms, inactivate the SERPINs (SERine Protease INhibitors) and generate soluble forms of a transmembrane receptor through shedding of the ectodomain.[18-21] MMPs are controlled at a transcriptional level depending on MMPs and on the tissue or cell type considered. Such a control is exerted by hormones, growth factors and cytokines as well as basigin or EMMPRIN (Extracellular Matrix metalloproteinase Inducer) which belongs to the immunoglobulin superfamily.[22]

The Adamalysin-Related Proteinases

This family includes the ADAMs which are cell-surface rather than secreted proteins that share a disintegrin and metalloproteinase domain. They are at least 32 ADAMs that have been cloned and sequenced, each containing a signal sequence followed in order by a pro-domain, a metalloproteinase or metalloproteinase-like domain, a disintegrin-like domain, a cysteine-rich domain, EGF-like repeats, a transmembrane domain, and a cytoplasmic tail. Accordingly, ADAMs potentially perform four distinct but complementary functions: proteolysis via the metalloproteinase domain, adhesion via the disintegrin domain, cell-cell fusion via a candidate hydrophobic fusion peptide in the cysteine-rich domain, and cell signaling via the intracellular domain. A large number of ADAMs show testis-specific expression and are mostly involved in sperm-egg recognition (Table 2).[23-25] ADAMTS are the soluble counterparts of the ADAMs. They do not contain a transmembrane domain, but instead contain thrombospondin-1 motifs that permit ECM-association. To date, 19 ADAMTSs have been identified in human tissues, and two of them display testis expression (ADAMTS-2 and -20; Table 2).

Table 2. General features of ADAMs and ADAMTS

ADAMs: 32 Full Length cDNAs	ADAMTS: 19 Human Genes
Active metalloproteases: 17 ADAMs (1, 8-10, 12, 13, 15-17, 19-21, 24-26, 28, 30)	Exhibit a metalloproteinase catalytic domain. However, most of them have been cloned based on structural organization and have unknown substrates (i.e., the orphan ADAMTSs: 6, 7, 10, 12, 16-19)
Inactive metalloproteases: 13 ADAMs (2-7, 11, 14, 16, 18, 22, 23, 28)	ADAMTS-1 and -8 are anti-angiogenic
Testis specific expression: 13 ADAMs (2, 3, 5, 16, 18, 20, 21, 24-26, 29, 30, 33)	ADAMTS (1, 4, 5, 8, 9, 15) are aggrecanases
Testis predominant expression: ADAMs (1, 4, 6, 31, 32)	ADAMTS (2, 3, 14) are pro-collagen N-proteinases
	ADAMTS (9, 20) have a GON domain
	ADAMTS-13 is a von Willebrand factor-cleaving protease

Note: When in testis, ADAMs are germinal cell products except ADAM 31 which is expressed in Leydig cells. Adapted from references 23-25.

The TIMPs

TIMPs are natural inhibitors of MMPs and inhibit the MMPs proteolytic activity by forming noncovalent 1:1 stoichiometric complexes resistant to heat denaturation and proteolytic degradation. Four TIMPs have been currently characterized and designated TIMP-1, -2, -3 and -4. They exhibit various N-glycosylation sites: two for TIMP-1, one for TIMP-3 and none for TIMPS -2 and -4. They are expressed in a variety of cell types and present in most tissues and body fluids. The TIMPs -1, 2 and 4 are secreted, whereas TIMP-3 is ECM-associated. TIMPs differ in many aspects including solubility, interaction with the proenzymes (proMMPs) and regulation of expression. TIMPs are 21-34 kDa proteins all possessing 12 conserved cycteine residues forming six disulfide bonds that fold the protein in two domains. The N-terminal domain of TIMP contains the MMP inhibitory domain. The C-terminal domain is involved in formation of complexes with the pro-enzymes, thereby regulating the MMP activation process.[26-28] TIMPs are multifunctional proteins. In addition to inhibiting target proteinases, TIMPs participate in the MMP activation process through their ability to form complexes with proMMPs. Further, evidences accumulated that TIMP-1 and TIMP-2 transduce an intracellular signalling, although to date no specific TIMP receptors have been characterized.[27-29] Originally, TIMP-1 was described for its erythroid-potentiating activity, and as such TIMP-1 plays a pivotal role in hematopoiesis.[26] TIMPs -1 and -2 have also been demonstrated to display antiapoptotic and anti-angiogenic activity in various cell lines depending or not on MMP inhibition.[29,30] The role of TIMP-3 has been deeply investigated mostly because inherited mutations in it lead to Sorbys fundus distrophy, a degenerative eye disease.[31,32] TIMP-4 has been less characterized but major functions for TIMP-4 have been described in implantation, heart function and ovulation.[27,28]

Serine Proteases and SERine Protease INhibitors (SERPINs)

The serine protease family is one of the earliest characterized and largest multigene proteolytic families, which has well characterized roles in diverse cellular activities including blood coagulation, platelet activation, fibrinolysis and thrombosis. The serine protease family can be further subdivided into 16 families including the plasminogen activators, the transmembrane-serine proteases and the kallikreins.[20]

Plasminogen Activators

In mammals, two major types of plasminogen activators have been identified, urokinase-type (uPA) and tissue-type (tPA). Even though both types of PAs catalyze the activation of plasminogen, the currently established functions of uPA-dependent plasminogen activation are mainly within physiological and pathological tissue remodeling processes involving degradation of matrix components and activation of latent proteinases or growth factors, whereas tPA is mainly involved in thrombolysis and neurobiology.[33,34] However, it has been observed in gene deficient mice that PAs could substitute each other.[34,35] Both PAs are released from cells as single chains with no (uPA) or low (tPA) activity, with cleavage of a polypeptide bond leading to the fully active two-chain forms. The most important feature of this system is the amplification loop achieved by the reciprocal activation of pro-PAs and plasminogen on the cell surface. Both plasmin-catalyzed conversion of pro-PA to active PA and the subsequent active PA-catalyzed conversion of plasminogen to plasmin are accelerated. Therefore, as long as pro-PAs and plasminogen are present, reciprocal proenzyme activation will maintain enzymatically active PAs and plasmin.[33,34,36] Another consideration is that although tPA and uPA are secreted proteases, both can bind to cell surface via specific cell surface receptors, being thus protected from the inhibitory actions of the abundant plasma inhibitors.

At least eight apparently distinct plasmin/plasminogen binding proteins have been proposed on various cell types, including α-enolase, amphoterin and annexin II.[37,38] Annexin II is a 36 kDa, calcium-dependent, phospholipid-binding protein found on the surface of many cell types, which exhibits specific, saturable binding for both plasminogen and tPA. In addition, it has the interesting property of independently binding tPA but not uPA, anchoring both tPA and plasminogen with high affinity in close proximity to each other on the cell surface, thus providing an environment in which plasmin production is greatly increased.[37,38] The receptor for uPA is a cysteine-rich, highly glycosylated protein, which is attached to the cell surface by a COOH-terminal glycosylphosphatidylinositol (GPI) anchor.[39-41] Both the inactive single-chain and the active two-chain uPA can bind to uPAR with high affinity. The receptor uPAR can also bind the serum and extracellular matrix protein vitronectin, which is a ligand of $\alpha v\beta 3$ integrin, an interaction that requires uPA. In contrast, plasminogen does not bind to uPAR. In addition to the membrane anchored form, cleavage of the GPI-anchor generates a soluble form of uPAR (suPAR). Although lacking a cytosolic domain, uPAR activates multiple intracellular signalling molecules through a connection with integrins, G-protein coupled receptors and caveolin. Signalling pathways induced by uPAR include cytosolic kinase pathways with the activation of intracellular tyrosine kinases, the Focal Adhesion Kinase (FAK) pathway leading to cytoskeletal reorganization, and intracellular calcium mobilization. It is also worth to note that both uPA (the aminoterminal fragment, ATF) and uPAR exhibit growth activities independant of their proteolytic activities.[40,41]

Type II Transmembrane Serine Proteases (TTSPs)

TTSPs constitute a rapidly expanding family of serine proteases defined by the presence of an N-terminal signal anchor and a C-terminal serine protease domain, separated by a stem region containing an array of protein domains that varies widely between individual TTSPs. These enzymes are ideally positioned to interact with other proteins on the cell surface as well as soluble proteins, matrix components, and proteins on adjacent cells. In addition, TTSPs have cytoplasmic N-terminal domains, suggesting possible functions in intracellular signal transduction. TTSPs are synthesized as single chains zymogens and are likely activated by cleavage following an arginine or lysine present in a highly conserved activation motif. TTSPs are likely to remain membrane-bound following activation. Altough a few of the TTSPs are expressed across several tissues and cell types, in general theses enzymes demonstrate relatively restricted expression patterns, indicating that they may have tissue-specific functions.[42]

Kallikreins

Kallikreins are represented by multigene families in humans and many animal species, especially in rat and mouse. Of particular interest are the glandular kallikreins, nowadays known as the tissue kallikreins. Kallikreins are expressed in a wide range of tissues including steroid-hormone producing or hormone-dependent tissues such as the prostate, breast, ovary and testis. Most, if not all, genes are under steroid hormone regulation, and there is a strong but circumstantial evidence linking kallikreins and cancer(s). Example is given with human kallikreins 2 and 3 (known as Prostate specific antigen) which are widely used tumor markers for prostate cancer. A total of 15 kallikrein genes is reported in the human genome versus at least 25 in the mouse species. Among them, 14 genes are presumed to encode serine proteases, the rest being pseudogenes. Interestingly, there are no homologs for human kallikreins 2 and 3 in the mouse or rat genomes. Tissue kallikreins are clustered at chromosome 19q13 in humans, 1q23 in rat and 7B2 in mouse. They share a similar genomic organization, being formed of five coding exons with very similar exon sizes. All kallikrein proteins are synthesized as prepro-peptides with a signal peptide at the N-terminus, followed by an activation peptide, and the mature protein. Certain ECM components such as fibronectin and laminin, IGFBPs (insulin growth factor binding proteins) and single chain tPA are substrates for kallikreins.[43,44]

Serpins

The serpins are a superfamily of proteins with full-length coding sequences known or predicted to be about one-half of a total of 500, which fold into a conserved tertiary structural domain. The name serpin derives from the fact that most of the first identified serpins were inhibitors of serine proteinases. Today, this name is clearly inappropriate because a high number of serpins display no inhibitory action against serine proteinases while others inhibit cysteine proteinases. Nevertheless, the HUGO gene nomenclature committee recommended retention of the name with classification into clades based on phylogenetic relationships.[45-48] For example, serpins in the A clade perform roles such as hormone transport i.e., thyroid-binding globulin (SERPINA6), corticosteroid-binding globulin (SERPINA7), and blood pressure regulation (angiotensinogen or SERPINA8) whereas serpins in the E clade are inhibitors of the plasminogen activators (SERPINE1 is plasminogen activator inhibitor 1 (PAI-1) and SERPINE2 is proteinase nexin 1(PN-1). However, SERPINA5 also known as Protein C Inhibitor (PCI) or plasminogen activator inhibitor 3 (PAI-3) binds retinoic acid and targets activated Protein C and the plasminogen activators.[49]

Serpins targeting serine proteinases have a unique suicide-substrate mechanism through an interaction with proteinases to form covalent complexes that are not dissociable when boiling in SDS but are sensitive to nucleophiles. Such a mechanism is based on a dramatic conformational change in the serpin. Thus the trapped complex is irreversible in nature. This feature is in marked contrast to what occurs with other classes of inhibitors, which instead used tight noncovalent association between the inhibitor and the proteinase, with little or no conformational change in either protein, to give a thermodynamically stable but reversible complex. Another specificity of serpins is that several of them including SERPINA5, SERPINE1 and SERPINE2 are activated by binding to heparin or other negatively charged glycosaminoglycans. The resulting enhancement in the rates of proteinase inhibition can be up to several 1000-fold suggesting that glycosaminoglycans are rate-limiting factors at sites of serpin action. In the case of the three serpins mentioned above, mechanism is a bridging mechanism in which glycosaminoglycans bind both serpin and proteinase to bring them in an appropriate interaction.[45-48]

An Overview of the Repertoire in Testis

MMPs and TIMPs

The occurrence of these molecules is highly dependent on the species, the developmental age of the testis and its endocrine environment, as summarized in Tables 3 and 4.[13,17,50-61] The MMP family has greatly expanded these last 20 years and a tissue distribution has generally been perfomed for each newly discovered MMP member using adult rat or mouse testes. Although the MMP-18, MMPs 23-26 and MMP-28 are present in the testis,[50,62-65] there is no indication relative to their cellular localisation. In fact, most of the information available are on the gelatinases MMP-2 and MMP-9 probably because of the avaibility of a rapid and simple biological test i.e., the gelatin zymography. The human fetal testis is also the site of expression of MMPs and TIMPs.[66] In the mouse, MMPs 2 and 9 are detected in fetal testes together with

Table 3. The relative mRNA levels for all mouse MMPs and TIMPs and several ADAMs in testicular tissue from newborn mice

mRNA Levels in Newborn Mouse Testes	Very High Levels	High Levels	Moderate Levels	Weak/Very Weak Levels
MMPs,	**MMPs:** 1, 11, 14, 15, 19, 23	**MMPs:** 2, 9, 28	**MMPs:** 3, 7, 8, 12, 13, 16, 24, 27	**MMPs:** 10, 17, 20, 21, 25
ADAMs	**ADAMs:** 10, 12, 15, 17, 19		**ADAM**-33	**ADAM**-28
TIMPs	**TIMPs** 2, 3, 4	**TIMP-1**		

Adapted from reference 50.

Table 4. Summary of the findings reported for MMPs and TIMPs in the testis

	Cellular Localization	Local /Hormonal Regulation	Fetal Testis	Developing and Adult Testis
TIMP-1	Sertoli cells, peritubular cells, but not in germ cells; adult Leydig cells	- FSH (↑) via cAMP, - IL1α(↑), TNFα, (↑) in Sertoli cell cultures	Sex-dimorphic pattern of expression; growth-promoting effect on the gonad	- Role in the assembly of adherens junctions - Role in the restructuring of the epithelium during spermiation and in the adhesion of germ cells to Sertoli cells - Facilitation of steroidogenesis
TIMP-2	20-day old rat Sertoli and peritubular cells, germ cells, adult Leydig cells	- FSH (↑) via cAMP - Cytokines (↑) in Sertoli cell cultures - TNFα opposes FSH-induced TIMP-2 expression	- No sex-dimorphic pattern of expression	- May have a role in activating proMMP-2 within Sertoli cells - Localization at the apical ectoplasmic specialization
TIMP-3	Sertoli cells, peritubular cells		Role in the migration of the mesonephros towards the urogenital ridge	Enhanced expression of a 30 kDa MW band correlates with enhanced Sertoli-peritubular cell interactions
MMP-9	Sertoli cells, peritubular cells	- TNFα (↑) in Sertoli cells - FGF2 (↑) in cocultures of Sertoli and peritubular cells	- No sex-dimorphic pattern of expression	- Participates in the regulation of Sertoli cell-tight junction dynamics in the rat testis - Induction of MMP-9 activity correlates with de novo cord formation
MT1-MMP	Ubiquitously expressed	- Not regulated by FSH	- No sex-dimorphic pattern of expression	- Activates pro-MMP2 together with TIMP-2
MMP-2	Sertoli, peritubular and Leydig cells but not germ cells	- FSH (↑) via cAMP, cytokine production inducers (↑) in Sertoli cell cultures	- No sex-dimorphic pattern of expression	- Together with MT1-MMP, may participate in germ cell migratory activity

Information is compiled from references 13,17,51-61.

the TIMPs 1-3 and EMMPRIN.[13] FSH regulation has been explored using 20-day old rat Sertoli cells, and it was shown that FSH regulated MMP-2 but not MMP-9 or MMP-14, and TIMP-1 and TIMP-2.[17,51,53-55,57-60,67,68] Cytokines largely involved in testicular physiology such as TNFα (tumor necrosis factor α), TGFβ3 (transforming growth factor β3) and FGF2 (basic fibroblast growth factor) have also been shown to regulate various MMPs and TIMPs in a culture or coculture model of testicular cells.[53-55,58,61] Leydig cells have been shown to express ADAM31,[69] as well as TIMP-2 throughout development.[70,71] It is yet unknown whether these proteins are under gonadotropin regulation in Leydig cells.

Serine Proteases and Serpins

PAs were the first serine proteases identified within the testis.[72] Plasminogen is also synthesized within the testis.[73] Originally, it was described that Sertoli cells were the site of synthesis of the two PAs, and FSH stimulates tPA while reducing uPA levels in the rat testis.[74,75] Expression of uPA is also under a retinoic acid control.[74,76] Pachytene and diakinetic spermatocytes exhibit immunoreactivity for tPA,[77] indicating that a tPA proteolytic event may occur at the spermatocyte surface level. It would be interesting to determine whether the immunoreactivity corresponded to a tPA binding protein or a tPA receptor present on germ cell surface. Annexin II is a good candidate, because it acts as a receptor for tPA and its mRNA is represented in a testis cDNA library.[78] By contrast, the receptor for urokinase has been identified on both Leydig cells and at Sertoli-germ cell contacts and/or germ cells,[79] indicating that proteolysis involving plasminogen may occur in the vicinity of Sertoli and germ cells and at the Leydig cell membrane. The receptor for uPA has also been identified on sperm but in that case, uPAR would be involved in sperm-egg recognition.[80] The binding of uPA to its receptor promotes cell adhesion by increasing the affinity of uPAR for vitronectin.[81] It is thus of interest that vitronectin has been identified in the cytoplasm of Leydig cells[82] and in germ cells,[83] and that PAI-1 is a Sertoli cell product as well as a peritubular product.[84,85] Indeed, PAI-1 might regulate cell adhesion or migration through competition with uPAR in binding to vitronectin.[81] PAI-1 is downregulated by cAMP analogs and FSH in Sertoli cells, and up-regulated by locally produced cytokines (TGFβ1, FGF2 and TNFα).[84-88] In contrast, PAI-3 or serpina5 is up-regulated by FSH and testosterone.[89-91] Of interest is the recent finding that other serpins produced by Sertoli cells are also regulated by androgens, including eppin and the serpins a3n and a12n.[91]

Germ cells are also a source of various serine proteases and inhibitors including the activated Protein C[92] and its inhibitor (serpina5),[79] the hepatocyte growth factor activator (HGFA) and its 2 specific inhibitors, the HAIs.[93] They also express the serpinb6b and testisin.[94,95] Testisin (also named TESP5) is a GPI-anchored protein expressed by premeiotic testicular germ cells and is a candidate tumor suppressor for testicular cancer.[95] Another TEStis Specific serine protease-1 TESSP-1 is a membrane-bound enzyme specifically expressed in type B spermatogonia and spermatocytes in the adult mouse.[96] It is not known whether these proteases act within the seminiferous epithelium or later in sperm-egg recognition events as shown with most ADAMs.[23]

Although few studies have explored the contribution of Leydig cells to the testicular protease repertoire, it is of interest that Leydig cells are known to express various serine proteases and serpins, and for some of these proteases, Leydig cells are the unique testicular site for their expression. For example, the serine protease originally named Leydin is in fact neurotrypsin.[18,97] Leydig cells are also the source of kallikreins 21, 24 and 27.[98-100] Interestingly, LH-hCG was found to regulate several serine proteases and serpins identified in Leydig cells (including urokinase, matriptase-2, kallikrein-21, HAI-2 and PCI),[93] indicative that common transcriptional signals may drive the expression of these molecules. Furthermore, kallikreins are regulated by testosterone and estradiol.[98-100] Table 5 recapitulates most of the data available on serine proteases and SERPINs expressed in testis.

Table 5. Serine proteases and serpins expressed in testis

	Name	Sertoli Cells	Germinal Cells	Leydig Cells
Plg Activators	uPA	FSH (↓) in rat	-	LH-hCG (↑) in mouse
	tPA	FSH (↑) in rat	+ (immunoreactivity)	Adult mouse Lc (weak)
HGF activator	HGFA	-	+	-
Protein C	aPC	-	+	+ (human testis)
TTSPs	Hepsin	+	-	-
	matriptase-2	-	-	LH-hCG (↓) in mouse
Kallikreins	Klk21, 24, 27	-	-	Steroid regulation
HGFA inhibitors	HAI-1/SPINT1	+	+	-
	HAI-2/SPINT-2	+	+ (truncated)	LH-hCG (↓) in mouse
PA inhibitors	PAI-1	FSH (↓) in rat	-	-
	PAI-2	+	-	+
	PAI-3 (PCI)	FSH, Testo. (↑)	+	LH-hCG (↓) in mouse
	PN-1	+	-	-
Other serpins	Serpinb6b	-	+	-
	SerpinA3N	Testo. (↑)	?	?
	SerpinA12N	Testo. (↑)	?	?
	Eppin	Testo. (↑)	?	?

(-), absent; (+), present; (↑), stimulation; (↓), inhibition; ?, not known; Testo, testosterone. Adapted from references 75,85,89-91,93-100.

The α2-Macroglobulin

Sertoli cells synthesize and secrete α2-macroglobulin, a protease inhibitor with a large spectrum of inhibitoy activities against proteinases of the thiol-, serine- metallo- and aspartic acid-families.[101] Such unique inhibition of proteinases by α2-macroglobulin is based on a « trap mechanism » in which α2-macroglobulin is organized as a noncovalently associated dimer of disulfide-linked dimers, and physically sequesters the proteinase inducing conformational changes in the proteinase. Thus binding of proteinases to α2-macroglobulin is irreversible.[102] In contrast to the hepatic protein, α2-macroglobulin is not an acute-phase protein in the rat testis,[103] and it may bind to various cytokines and growth factors thus regulating their bioavaibility.

What Potential Functions in Testicular Physiology?

Growth Factor and Receptor Activation and/or Receptor Shedding

Based on the described functions of proteases and inhibitors and considering testicular architecture and physiology, proteases and antiproteases may have a unique function in delivering growth factors trapped in the ECM , in activating growth factors or growth factor receptors, or in the shedding of transmembrane receptors generating soluble forms that woud act as dominant negative and impede normal signal transducing pathway following ligand binding to its receptor. ECM is known to function as a reservoir of endogeneous growth factors, sequestering them in an inactive state and protecting them from proteolytic degradation. For example FGF2 which is deeply involved in testicular physiology[61] does not contain a sequence signal for secretion, and it has been proposed that following environmental stimuli, FGF2 is released from the ECM through the action of proteases allowing it to bind to specific transmembrane FGF receptors and transduce a signal.[104] In addition to release growth factors stored in the ECM, proteases activate growth factors synthesised as inactive pro-factors. For example, uPA activates (at least in seminiferous tubules) pro-TGF-beta and pro-HGF,[18-20] two decisive growth factors in testicular physiology.[105-106] In addition, HGFA and hepsin are two serine proteinases recently identified in the mouse testis, in germinal cells and in peritubular or Sertoli cells, respectively.[93] This is indicative that the pro-HGF produced by peritubular cells throughout development[106] may be activated by hepsin whereas pro-HGF produced by adult Sertoli cells[107] would be activated by either HGFA or hepsin, fueling the concept of paracriny between germ cells and Sertoli cells.[1-4] Further, the testis is also the source for inhibitors of HGFA and hepsin, and one such inhibitor, HAI-2 (HGFA inhibitor type 2) is downregulated by LH-hCG in Leydig cells.[93] Therefore, a proteolytic level of regulation probably exists together with a transcriptional level of regulation in the testis. However, its relative importance versus the transcriptional level of regulation is unknown. In this context, it should be mentioned that c-MET but also FGFR-1 may be specific targets for metalloproteases on the cell surface, yielding soluble receptors that may modulate the biological activities of their respective ligands.[108,109]

ECM Matrix Remodeling

One of the most described roles for proteases and inhibitors relates to the degradation of extra-cellular matrix that forms a physical barrier for cells to invade. In a very comprehensive review[110] on basement membrane and its testicular composition, ECM matrix remodeling is presented as a major event during organogenesis and growth whereas adulthood is characterized by a very low index in the turnover of extracellular matrix components. Furthermore, human pathological testes exhibit a hyalinisation of the seminiferous tubules that is accompanied by a lower sperm production ability and such a feature is also the hallmark of the testicular phenotype in the klinefeleter syndrome.[111,112] Thus, a physiological link is likely to exist between ECM and sperm production.

Testis Cord Formation

ECM consitutes a pathway along which cells may migrate, for instance during the migration of primordial germ cells. Indeed, PGCs express several integrins that may act as receptors for fibronectin and laminin that pave the PGC pathway toward the genital ridge.[113,114] Another very important involvement of ECM proteins during testis organogenesis consists of the formation of a basement membrane between the epithelializing Sertoli cells and the mesenchymal peritubular cells.[110,115-119] Originally, the genital ridge is composed of primordial germ cells and a thickened layer of coelomic epithelium. When the indifferent gonad has a XY genotype, SRY induces a cascade of gene expression which results initially in the migration of mesenchymal cells as well as endothelial cells from the adjacent mesonephros. No migration occurs in case of a XX gonad.[120,121] Such a migration is accompanied by extensive restructuring which underlines a crucial need for balancing the proteinases/inhibitors ratio. Accordingly, major sex-related differences in the ECM components distribution[122-126] and the expression of proteases and inhibitors have been reported.[11-13,127-131] Knowledge in this area has greatly been enhanced with the development of microarray studies dedicated to the identification of genes expressed in a sex-dimorphic fashion during the initial phases of testicular differentiation.[130,131] Table 6 summarizes data on the proteinases and inhibitors.

Investigations on the desert hedgehog (dhh) classified in the cysteine proteinases family,[19,20] have also greatly increased our understanding on the role of the basement membrane in testis compartimentation.[132-135] Sertoli cells are the source of Dhh whereas receptors are localized on peritubular cells and possibly Leydig cells. Interestingly, Dhh expression levels increase more than 45-fold at the time of testicular differentiation,[130,131] and Dhh-null testes exhibit disorganized cords with occasional germ cells seen outside cords and abnormal Leydig cell development. It was concluded that these defects likely stemmed from abnormal peritubular stimulation due to the

Table 6. Fold-increase in proteinases and inhibitors in fetal testes versus time-matched fetal ovaries

Name	1.5 < Fold Change <5	Fold Change >5
Serine proteinases	Masp 1 $^{E12.5}$ Neurotrypsin$^{E12.5,E13.5}$	Neurotrypsin$^{E11.5}$
Aspartic proteinases		Renin 1$^{E11.5,E12.5,E13.5}$
Cysteine proteinases	Caspase 7$^{E12.5}$ Cathepsin L$^{E13.5}$	Dhh$^{E12.5,E13.5}$
Metallo-proteinases	ADAMTS7$^{E11.5}$ ADAMTS 2, 5, 16$^{E12.5}$ ADAMTS 2, 5, 7$^{E13.5}$ ADAM 12, 19$^{E13.5}$	ADAMTS16$^{E11.5}$
Serpin	(Serpin B1a, serpin A3g, SPINT-2)$^{E12.5}$ (Serpin B1a, Serpin A 3g)$^{E13.5}$	Serpin E2 $^{E11.5}$ Serpin E2 $^{E12.5}$ (Serpin A5, Serpin E2)$^{E13.5}$
Cystatin	(Cystatin 8, cystatin C)$^{E12.5,13.5}$	Cystatin 9$^{E11.5,E12.5,E13.5}$
Tissue Inhibitor of MMPs	TIMP-1$^{E13.5}$	

E11.5, E12.5, E13.5, indicate the age at which the fold-change was registered. Data are from microarray studies of two laboratories.[130,131]

lack of Dhh.[132-135] Therefore, it would be of high interest to determine which proteinases and inhibitors may lie downstream of the Dhh/receptor complex.

Testis Growth and Lumen Formation

The prepubertal period is characterized by a rapid growth of the testis, the transformation of the seminiferous cords into tubules and the initiation of spermatogenesis. Specifically, tight junctions are formed between neighboring Sertoli cells thus creating the blood-testis barrier, and cords developed a lumen becoming tubules. Accordingly, Sertoli cells reorganize their cytoskeleton to support additional spermatogenic cell types as spermatogenesis is initiated, and tubules increase in diameter as well as in length. Several in vitro observations raise the possibility that proteases and inhibitors in response to hormonal (mainly FSH) and local stimuli such as HGF and FGF2 are critically involved in these substantial prepubertal changes.

For instance, using prepubertal rat Sertoli cells cultured in a two-chambered assembly to mimick the Sertoli cell barrier, it was demonstrated that proteases were implicated in the changes in the Sertoli cell cytoskeleton elicited by FSH and in modulation of the formation and maintenance of the Sertoli cell barrier. The nature of the protease(s) is not fully identified, but α2-macroglobulin opposed its(their) action and increased integrity of the Sertoli cell barrier.[67,136] MMP-2 and tPA are good candidates because they are Sertoli cell products and under FSH control.[55,74,75] A second set of experiments was designed to examine cord and lumen formation by Sertoli cells cocultured with rat prepubertal peritubular cells or Sertoli cells cultured on a reconstituted ECM. These models have been extremely fruitful in evidencing cooperativity between Sertoli cells and testicular peritubular cells in the production and deposition of extracellular matrix components,[137] and in highlighting the role of laminin in the morphognetic cascade resulting in the formation of tubule-like structure.[138,139] Other experiments also suggested that ECM components regulated the expression of tight junction proteins and the formation of a lumen.[58,60] Inasmuch as MMPs and PAs degrade laminin, fibronectin and collagen

IV i.e., the major ECM components of the testicular basement membrane, any remodeling necessary to support the rapid and extensive growth of the prepubertal testis is thus expected to involve a delicate interplay between proteases and inhibitors, and certain growth factors. Indeed, various growth factors promote formation of cord-like structures by Sertoli cells in vitro. For instance, FGF2 which mediates mesenchymal-epithelial interactions of peritubular cells and Sertoli cells in the rat testis, promoted de novo testis cord formation and enhanced MMP-9, the 30 kDa glycosylated form of TIMP3 and PAI-1 in the cocultures.[61] It would be of interest to investigate the expression pattern of proteases and inhibitors in the HGF-treated cultures because HGF is a powerful morphogen for Sertoli cells cultured on a reconstituted basement membrane. It not only promotes cords but also their further remodeling into tubules.[107,140] Additionally, the antisense strategy would constitute an elegant means to link morphogen cytokines, ECM components, restructuring events and involvement of proteases.

Few data are yet available in vivo to support these in vitro experiments. However, a recent study highlighted the role of laminin during the prepubertal period. Indeed, it was shown that male mice deficient for laminin alpha2 chain exhibited abnormal testicular basement membranes and displayed a defect in the timing of lumen formation, resulting in production of fewer spermatids. Furthermore, the authors demonstrated that laminin alpha1 chain corrected male infertility caused by absence of laminin alpha2 chain.[141]

Spermatogenesis and the Apical Migration of Germ Cells towards the Lumen

Different authors have been interested in understanding the dynamics of spermatogenesis which relies on the passage of the blood-testis barrier and the release of the elongated spermatids at the apex (spermiation). The description of the testis barrier is beyond the scope of this chapter and is treated in a recent and excellent review.[16] However, it is noteworthy that the testis barrier is unique when compared to other blood-tissue barriers (e.g., blood-brain and blood-retina barriers) that it is composed of gap junctions, desmosomes, tight junctions and ectoplasmic specializations, precluding that the passage of germ cells requires a finely tuned process to allow its spatiotemporal opening and closing, not disturbing the integrity of the testis barrier which would provoke a pathological arrest of spermatogenesis. Because this situation is reminiscent of cell migation across ECM, different authors have concentrated their efforts in determining the composition of the junctions, most specifically those that are restricted to testis i.e., the ectoplasmic specialisations, and the way junctional proteins are transcriptionally and post-transcriptionally regulated. It was also reasonable to think that proteases which act like scissors would help germ cells in migrating along Sertoli cell membranes, and that specific inhibitors would restrict the activity of the proteases in a finely tuned regulatory fashion to preserve homeostasis. Therefore, a list of the cytokines, proteases and inhibitors present at the right time and at the right place has been tentatively established.[142,143]

First evidences came from the demonstration that the plasminogen activators were expressed as a function of the stages of the seminiferous epithelium, and an increased PA activity was found at the time of elongating spermatid translocation and spermiation at the stages VII-VIII.[74,77,144,145] Interestingly, the expression of α2-macroglobulin fluctuates with the stages of the seminiferous epithelium, and immunostaining concentrated at stages I-VI, thus prior spermiation indicative that α2-macroglobulin may protect the integrity of the seminiferous epithelium against excessive proteolysis.[146] Furthermore, it was shown that addition of germ cells to Sertoli cell cultures resulted in an enhancement of PA activity[147] (and also of cathepsin L, a cysteine protease)[148,149] and that this correlated in time with the dynamics of assembly/desassembly of the de novo adherens junctions formation between the cultured Sertoli cells. Furthermore, the expression of α2-macroglobulin but also of cystatin (a cathepsin L inhibitor) in the coculture model was consistent with the idea that proteases and their corresponding inhibitors were working synergistically supporting the evidence that they may be involved in the adherence of germ cells to Sertoli cells and the subsequent formation of intercellular junctions.[150-152]

Spermiation i.e., extrusion of elongated spermatids into the lumen, is the alternate major event occurring during stages VII-VIII. It is followed by the phagocytosis of the cytoplasts shed from the elongated spermatids, which are called the residual bodies.[1,153,154] Interestingly, phagocytosis of residual bodies resulted in an increase PA activity[155] in an in vitro model of coculture of Sertoli cells and residual bodies.[156] Further, the addition of an anti-interleukin 1α antibody prevented the RB-induced enhancement of PA activity,[155] thus emphasizing the role of this cytokine in the process of spermiation.[157,158] Furthermore, given that the increased PA activity may facilitate the passage of germ cells accross the testis barrier, it was suggested that a proteolysis-dependent message would participate in the synchronisation process of the spermatogenesis cycle,[155] supporting the pionnering hypothesis of Regaud and Roosen-Runge.[153,154] Two other cytokines have proven to be essential at least in the passage of the testis barrier by preleptotene spermatocytes. These are TGFβ3 and TNFα and the readers are encouraged to read recent reviews on the subject.[16,143,152]

Interestingly, stages VII-VIII are highly testosterone-dependent as demonstrated in models with testosterone deficiency in which a premature detachment of germ cells in the lumens of the tubules is described.[159-162] In addition, androgens inhibit PA activity secreted by Sertoli cells in culture in a two-chambered assembly.[163] Thus serpinA5 is of tremendous interest because it is upregulated by testosterone,[90,91] it opposed PA activity and deficient mice develop male sterility.[164] Specifically, lumens are filled with immature germ cells because of an unopposed proteolytic activity of the urokinase type.[164] Such a testicular phenotype is reminiscent of the testicular phenotype described in mice deficient for claudin 11.[165] Claudin 11 as well as claudin 1 and 3 are essential components of the testis barrier,[165,166] and they are up-regulated by testosterone.[166-168] In addition, claudins contribute together with MT1-MMP and TIMP-2 in activating MMP-2 secreted as a pro-form.[169] MMPs may also be activated by urokinase. Thus, the germ cell enhancement of MMP-2 activity[17] may in part, result from the increase in the activity of the PAs observed in Sertoli cell-germ cell cocultures and discussed above. In that context, it would be of interest to determine whether claudins are substrates for either PAs or MMPs, and to investigate claudin expression in the serpinA5-deficient testes and vice-versa.

Collectively, it appears that germ cells which do not bear classic characteristics of migrating cells regulate their own progression within the seminiferous epithelium, through a modulation of the expression pattern of the proteases and inhibitors produced by Sertoli cells, supporting the hypothesis that Sertoli cells act as facilitators of migration, and adding a new function to these nurse cells. Future experiments aiming at dissecting the kinetics of the reliant events of spermiation and translocation would be useful in deciphering such integrated system with hormones and local environment.

Proteolysis and Steroidogenesis

Because Leydig cells exhibit a specific repertoire of proteases and inhibitors and that several (if not all) of them are under gonadotropin regulation via cAMP,[93] the question arises as to whether a link exists between steroidogenesis and proteolysis. Different arguments emphasize a role of ECM in the capacity of Leydig cells to respond to LH-hCG, and thus indirectly of proteases and inhibitors. For instance, it was shown that fibronectin and collagen IV induce downregulation of steroidogenic response to gonadotropins.[170,171] Furthermore, TGFβ which is known to cause augmented fibronectin deposition[172] and to elicit cytoskeletal changes in Leydig cells similar to those evidenced when these cells are cultured on plates precoated with fibronectin,[173] inhibits DNA synthesis and antagonizes gonadotropin steroidogenic action in Leydig cells.[173,174] However, direct evidences for involvement of proteases are still lacking.

Lessons from Transgenic Mice

Inasmuch as proteases and inhibitors are extremely abundant and redundant in their spectrum of actions, it is not surprising that very little knockout mouse models have to date contributed to our understanding on their roles in testicular function (Table 7). However, it should be

Table 7. Data obtained from the generation of transgenic mice with reduced fertility

Transgenic Mice	Phenotype of the Deficient Male Mice
ADAMTS-2	Infertile with few sperms and large number of round spermatids but few elongate spermatids.[182]
Cathepsin-L	Furless mice. Tubules contain 32% fewer spermatids per Sertoli cell than the average tubule number of control mice, as a result of reduced formation of preleptotene spermatocytes and their differentiation into pachytene spermatocytes.[177]
EMMPRIN	Male mice are azoospermic because spermatogenesis is arrested at the metaphase of the first meiotic division, and the lumens are filled with round degenerated cells.[179]
Matrilysin	Overproduction causes reduced sperm production beginning at 8 months of age. The architecture of the testes is altered.[183]
MT1-MMP	Dwarfs with craniofacial and skeletal abnormalities ; show no signs of sexual maturation.[178]
Protease nexin-1 (SerpinE2)	Sterility results from a defect in semen protein composition, which leads to inadequate semen coagulation and deficient vaginal plug formation.[179]
Protein C Inhibitor (Serpina5)	Sterility would be due to a destruction of the BHT because of increase urokinase activity within the seminiferous epithelium resulting in premature detachment of germ cells into the lumen.[164]

stated that most of the time no systematic analysis of the testes of the deficient mice had been undertaken unless the authors experienced reproductive difficulties. For example, male mice deficient in PAI-1,[175] TIMP-1[176] or cathepsin L[177] may still reproduce. However because several pieces of evidences supported a role for cathepsin L in germ cell movement during spermatogenesis, testes from deficient mice were carefully investigated and tubules were found to contain 32% fewer spermatids than the average tubule number of control mice.[177] Such a study should be done on the MT1-MMP-deficient male mice which showed "no signs of sexual maturation", as stated in the original publication.[178] In other cases, the testis may not be the primary target as shown with male mice deficient in serpinE2 which are sterile because of altered semen protein composition.[179] The different cases reported in Table 7 should be more informative with respect to the role of proteinases in testicular physiology, provided that an extensive study of the male reproductive system is done. Indeed, male mice deficient for EMMPRIN are azoospermic. Specifically, spermatogenesis is arrested at the metaphase of the first meiotic division, and the lumens are filled with round degenerated cells.[180] Given that the expression of EMMPRIN correlates in time with the appearance of spermatocytes in the seminiferous epithelium, it is predicted that EMMPRIN is involved in the interactions between Sertoli cells and germ cells.[180,181] However, no studies have yet reported the expression pattern of the MMPs known to be under EMMPRIN control in the deficient testes. Male sterility is also observed in transgenic mice with inactive alleles for ADAMTS-2,[182] overexpression of MMP-7[183] and deficiency for serpina5,[164] but the exact nature of the disorder remains to be fully characterized.

Conclusions and Future Directions

We herein provided a series of evidences highlighting that proteases may be active partners in establishing and maintaining testicular architecture, and in facilitating germ cell migration which constitutes a prerequisite for germ cell progression throughout the spermatogenic process. Therefore, it may be worth to revisit the phenotypes of transgenic male mice deficient for a proteinase or an inhibitor proven to be expressed at the time of translocation and/or spermiation. Furthermore inasmuch as various proteases, inhibitors, junctional components (e.g., claudins, occludins, JAMs) are under a complex hormonal regulation via gonadotropins and/or testosterone, and local regulatory control involving cytokines and growth factors, models with reduced testosterone bioavaibility or with limited FSH or LH action coupled to microarray studies, as those recently published[89,91] should be of tremendous benefit to fully understand the mechanisms that underpin the role of proteases and inhibitors in testis development and function.

Acknowledgements

M.G. Forest is thanked for her contribution in carefully reading the manuscript. J. Bois and M.A. Dicarlo are thanked for their help in typing the manuscript.

References

1. Russell LD. Sertoli-germ cell interrelations: A review. Gamete Res 1980; 3:79-202.
2. Jegou B, Sharpe RM. Paracrine mechanisms in testicular control. In: de Kretser DM, ed. Molecular Biology of the Male Reproductive System. San Diego: Academic Press, 1993:271-310.
3. de Kretser DM, Loveland KL, Meinhardt A et al. Spermatogenesis. Hum Reprod 1998; 13(Suppl. 1):1-8.
4. Griswold MD. The central role of Sertoli cells seminiferous epithelium. Semin Cell Dev Biol 1998; 9:411-416.
5. McElreavey K, Fellous M. Sex determination and the Y chromosome. Am J Med Genet 1999; 89(4):176-185.
6. Swain A, Lovell-Badge R. Mammalian sex determination: A molecular drama. Genes Dev 1999; 13:755-767.
7. Josso N, Racine C, Di Clemente N et al. The role of anti-Müllerian hormone in gonadal development. Mol Cell Endocrinol 1998; 145:3-7.
8. Yao HH, Tilmann C, Zhao GO et al. The battle of the sexes: Opposing pathways in sex determination. In: Chadwick D, Goode J, eds. Symposium on the Genetics and Biology of Sex Determination. London: Novartis Foundation, 2002:187-198.
9. Brennan J, Capel B. One tissue, two fates: Molecular genetic events that underlie testis versus ovary development. Nat Rev Genet 2004; 5(7):509-521.
10. Koopman P. Sex determination: A tale of two Sox genes. Trends Genet 2005; 21(7):367-370.
11. Töhönen V, Osterlund C, Nordqvist K. Testatin: A cystatin-related gene expressed during early testis development. Proc Natl Acad Sci USA 1998; 95(24):14208-14213.
12. Grimmond S, Van Hateren N, Siggers P et al. Sexually dimorphic expression of protease nexin-1 and vanin-1 in the developing mouse gonad prior to overt differentiation suggests a role in mammalian sexual development. Hum Mol Genet 2000; 9(10):1553-1560.
13. Guyot R, Magre S, Leduque P et al. Differential expression of tissue inhibitor of metalloproteinases type 1 (TIMP-1) during mouse gonad development. Dev Dyn 2003; 227(3):357-366.
14. Fritz IB, Tung PS, Ailenberg M. Proteases and antiproteases in the seminiferous tubules. In: Russell LD, Griswold MD, eds. The Sertoli Cell. Clearwater: Cache River Press, 1993:217-235.
15. Charron M, Wright WW. Proteases and protease inhibitors. In: Skinner MK, Griswold MD, eds. Sertoli Cell Biology. London: Elsevier Academic Press, 2005:121-152.
16. Wong CH, Cheng CY. The blood-testis barrier: Its biology, regulation, and physiological role in spermatogenesis. Curr Top Dev Biol 2005; 71:263-296.
17. Longin J, Guillaumot P, Chauvin MA et al. MT1-MMP in rat testicular development and the control of Sertoli cell proMMP-2 activation. J Cell Science 2001; 114(Pt 11):2125-2134.
18. Vu TH, Werb Z. Matrix metalloproteinases: Effectors of development and normal physiology. Genes Dev 2000; 14(17):2123-2133.
19. Puente XS, Sanchez LM, Overall CM et al. Human and mouse proteases: A comparative genomic approach. Nat Rev Genet 2003; 4(7):544-558.
20. Puente XS, Lopez-Otin C. A genomic analysis of rat proteases and protease inhibitors. Genome Res 2004; 4(4):609-622.
21. Curry TEJ, Osteen KG. The matrix metalloproteinase system: Changes, regulation, and impact throughout the ovarian and uterine reproductive cycle. Endocr Rev 2003; 24(4):428-465.
22. Gabison EE, Hoang-Xuan T, Mauviel A et al. EMMPRIN/CD147, an MMP modulator in cancer, development and tissue repair. Biochimie 2005; 87(3-4):361-368.
23. Primakoff P, Myles DG. The ADAM gene family: Surface proteins with adhesion and protease activity. Trends Genet 2000; 6(2):83-87.

24. Apte SS. A disintegrin-like and metalloprotease (reprolysin type) with thrombospondin type 1 motifs: The ADAMTS family. Int J Biochem Cell Biol 2004; 36(6):981-985.
25. Porter S, Clark IM, Kevorkian L et al. The ADAMTS metalloproteinases. Biochem J 2005; 386(Pt 1):15-27.
26. Edwards DR, Waterhouse P, Holman ML et al. A growth-responsive gene (16C8) in normal mouse fibroblasts homologous to a human collagenase inhibitor with erythroid-potentiating activity: Evidence for inducible and constitutive transcripts. Nucleic Acids Res 1986; 14(22):8863-8878.
27. Woessner JFJ. MMPs and TIMPs—An historic perspective. Mol Biotechnol 2002; 22(1):33-49.
28. Lambert E, Dasse E, Haye B et al. TIMPs as multifacial proteins. Crit Rev Oncol Hematol 2004; 49(3):187-198.
29. Stetler-Stevenson WG, Seo DW. TIMP-2: An endogenous inhibitor of angiogenesis. Trends Mol Med 2005; 11(3):97-103.
30. Mannello F, Gazzanelli G. Tissue inhibitors of metalloproteinases and programmed cell death: Conundrums, controversies and potential implications. Apoptosis 2001; 6(6):479-482.
31. Weber BH, Vogt G, Pruett RC et al. Mutations in the tissue inhibitor of metalloproteinases-3 (TIMP-3) in patients with Sorsby's fundus dystrophy. Nat Genet 1994; 8(4):352-356.
32. Fata JE, Leo KJ, Voura EB et al. Accelerated apoptosis in the Timp-3-deficient mammary gland. J Clin Invest 2001; 108(6):831-841.
33. Carmeliet P, Collen D. Development and disease in proteinase-deficient mice: Role of the plasminogen, matrix metalloproteinase and coagulation system. Thromb Res 1998; 91(6):255-285.
34. Dano K, Behrendt N, Hoyer-Hansen G et al. Plasminogen activation and cancer. Thromb Haemost 2005; 93(4):676-681.
35. Leonardsson G, Peng XR, Liu K et al. Ovulation efficiency is reduced in mice that lack plasminogen activator gene function: Functional redundancy among physiological plasminogen activators. Proc Natl Acad Sci USA 1995; 92(26):12446-12450.
36. Ny T, Wahlberg P, Brandstrom IJ. Matrix remodeling in the ovary: Regulation and functional role of the plasminogen activator and matrix metalloproteinase systems. Mol Cell Endocrinol 2002; 187(1-2):29-38.
37. Hajjar KA. Cellular receptors in the regulation of plasmin generation. Thromb Haemost 1995; 74(1):294-301.
38. Kim J, Hajjar KA. Annexin II: A plasminogen-plasminogen activator coreceptor. Front Biosci 2002; 7:d341-d348.
39. Solberg H, Lober D, Eriksen J et al. Identification and characterization of the murine cell surface receptor for the urokinase-type plasminogen activator. Eur J Biochem 1992; 205(2):451-458.
40. Blasi F, Carmeliet P. uPAR: A versatile signalling orchestrator. Nat Rev Mol Cell Biol 2002; 3(12):932-943.
41. Alfano D, Franco P, Vocca I et al. The urokinase plasminogen activator and its receptor: Role in cell growth and apoptosis. Thromb Haemost 2005; 93(2):205-211.
42. Hooper JD, Clements JA, Quigley JP et al. Type II transmembrane serine proteases. Insights into an emerging class of cell surface proteolytic enzymes. J Biol Chem 2001; 276(2):857-860.
43. Diamandis EP, Yousef GM. Human tissue kallikreins: A family of new cancer biomarkers. Clin Chem 2002; 48(8):1198-1205.
44. Diamandis EP, Yousef GM, Olsson AY. An update on human and mouse glandular kallikreins. Clin Biochem 2004; 37(4):258-260.
45. Potempa J, Korzus E, Travis J. The serpin superfamily of proteinase inhibitors: Structure, function, and regulation. J Biol Chem 1994; 269(23):15957-15960.
46. Silverman GA, Bird PI, Carrell RW et al. The serpins are an expanding superfamily of structurally similar but functionally diverse proteins. Evolution, mechanism of inhibition, novel functions, and a revised nomenclature. J Biol Chem 2001; 276(36):33293-33296.
47. Gettins PG. Serpin structure, mechanism, and function. Chem Rev 2002; 102(12):4751-4804.
48. Pike RN, Buckle AM, Le Bonniec BF et al. Control of the coagulation system by serpins. Getting by with a little help from glycosaminoglycans. FEBS J 2005; 272(19):4842-4851.
49. Jerabek I, Zechmeister-Machhart M, Binder BR et al. Binding of retinoic acid by the inhibitory serpin protein C inhibitor. Eur J Biochem 2001; 268(22):5989-5996.
50. Nuttall RK, Sampieri CL, Pennington CJ et al. Expression analysis of the entire MMP and TIMP gene families during mouse tissue development. FEBS Lett 2004; 563(1-3):129-134.
51. Ulisse S, Farina AR, Piersanti D et al. Follicle-stimulating hormone increases the expression of tissue inhibitors of metalloproteinases TIMP-1 and TIMP-2 and induces TIMP-1 AP-1 site binding complex(es) in prepubertal rat Sertoli cells. Endocrinology 1994; 135(6):2479-2487.
52. Boujrad N, Ogwuegbu SO, Garnier M et al. Identification of a stimulator of steroid hormone synthesis isolated from testis. Science 1995; 268(5217):1609-1612.

53. Hoeben E, Van Haelst I, Swinnen JV et al. Gelatinase A secretion and its control in peritubular and Sertoli cell cultures: Effects of hormones, second messengers and inducers of cytokine production. Mol Cell Endocrinol 1996; 118(1-2):37-46.
54. Gronning LM, Wang JE, Ree AH et al. Regulation of tissue inhibitor of metalloproteinases-1 in rat Sertoli cells: Induction by germ cell residual bodies, interleukin-1alpha, and second messengers. Biol Reprod 2000; 62(4):1040-1046.
55. Longin J, Le Magueresse-Battistoni B. Evidence that MMP-2 and TIMP-2 are at play in the FSH-induced changes in Sertoli cells. Mol Cell Endocrinol 2002; 189(1-2):25-35.
56. Nishino K, Yamanouchi K, Naito K et al. Matrix metalloproteinases regulate mesonephric cell migration in developing XY gonads which correlates with the inhibition of tissue inhibitor of metalloproteinase-3 by Sry. Dev Growth Differ 2002; 44(1):35-43.
57. Mruk DD, Siu MK, Conway AM et al. Role of tissue inhibitor of metalloproteases-1 in junction dynamics in the testis. J Androl 2003; 24(4):510-523.
58. Siu MK, Lee WM, Cheng CY. The interplay of collagen IV, tumor necrosis factor-α, gelatinase B (matrix metalloprotease-9), and tissue inhibitor of metalloproteases-1 in the basal lamina regulates Sertoli cell-tight junction dynamics in the rat testis. Endocrinology 2003; 144(1):371-387.
59. Siu MK, Cheng CY. Interactions of proteases, protease inhibitors, and the beta1 integrin/laminin gamma3 protein complex in the regulation of ectoplasmic specialization dynamics in the rat testis. Biol Reprod 2004; 70(4):945-964.
60. Siu MK, Cheng CY. Dynamic cross-talk between cells and the extracellular matrix in the testis. Bioessays 2004; 26(9):978-992.
61. El Ramy R, Vérot A, Mazaud S et al. Fibroblast growth factor (FGF) 2 and FGF9 mediate mesenchymal-epithelial interactions of peritubular and Sertoli cells in the rat testis. J Endocrinol 2005; 187(1):135-147.
62. Bernal F, Hartung HP, Kieseier BC. Tissue mRNA expression in rat of newly described matrix metalloproteinases. Biol Res 2005; 38(2-3):267-271.
63. Cossins J, Dudgeon TJ, Catlin G et al. Identification of MMP-18, a putative novel human matrix metalloproteinase. Biochem Biophys Res Commun 1996; 228(2):494-498.
64. Velasco G, Pendas AM, Fueyo A et al. Cloning and characterization of human MMP-23, a new matrix metalloproteinase predominantly expressed in reproductive tissues and lacking conserved domains in other family members. J Biol Chem 1999; 274(8):4570-4576.
65. Lohi J, Wilson CL, Roby JD et al. Epilysin, a novel human matrix metalloproteinase (MMP-28) expressed in testis and keratinocytes and in response to injury. J Biol Chem 2001; 276(13):10134-10144.
66. Robinson LL, Sznajder NA, Riley SC et al. Matrix metalloproteinases and tissue inhibitors of metalloproteinases in human fetal testis and ovary. Mol Hum Reprod 2001; 7(7):641-648.
67. Ailenberg M, Fritz IB. Influences of follicle-stimulating hormone, proteases, and antiproteases on permeability of the barrier generated by Sertoli cells in a two-chambered assembly. Endocrinology 1989; 124(3):1399-1407.
68. Ailenberg M, Stetler-Stevenson WG, Fritz IB. Secretion of latent type IV procollagenase and active type IV collagenase by testicular cells in culture. Biochem J 1991; 279(Pt 1):75-80.
69. Liu L, Smith JW. Identification of ADAM 31: A protein expressed in Leydig cells and specialized epithelia. Endocrinology 2000; 141(6):2033-2042.
70. Blavier L, DeClerck YA. Tissue inhibitor of metalloproteinases-2 is expressed in the interstitial matrix in adult mouse organs and during embryonic development. Mol Biol Cell 1997; 8(8):1513-1527.
71. Ge RS, Dong O, Sottas CM et al. Gene expression in rat Leydig cells during development from the progenitor to adult stage: A cluster analysis. Biol Reprod 2005; 72(6):1405-1415.
72. Lacroix M, Smith FE, Fritz IB. Changes in levels of plasminogen activator activity in normal and germ-cell-depleted testes during development. Mol Cell Endocrinol 1982; 26(3):259-267.
73. Saksela O, Vihko KK. Local synthesis of plasminogen by the seminiferous tubules of the testis. FEBS Lett 1986; 204(2):193-197.
74. Vihko KK, Penttila TL, Parvinen M et al. Regulation of urokinase- and tissue-type plasminogen activator gene expression in the rat seminiferous epithelium. Mol Cell Endocrinol 1989; 31(1):52-59.
75. Tolli R, Monaco LDB, Di Bonito P et al. Hormonal regulation of urokinase- and tissue- type plasminogen activator in rat Sertoli cells. Biol Reprod 1995; 53(1):193-200.
76. Canipari R, Galdieri M. Retinoid modulation of plasminogen activator production in rat Sertoli cells. Biol Reprod 2000; 63(2):544-550.
77. Vihko KK, Kristensen P, Dano K et al. Immunohistochemical localization of urokinase-type plasminogen activator in Sertoli cells and tissue-type plasminogen activator in spermatogenic cells in the rat seminiferous epithelium. Dev Biol 1988; 126(1):150-155.

78. O'Shaughnessy PJ, Fleming L, Baker PJ et al. Identification of developmentally regulated genes in the somatic cells of the mouse testis using serial analysis of gene expression. Biol Reprod 2003; 69(3):797-808.
79. Odet F, Guyot R, Leduque P et al. Evidence for similar expression of protein C inhibitor and the urokinase-type plasminogen activator system during mouse testis development. Endocrinology 2004; 145:1481-1489.
80. Huarte J, Belin D, Bosco D et al. Plasminogen activator and mouse spermatozoa: Urokinase synthesis in the male genital tract and binding of the enzyme to the sperm cell surface. J Cell Biol 1987; 104(5):1281-1289.
81. Dellas C, Loskutoff DJ. Historical analysis of PAI-1 from its discovery to its potential role in cell motility and disease. Thromb Haemost 2005; 93(4):631-640.
82. Sawada H, Sugawara I, Kitami A et al. Vitronectin in the cytoplasm of Leydig cells in the rat testis. Biol Reprod 1996; 54(1):29-35.
83. Nuovo GJ, Preissner KT, Bronson RA. PCR-amplified vitronectin mRNA localizes in situ to spermatocytes and round spermatids in the human testis. Hum Reprod 1995; 10(8):2187-2191.
84. Hettle JA, Balekjian E, Tung PS et al. Rat testicular peritubular cells in culture secrete an inhibitor of plasminogen activator activity. Biol Reprod 1988; 38(2):359-371.
85. Le Magueresse-Battistoni B, Pernod G, Sigillo F et al. Plasminogen activator inhibitor-1 is expressed in cultured rat Sertoli cells. Biol Reprod 1998; 59(3):591-598.
86. Nargolwalla C, McCabe D, Fritz IB. Modulation of levels of messenger RNA for tissue-type plasminogen activator in rat Sertoli cells, and levels of messenger RNA for plasminogen activator inhibitor in testis peritubular cells. Mol Cell Endocrinol 1990; 70(1):73-80.
87. Le Magueresse-Battistoni B, Pernod G, Kolodie L et al. Plasminogen activator inhibitor-1 regulation in cultured rat peritubular cells by basic fibroblast growth factor and transforming growth factor-alpha. Endocrinology 1996; 137(10):4243-4249.
88. Le Magueresse-Battistoni B, Pernod G, Kolodie L et al. Tumor necrosis factor-alpha regulates plasminogen activator inhibitor-1 in rat testicular peritubular cells. Endocrinology 1997; 138(3):1097-1105.
89. Meachem SJ, Ruwanpura SM, Ziolkowski J et al. Developmentally distinct in vivo effects of FSH on proliferation and apoptosis during testis maturation. J Endocrinol 2005; 186(3):429-446.
90. Anway MD, Show MD, Zirkin BR. Protein C inhibitor expression by adult rat Sertoli cells: Effects of testosterone withdrawal and replacement. J Androl 2005; 26(5):578-585.
91. Denolet E, De Gendt K, Allemeersch J et al. The effect of a Sertoli cell-selective knockout of the androgen receptor on testicular gene expression in prepubertal mice. Mol Endocrinol 2006; 20:321-334.
92. Yamamoto K, Loskutoff DJ. Extrahepatic expression and regulation of protein C in the mouse. Am J Pathol 1998; 153(2):547-555.
93. Odet F, Vérot A, Le Magueresse-Battistoni B. The mouse testis is the source of various serine proteases and SERine Proteinase INhibitors (SERPINs). Serine proteases and SERPINs identified in Leydig cells are under gonadotropin regulation. Endocrinology 2006; 147(9):4374-83.
94. Charron Y, Madani R, Nef S et al. Expression of Serpinb6 serpins in germ and somatic cells of mouse gonads. Mol Reprod Dev 2006; 73(1):9-19.
95. Honda A, Yamagata K, Sugiura S et al. A mouse serine protease TESP5 is selectively included into lipid rafts of sperm membrane presumably as a glycosylphosphatidylinositol-anchored protein. J Biol Chem 2002; 277(19):16976-16984.
96. Takano N, Matsui H, Takahashi T. TESSP-1: A novel serine protease gene expressed in the spermatogonia and spermatocytes of adult mouse testes. Mol Reprod Dev 2005; 70(1):1-10.
97. Poorafshar M, Hellman L. Cloning and structural analysis of leydin, a novel human serine protease expressed by the Leydig cells of the testis. Eur J Biochem 1999; 261(1):244-250.
98. Matsui H, Moriyama A, Takahashi T. Cloning and characterization of mouse klk27, a novel tissue kallikrein expressed in testicular Leydig cells and exhibiting chymotrypsin-like specificity. Eur J Biochem 2000; 267(23):6858-6865.
99. Matsui H, Takahashi T. Mouse testicular Leydig cells express Klk21, a tissue kallikrein that cleaves fibronectin and IGF-binding protein-3. Endocrinology 2001; 142:4918-4929.
100. Matsui H, Takano N, Takahashi T. Characterization of mouse glandular kallikrein 24 expressed in testicular Leydig cells. Int J Biochem Cell Biol 2005; 37(11):2333-2343.
101. Cheng CY, Grima J, Stahler MS et al. Sertoli cell synthesizes and secretes a protease inhibitor, α2-macroglobulin. Biochemistry 1990; 29(4):1063-1068.
102. Gettins PG. Thiol ester cleavage-dependent conformational change in human α2-macroglobulin. Influence of attacking nucleophile and of Cys949 modification. Biochemistry 1995; 34(38):12233-12240.

103. Stahler MS, Schlegel P, Bardin CW et al. Alpha 2-macroglobulin is not an acute-phase protein in the rat testis. Endocrinology 1991; 128(6):2805-2814.
104. Powers CJ, McLeskey SW, Wellistein A. Fibroblast growth factors, their receptors and signalling. Endocr Relat Cancer 2000; 7(3):165-197.
105. Loveland KL, Hime G. TGFbeta superfamily members in spermatogenesis: Setting the stage for fertility in mouse and Drosophila. Cell Tissue Res 2005; 322(1):141-146.
106. Catizone A, Ricci G, Arista V et al. Hepatocyte growth factor and c-MET are expressed in rat prepuberal testis. Endocrinology 1999; 140(7):3106-3113.
107. Catizone A, Ricci G, Galdieri M. Expression and functional role of hepatocyte growth factor receptor (C-MET) during postnatal rat testis development. Endocrinology 2001; 142(5):1828-1834.
108. Wajih N, Walter J, Sane DC. Vascular origin of a soluble truncated form of the hepatocyte growth factor (c-met). Circ Res 2002; 90(1):46-52.
109. Levi E, Fridman R, Hiao HQ et al. Matrix metalloproteinase 2 releases active soluble ectodomain of fibroblast growth factor receptor 1. Proc Natl Acad Sci USA 1996; 93(14):1069-7074.
110. Dym M. Basement membrane regulation of Sertoli cells. Endocr Rev 1994; 15(1):102-115.
111. de Kretser DM, Kerr JB, Paulsen CA. The peritubular tissue in the normal and pathological human testis. An ultrastructural study. Biol Reprod 1975; 12(3):317-324.
112. Aksglaede L, Wikstrom AM, Rajpert-De Meyts E et al. Natural history of seminiferous tubule degeneration in Klinefelter syndrome. Hum Reprod 2006; 12(1):39-48.
113. Anderson R, Fassler R, Georges-Labouesse E et al. Mouse primordial germ cells lacking beta1 integrins enter the germline but fail to migrate normally to the gonads. Development 1999; 126(8):1655-1664.
114. De Felici M, Scaldaferri ML, Farini D. Adhesion molecules for mouse primordial germ cells. Front Biosci 2005; 10:542-551.
115. Pelliniemi LJ, Paranko J, Grund SK et al. Extracellular matrix in testicular differentiation. Ann NY Acad Sci 1984; 438:405-416.
116. Magre S, Jost A. Dissociation between testicular organogenesis and endocrine cytodifferentiation of Sertoli cells. Proc Natl Acad Sci USA 1984; 81(24):7831-7834.
117. Kuopio T, Paranko J, Pelliniemi LJ. Basement membrane and epithelial features of fetal-type Leydig cells in rat and human testis. Differentiation 1989; 40(3):198-206.
118. Kanai Y, Hayashi Y, Kawakami H et al. Effect of tunicamycin, an inhibitor of protein glycosylation, on testicular cord organization in fetal mouse gonadal explants in vitro. Anat Rec 1991; 230(2):199-208.
119. Mackay S. Gonadal development in mammals at the cellular and molecular levels. Int Rev Cytol 2000; 200:47-99.
120. Merchant-Larios H, Moreno-Mendoza N, Buehr M. The role of the mesonephros in cell differentiation and morphogenesis of the mouse fetal testis. Int J Dev Biol 1993; 37(3):407-415.
121. Capel B. The battle of the sexes. Mech Dev 2000; 92(1):89-103.
122. Paranko J. Expression of type I and III collagen during morphogenesis of fetal rat testis and ovary. Anat Rec 1987; 219(1):91-101.
123. Frojdman K, Paranko J, Kuopio T et al. Structural proteins in sexual differentiation of embryonic gonads. Int J Dev Biol 1989; 33(1):99-103.
124. Fridmacher V, Locquet O, Magre S. Differential expression of acidic cytokeratins 18 and 19 during sexual differentiation of the rat gonad. Development 1992; 115(2):503-517.
125. Frojdman K, Paranko J, Virtanen I et al. Intermediate filaments and epithelial differentiation of male rat embryonic gonad. Differentiation 1992; 50(2):113-123.
126. Pelliniemi LJ, Frojdman K. Structural and regulatory macromolecules in sex differentiation of gonads. J Exp Zool 2001; 290(5):523-528.
127. Griffin JK, Blecher SR. Extracellular matrix abnormalities in testis and epididymis of XXSxr ("sex-reversed") mice. Mol Reprod Dev 1994; 38(1):1-7.
128. Perera EM, Martin H, Seeherunvong T et al. Tescalcin, a novel gene encoding a putative EF-hand Ca(2+)-binding protein, Col9a3, and renin are expressed in the mouse testis during the early stages of gonadal differentiation. Endocrinology 2001; 142(1):455-163.
129. Mazaud S, Guyot R, Guigon CJ et al. Basal membrane remodeling during follicle histogenesis in the rat ovary: Contribution of proteinases of the MMP and PA families. Dev Biol 2005; 277(2):403-416.
130. Nef S, Schaad O, Stallings NR et al. Gene expression during sex determination reveals a robust female genetic program at the onset of ovarian development. Dev Biol 2005; 287(2):361-377.
131. Beverdam A, Koopman P. Expression profiling of purified mouse gonadal somatic cells during the critical time window of sex determination reveals novel candidate genes for human sexual dysgenesis syndromes. Hum Mol Genet 2006; 15(3):417-431.

132. Bitgood MJ, Shen L, McMahon AP. Sertoli cell signaling by Desert hedgehog regulates the male germline. Curr Biol 1996; 6(3):298-304.
133. Clark AM, Garland KK, Russell LD. Desert hedgehog (Dhh) gene is required in the mouse testis for formation of adult-type Leydig cells and normal development of peritubular cells and seminiferous tubules. Biol Reprod 2000; 63(6):1825-1838.
134. Pierucci-Alves F, Clark AM, Russell LD. A developmental study of the Desert hedgehog-null mouse testis. Biol Reprod 2001; 65(5):1392-1402.
135. Yao HH, Capel B. Disruption of testis cords by cyclopamine or forskolin reveals independent cellular pathways in testis organogenesis. Dev Biol 2002; 246(2):356-365.
136. Tung PS, Burdzy K, Fritz IB. Proteases are implicated in the changes in the Sertoli cell cytoskeleton elicited by follicle-stimulating hormone or by dibutyryl cyclic AMP. J Cell Physiol 1993; 155(1):139-148.
137. Skinner MK, Tung PS, Fritz IB. Cooperativity between Sertoli cells and testicular peritubular cells in the production and deposition of extracellular matrix components. J Cell Biol 1985; 100(6):1941-1947.
138. Hadley MA, Weeks BS, Kleinman HK et al. Laminin promotes formation of cord-like structures by Sertoli cells in vitro. Dev Biol 1990; 40(2):318-327.
139. Tung PS, Fritz IB. Role of laminin in the morphogenetic cascade during coculture of Sertoli cells with peritubular cells. J Cell Physiol 1994; 161(1):77-88.
140. van der Wee K, Hofmann MC. An in vitro tubule assay identifies HGF as a morphogen for the formation of seminiferous tubules in the postnatal mouse testis. Exp Cell Res 1999; 252(1):175-185.
141. Hager M, Gawlik K, Nystrom A et al. Laminin {alpha}1 chain corrects male infertility caused by absence of laminin {alpha}2 chain. Am J Pathol 2005; 167(3):823-833.
142. Lui WY, Mruk D, Lee WM et al. Sertoli cell tight junction dynamics: Their regulation during spermatogenesis. Biol Reprod 2003; 68(4):1087-1097.
143. Xia W, Mruk DD, Lee WM et al. Cytokines and junction restructuring during spermatogenesis—A lesson to learn from the testis. Cytokine Growth Factor Rev 2005; 16(4-5):469-493.
144. Penttila TL, Kaipia A, Toppari J et al. Localization of urokinase- and tissue-type plasminogen activator mRNAs in rat testes. Mol Cell Endocrinol 1994; 105(1):55-64.
145. Toppari J, Vihko KK, Rasanen KG et al. Regulation of stages VI and VIII of the rat seminiferous epithelial cycle in vitro. J Endocrinol 1986; 108(3):417-422.
146. Zhu LJ, Cheng CY, Phillips DM et al. The immunohistochemical localization of alpha 2-macroglobulin in rat testes is consistent with its role in germ cell movement and spermiation. J Androl 1994; 15:575-582.
147. Mruk D, Zhu LJ, Silvestrini B et al. Interactions of proteases and protease inhibitors in Sertoli-germ cell cocultures preceding the formation of specialized Sertoli-germ cell junctions in vitro. J Androl 1997; 18(6):612-622.
148. Wright WW, Zabludoff SD, Penttila TL et al. Germ cell-Sertoli cell interactions: Regulation by germ cells of the stage-specific expression of CP-2/cathepsin L mRNA by Sertoli cells. Dev Genet 1995; 16(2):104-113.
149. Zabludoff SD, Charron M, DeCerbo JN et al. Male germ cells regulate transcription of the cathepsin l gene by rat Sertoli cells. Endocrinology 2001; 142(6):2318-2327.
150. Braghiroli L, Silvestrini B, Sorrentino C et al. Regulation of alpha2-macroglobulin expression in rat Sertoli cells and hepatocytes by germ cells in vitro. Biol Reprod 1998; 59(1):111-123.
151. Wong CC, Chung SS, Grima J et al. Changes in the expression of junctional and nonjunctional complex component genes when inter-Sertoli tight junctions are formed in vitro. J Androl 2000; 21(2):227-237.
152. Mruk D, Cheng CY. Sertoli-Sertoli and Sertoli-germ cell interactions and their significance in germ cell movement in the seminiferous epithelium during spermatogenesis. Endocr Rev 2004; 25(5):747-806.
153. Regaud C. Etudes sur la structure des tubes séminifères et sur la spermatogenèse chez les mammifères. Arch Anat Microscop Morphol Exp 1901; 4:101-156, 231-280.
154. Roosen-Runge EC. Kinetics of spermatogenesis in mammals. Ann NY Acad Sci 1952; 55(4):574-584.
155. Sigillo F, Pernod G, Kolodie L et al. Residual bodies stimulate rat Sertoli cell plasminogen activator activity. Biochem Biophys Res Commun 1998; 250(1):59-62.
156. Pineau C, Le Magueresse B, Courtens JL et al. Study in vitro of the phagocytic function of Sertoli cells in the rat. Cell Tissue Res 1991; 264(3):589-598.
157. Gerard N, Syed V, Jegou B. Lipopolysaccharide, latex beads and residual bodies are potent activators of Sertoli cell interleukin-1 alpha production. Biochem Biophys Res Commun 1992; 185(1):154-161.

158. Syed V, Stephan JP, Gerard N et al. Residual bodies activate Sertoli cell interleukin-1α (IL-1α) release, which triggers IL-6 production by an autocrine mechanism, through the lipoxygenase pathway. Endocrinology 1995; 136(7):3070-3078.
159. Sharpe RM, Maddocks S, Millar M et al. Testosterone and spermatogenesis. Identification of stage-specific, androgen-regulated proteins secreted by adult rat seminiferous tubules. J Androl 1992; 13(2):172-184.
160. O'Donnell L, McLachlan RI, Wreford NG et al. Testosterone withdrawal promotes stage-specific detachment of round spermatids from the rat seminiferous epithelium. Biol Reprod 1996; 55(4):895-901.
161. Zirkin BR. Spermatogenesis: Its regulation by testosterone and FSH. Semin Cell Dev Biol 1998; 9(4):417-421.
162. Hill CM, Anway MD, Zirkin BR et al. Intratesticular androgen levels, androgen receptor localization, and androgen receptor expression in adult rat Sertoli cells. Biol Reprod 2004; 71(4):1348-1358.
163. Ailenberg M, McCabe D, Fritz IB. Androgens inhibit plasminogen activator activity secreted by Sertoli cells in culture in a two-chambered assembly. Endocrinology 1990; 126(3):1561-1568.
164. Uhrin P, Dewerchin M, Hilpert M et al. Disruption of the protein C inhibitor gene results in impaired spermatogenesis and male infertility. J Clin Invest 2000; 106(12):1531-1539.
165. Gow A, Southwood CM, Li JS et al. CNS myelin and Sertoli cell tight junction strands are absent in Osp/claudin-11 null mice. Cell 1999; 99(6):649-659.
166. Meng J, Holdcraft RW, Shima JE et al. Androgens regulate the permeability of the blood-testis barrier. Proc Natl Acad Sci USA 2005; 102(46):16696-16700.
167. Gye MC. Changes in the expression of claudins and transepithelial electrical resistance of mouse Sertoli cells by Leydig cell coculture. Int J Androl 2003; 26:271-278.
168. Florin A, Maire M, Bozec A et al. Androgens and postmeiotic germ cells regulate claudin-11 expression in rat Sertoli cells. Endocrinology 2005; 146(3):1532-1540.
169. Miyamori H, Takino T, Kobayashi Y et al. Claudin promotes activation of pro-matrix metalloproteinase-2 mediated by membrane-type matrix metalloproteinases. J Biol Chem 2001; 276(30):28204-28211.
170. Diaz ES, Pellizzari E, Meroni S et al. Effect of extracellular matrix proteins on in vitro testosterone production by rat Leydig cells. Mol Reprod Dev 2002; 61(4):493-503.
171. Diaz ES, Pellizzari E, Casanova M et al. Type IV collagen induces downregulation of steroidogenic response to gonadotropins in adult rat Leydig cells involving mitogen-activated protein kinase. Mol Reprod Dev 2005; 72(2):208-215.
172. Leask A, Abraham DJ. TGF-β signaling and the fibrotic response. FASEB J 2004; 18(7):816-827.
173. Dickson C, Webster DR, Johnson H et al. Transforming growth factor-β effects on morphology of immature rat Leydig cells. Mol Cell Endocrinol 2002; 195(1-2):65-77.
174. Gnessi L, Fabbri A, Spera G. Gonadal peptides as mediators of development and functional control of the testis: An integrated system with hormones and local environment. Endocr Rev 1997; 18(4):541-609.
175. Carmeliet P, Kieckens L, Schoonjans L et al. Plasminogen activator inhibitor-1 gene-deficient mice. I. Generation by homologous recombination and characterization. J Clin Invest 1993; 92(6):2746-2755.
176. Nothnick WB, Soloway PD, Curry TEJ. Pattern of messenger ribonucleic acid expression of tissue inhibitors of metalloproteinases (TIMPs) during testicular maturation in male mice lacking a functional TIMP-1 gene. Biol Reprod 1998; 59(2):364-370.
177. Wright WW, Smith L, Kerr C et al. Mice that express enzymatically inactive cathepsin L exhibit abnormal spermatogenesis. Biol Reprod 2003; 68:680-687.
178. Holmbeck K, Bianco P, Caterina J et al. MT1-MMP-deficient mice develop dwarfism, osteopenia, arthritis, and connective tissue disease due to inadequate collagen turnover. Cell 1999; 99(1):81-92.
179. Murer V, Spetz JF, Hengst U et al. Male fertility defects in mice lacking the serine protease inhibitor protease nexin-1. Proc Natl Acad Sci USA 2001; 98(6):3029-3033.
180. Toyama Y, Maekawa M, Kadomatsu K et al. Histological characterization of defective spermatogenesis in mice lacking the basigin gene. Anat Histol Embryol 1999; 28:205-213.
181. Maekawa M, Suzuki-Toyota F, Toyama Y et al. Stage-specific localization of basigin, a member of the immunoglobulin superfamily, during mouse spermatogenesis. Arch Histol Cytol 1998; 61(5):405-415.
182. Li SW, Arita M, Fertala A et al. Transgenic mice with inactive alleles for procollagen N-proteinase (ADAMTS-2) develop fragile skin and male sterility. Biochem J 2001; 355(Pt 2):271-278.
183. Rudolph-Owen LA, Cannon P, Matrisian LM. Overexpression of the matrix metalloproteinase matrilysin results in premature mammary gland differentiation and male infertility. Mol Biol Cell 1998; 9:421-435.

CHAPTER 9

Antioxidant Systems and Oxidative Stress in the Testes

R. John Aitken* and Shaun D. Roman

Introduction

Spermatogenesis is an extremely active replicative process capable of generating approximately 1,000 sperm a second. The high rates of cell division inherent in this process imply correspondingly high rates of mitochondrial oxygen consumption by the germinal epithelium. However, the poor vascularization of the testes means that oxygen tensions in this tissue are low[1] and that competition for this vital element within the testes is extremely intense. Since both spermatogenesis[2] and Leydig cell steroidogenesis[3,4] are vulnerable to oxidative stress, the low oxygen tension that characterizes this tissue may be an important component of the mechanisms by which the testes protects itself from free radical-mediated damage. In addition, the testes contain an elaborate array of antioxidant enzymes and free radical scavengers to ensure that the twin spermatogenic and steroidogenic functions of this organ are not impacted by oxidative stress. These antioxidant defence systems are of major importance because peroxidative damage is currently regarded as the single most important cause of impaired testicular function underpinning the pathological consequences of a wide range of conditions from testicular torsion to diabetes and xenobiotic exposure. This chapter sets out the specific nature of these antioxidant defence systems and also reviews the factors that have been found to impair their activity, precipitating a state of oxidative stress in the testes and impairing the latter's ability to produce viable spermatozoa capable of initiating and supporting embryonic development.

Antioxidant Enzymes

Despite the low oxygen tensions that characterize the testicular micro-environment, this tissue remains vulnerable to oxidative stress due to the abundance of highly unsaturated fatty acids (particularly 20:4 and 22:6) and the presence of potential reactive oxygen species (ROS)-generating systems. ROS generation can be from the mitochondria and a variety of enzymes including the xanthine- and NADPH- oxidases,[5,6] and the cytochrome P450s.[7] These enzymes specialize in the professional generation of ROS or produce these toxic metabolites as an inadvertent consequence of their biochemical activity. In order to address this risk, the testes have developed a sophisticated array of antioxidant systems comprising both enzymatic and non-enzymatic constituents. Concerning the enzymatic constituents of this defence system, the induction of oxidative stress in the testes precipitates a response characterized by the NF-κB mediated induction of mRNA species for superoxide dismutase (SOD), glutathione peroxi-

*Corresponding Author: R. John Aitken—ARC Centre of Excellence in Biotechnology and Development, Discipline of Biological Sciences, University of Newcastle, Callaghan, NSW 2308, Australia. Email: john.aitken@newcastle.edu.au

Molecular Mechanisms in Spermatogenesis, edited by C. Yan Cheng. ©2008 Landes Bioscience and Springer Science+Business Media.

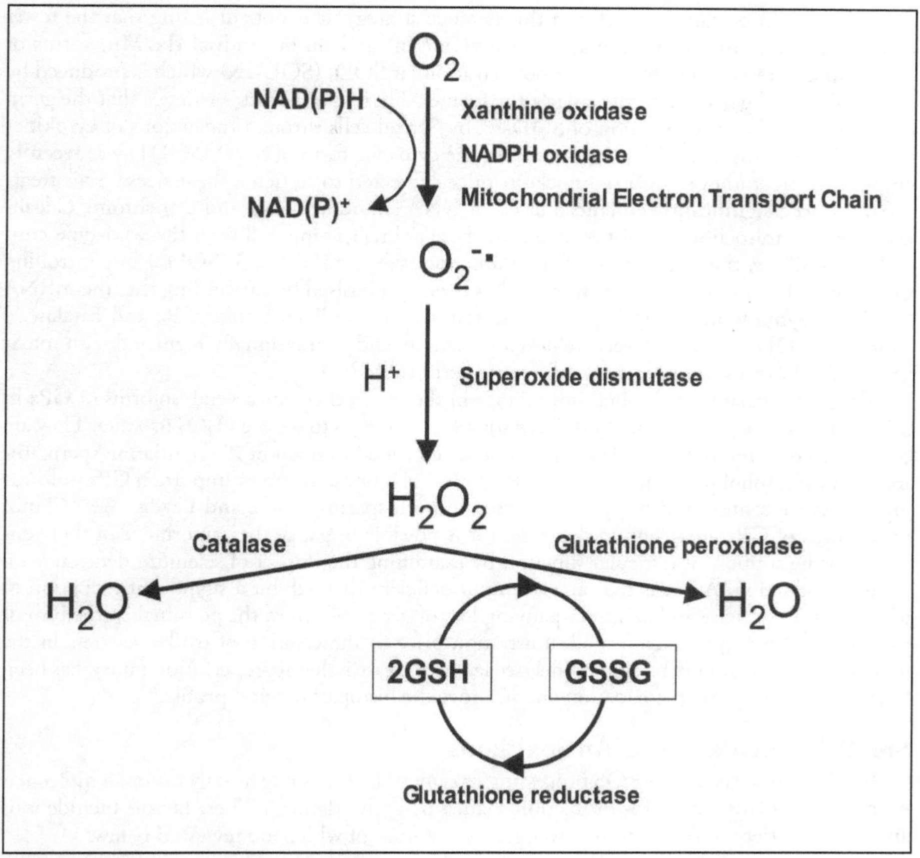

Figure 1. Major pathways of reactive oxygen species generation and metabolism. Superoxide can be generated by specialized enzymes, such as the xanthine or NADPH oxidases, or as a by-product of cellular metabolism, particularly the mitochondrial electron transport chain. Superoxide dismutase then converts the superoxide to hydrogen peroxide which has to be rapidly removed from the system. This is generally achieved by catalase or peroxidases, such as the glutathione peroxidases which use reduced glutathione (GSH) as the electron donor.

dase (GPx) and glutathione-S-transferase (GST) activities.[8] The fundamental biochemistry of these antioxidant enzymes is summarized in (Fig. 1) and involves the rapid conversion of superoxide anion ($O_2^{-\cdot}$) to hydrogen peroxide (H_2O_2) in the presence of SOD in order to prevent the former from participating in the formation of highly pernicious hydroxyl radicals. The H_2O_2 generated in this manner is a powerful membrane permeant oxidant in its own right that has to be rapidly eliminated from the cell in order to prevent the induction of oxidative damage to lipids, proteins and DNA. The elimination of H_2O_2 is either effected by catalase or glutathione peroxidase, with the latter predominating in the case of the testes.[9,10] GST on the other hand involves a large and complex family of proteins that catalyse the conjugation of reduced glutathione via the sulfhydryl group to electrophilic centres on a wide variety of substrates in preparation for excretion from the cell. This activity is critical in the detoxification of peroxidised lipids as well as the metabolism of xenobiotics.

Given the importance of SOD in this defence strategy, it is not surprising that the testes contain not only the conventional cytosolic (Cu/Zn) and mitochondrial (Fe/Mn) forms of SOD but also feature an unusual form of extracellular SOD, (SOD-Ex) which is produced by both Sertoli and germ cells, particularly the former. There is also some evidence that the germ cells may stimulate the secretion of SOD-Ex by Sertoli cells through the actions of cytokines such as interleukin-1α.[11] The importance of the cytosolic form of SOD (SOD1) was recently emphasised in studies of SOD1-knockout mice subjected to testicular heat stress. This treatment induced significantly enhanced levels of DNA strand breakage and cytochrome C leakage from the mitochondria of germ cells in these animals compared with the wild-type controls.[12] Similarly, the importance of the mitochondrial form of SOD (SOD2) in controlling $O_2^{-\cdot}$ leakage from testicular mitochondria has been emphasised by the finding that the mRNA for this enzyme is markedly higher in the testes than the liver, unlike GPx and catalase.[13] Moreover, SOD-2 mRNA levels are developmentally and translationally regulated with maximal levels of expression in early post-meiotic germ cells.[13]

Although catalase is of limited importance in the testes, there are several isoforms of GPx in this tissue that use glutathione (GSH) as a source of electrons to reduce H_2O_2 to water. They are concentrated in the mitochondria, nucleus and acrosomal domain of differentiating spermatozoa.[14] The phospholipid hydroperoxide GPx (PHGPx) is one of the most important GPx isoforms in a testicular context and is highly expressed in both spermatogenic and Leydig cells.[15] Since most forms of GPx are selenium dependent it is possible to gauge the importance of these enzymes in the support of testicular function by examining the impact of selenium deficiency on male reproduction. Animals fed on a selenium deficient diet exhibit a significant reduction of testicular GPx activity and an accompanying loss of germ cells from the germinal epithelium of the testes.[16] Moreover, selenium administration prior to the creation of oxidative stress in the testes using the torsion/detorsion model (see later) to create ischemia-reperfusion injury, has been found to suppress lipid peroxidation and improve the histopathological profile.[17]

Small Molecular Mass Antioxidants

In addition to the major ROS processing enzymes, the testes rely heavily on small molecular weight antioxidant factors for protection against oxidative damage. These factors include ions and a wide variety of free radical scavengers, the nature of which are reviewed below.

Zinc

Zinc is an acknowledged antioxidant factor that as well as being a core constituent of free radical scavenging enzymes such as SOD and a recognized protector of sulfhydryl groups, is also thought to impair lipid peroxidation by displacing transition metals such as iron and copper from catalytic sites.[18] In keeping with such a central antioxidant role, this element has a profound effect on the level of oxidative stress experienced by the testes. Thus rats fed a zinc deficient diet experience a decrease in testicular antioxidant potential and a concomitant increase of lipid peroxidation in this tissue.[19] Conversely, zinc administration will counteract the oxidative stress created in the testes by exposure to lead.[20-21] as well as the peroxidative damage induced by ischemia-reperfusion as a consequence testicular torsion-detorsion.[22] Zinc administration has also been shown to attenuate the testicular oxidative DNA damage induced by cadmium as well as the decline in sperm production and testosterone secretion induced by this heavy metal.[23]

Vitamins C and E

It has been recognized since the 1940s that vitamin E (α-tocopherol) is a powerful lipophilic antioxidant that is absolutely vital for the maintenance of mammalian spermatogenesis.[24] It is present in particularly high amounts in Sertoli cells and pachytene spermatocytes and to a lesser extent round spermatids.[25] Vitamin C (ascorbic acid) also contributes to the support of spermatogenesis at least in part through its capacity to reduce α-tocopherol and maintain this antioxidant in an active state. Vitamin C is itself maintained in a reduced state by a GSH-dependent dehydroascorbate reductase, which is abundant in the testes.[26] Deficiencies of vitamins C or E leads to a state of oxidative stress in the testes that disrupts both spermatogenesis and the production of testosterone.[24] Conversely, ascorbate administration to normal animals stimulates both sperm production and testosterone secretion.[27] This vitamin also counteracts the testicular oxidative stress induced by exposure to pro-oxidants such as arsenic, PCBs (Arochlor 1254), cadmium, endosulfan and alcohol.[28-32] Furthermore, endogenous ascorbate levels decrease dramatically when oxidative stress is induced in the testes by, for example, chronic exposure to lead, chromium, cadmium or aflatoxin.[33-25] Vitamin E has also been shown to suppress lipid peroxidation in testicular microsomes and mitochondria[36,37] and to reverse the detrimental effects of oxidative stress on testicular function mediated by exposure to such factors as ozone, iron overload, intensive exercise or exposure to aflatoxin, PCB, cyclophosphamide and formaldehyde.[28,32,33,38-42] Furthermore testicular vitamin E levels have also been shown to fall significantly when oxidative stress is induced by exposure to pro-oxidant stimuli such as chromium.[34]

Melatonin and Cytochrome C

The pineal hormone melatonin (N -acetyl, 5-methoxytryptamine) also plays a major role in protecting the testes from oxidative stress, given the significant stimulatory effect of pinealectomy on the oxidative damage recorded in the testes as a consequence of induced hyperthyroidism.[43] Melatonin has two major attributes that set it apart from most other antioxidants. Firstly, it undergoes a two electron oxidation when acting as antioxidant, rather than the one electron oxidation favoured by many free radical scavengers. As a result, this compound cannot redox cycle and inadvertently generate free radicals. Secondly, melatonin is readily soluble in both lipid and aqueous environments and can readily cross the blood-testes barrier to protect the germinal epithelium. Melatonin levels in seminal plasma are depressed in infertile patients exhibiting poor motility, leukocytospermia, varicocele and non-obstructive azoospermia, all of which are conditions associated with oxidative stress in the male tract.[44] Moreover, the intraperitoneal injection of melatonin has been shown to alleviate oxidative stress in the testes following the experimental induction of a left sided varicocele.[45]

Another small molecular mass free radical scavenger that has recently been shown to play a major role in reducing H_2O_2 is a testes-specific form of cytochrome C. This cytochrome C isoform is also a powerful activator of apoptosis, providing additional protection to the testes by virtue of its ability to facilitate the depletion of damaged germ cells.[46]

Disruption of the Antioxidant Status of the Testes

Notwithstanding the antioxidant protection afforded to the testes in order to support its dual functions of steroidogenesis and sperm production, a wide variety of endogenous and exogenous factors are known to perturb these defences and generate a state of oxidative stress. In the following section, some of these factors are reviewed.

Cryptorchidism

The elevated temperatures associated with experimental cryptorchidism are associated with oxidative stress in the testes and a reduction in SOD and catalase activities.[47] Consistent with these findings, direct exposure of spermatogenic cells to elevated temperatures was found to induce high rates of apoptosis via mechanisms that were associated with elevated levels of H_2O_2 generation and could be ameliorated by the addition of catalase.[48] Moreover the consequence of heat stress on spermatogenic cells was exacerbated in SOD1-knock out mice via mechanisms that could be reversed by the addition of Tiron, a superoxide anion radical scavenger.[49] The clinical significance of this finding can be seen in the high levels of DNA damage and ROS generation seen in the spermatozoa of patients with a history of cryptorchidism.[50]

Testicular Torsion

Testicular torsion is a relatively common, painful condition that must be treated rapidly if the testes are not to suffer permanent damage. Prolonged torsion leads to testicular ischaemia and high levels of oxidative stress in the ipsilateral testes associated with NO and H_2O_2 production, increased lipid peroxide formation, isoprostane accumulation, antioxidant enzyme depletion and increased rates of mitochondria-mediated apoptosis in the germ line.[51-53] Even short periods of ischaemia, for 3 hours or less, can lead to a high levels of oxidative stress in the testes, depletion of testicular glutathione levels and the consequent disruption of spermatogenesis. Significantly, the level of peroxidative damage observed in testicular tissue increases following detorsion, indicating the induction of reperfusion injury.[54] The biochemical basis for reperfusion injury is thought to involve a key metabolic enzyme, xanthine dehydrogenase, which becomes converted to a xanthine oxidase during ischaemia, due to oxidation of essential -SH groups and/or a limited proteolytic clip. As soon as the tissue is reperfused with blood, the xanthine oxidase is suddenly presented with oxidizable substrate in the form of xanthine/hypoxanthine and starts to generate copious amounts of ROS. The latter then induce high levels of peroxidative damage via mechanisms that are enhanced by the local release of transition metals. Although this scheme of events was developed to explain the tissue injury associated with conditions such as myocardial infarction, it also applies to the testicular injury associated with torsion-detorsion. The general notion that the testicular damage precipitated by temporary ischaemia is associated with oxidative stress is supported by the sudden induction of lipid peroxidation and the concomitant suppression of endogenous antioxidant activities including SOD, catalase and glutathione peroxidase.[17,55-57] In addition, the tissue injury induced by testicular torsion/detorsion can be dramatically alleviated by pretreatment with exogenous antioxidants such as selenium, resveratrol, L-carnitine, caffeic acid phenethyl ester and garlic extract.[17,57-60] Finally the enzyme purportedly associated with reperfusion injury, xanthine oxidase, can be inhibited by allopurinol and the latter is known to reduce the testicular damage associated with testicular torsion.[56] Notwithstanding the importance of xanthine oxidase-mediated oxidative stress it should also be noted that neutrophil infiltration into the testes following torsion may represent yet another source of uncontrolled free radical generation responsible for mediating the pathophysiological consequences of temporary testicular ischaemia.[61]

One of the major issues associated with the clinical management of unilateral testicular torsion is whether the ipsilateral testis should be removed in order to preserve the contralateral testis. In animal models prolonged testicular torsion results in excessive ROS generation, depletion of antioxidant enzymes and the appearance of oxidative damage in the contralateral testes.[62-64] In light of these data, surgical removal of the ipsilateral testes would seem warranted if the period of ischaemia has been extensive.

Varicocele

The impaired venous drainage to the testes seen with varicocele is also associated with the disruption of spermatogenesis via mechanisms involving the induction of oxidative stress. In clinical studies, the presence of a varicocele has been shown to correlate with excess ROS generation by the spermatozoa, high rates of DNA damage in these cells and depleted antioxidant levels in the seminal plasma.[65-67] In a recent study, surgical correction of left sided varicocele was shown to significantly improve sperm concentration, total count, morphology and motility in concert with significant improvements in the antioxidant status of the spermatozoa and seminal plasma.[68] This reduction in oxidative stress secondary to varicocele excision was accompanied by a reduction in both protein carbonyl expression and DNA damage in the spermatozoa.[68] Independent studies have also shown that the testicular expression of 4-hydroxy-2-nonenal modified proteins (another marker of oxidative stress) is significantly higher in patients that responded positively to varicocelectomy, suggesting that surgical treatments are capable of reducing oxidative stress in the testes.[69] Immunocytochemical analyses of 8-hydroxy-2'-deoxyguanosine expression in the testes of varicocele patients also revealed particularly high levels of oxidative DNA damage in the spermatogonia and spermatocytes that correlated well with the severity of the varicosity.[70] The general concept that testicular pathologies associated with varicocele are linked with the induction of oxidative stress has been confirmed in animal models. Thus, creation of experimental bilateral varicocele in rats is associated with increases in lipid peroxidation and NO generation and a corresponding decrease in testicular antioxidant status.[71] Moreover, the pathological consequences of experimental varicocele induction can be significantly reversed by the concomitant administration of an antioxidant, melatonin.[45]

The site of free radical generation in varicocele patients is still open to conjecture. On the one hand, enhanced free radical generation by the spermatozoa and/or precursor germ cells has been repeatedly suggested,[65,72,73] on the other, there is evidence to suggest that excess free radical generation may involve the spermatic vein itself.[74] The excess generation of free radicals by the spermatozoa may be an indirect consequence of impaired spermatogenesis/epididymal function resulting in the retention of excess residual cytoplasm. The presence of excess cytoplasm has been positively correlated with the generation of ROS by human spermatozoa, via mechanisms involving the facilitated supply NADPH to oxidases in the sperm plasma membrane.[75] These enzymes, including NOX5 and DUOX, both of which have been identified in human spermatozoa,[5,76] are normally deprived of sufficient NADPH to drive free radical generation; what hexose monophosphate shunt activity there is, being largely devoted to the maintenance of glutathione reductase activity.[77] However, when excess residual cytoplasm is present the limited substrate availability is no longer an issue and free radical generation can be initiated. The relevance of this model to the oxidative stress detected in cases of varicocele is clearly suggested by the effects of varicocelectomy. Thus, not only do the spermatozoa produced by such patients exhibit high levels of ROS in association with cytoplasmic retention but also surgical correction of this condition both prevents cytoplasmic retention and suppresses ROS generation.[73,78,79] A causative association between these events therefore seems likely.

Hyperthyroidism

The induction of hyperthyroidism in rats is associated with oxidative stress in the testes as reflected by increased lipid peroxidation, elevated GSH levels and induction of antioxidant enzymes. The oxidative stress appears to be associated with a thyroxine dependent increase in mitochondrial activity and concomitant leakage of electrons from the mitochondrial electron transport chain.[80,81] The oxidative stress precipitated by hyperthyroidism can be exacerbated by pinealectomy removing melatonin, an important testicular antioxidant, from the redox equation.[43] These data resonate with clinical studies indicating that hyperthyroidism is associated with poor semen quality, particularly impaired motility, that normalize when the patients' thyroid dysfunction is corrected and euthyroidism established.[82] It should also be noted that hypothyroidism can induce oxidative stress in the testes as reflected by enhanced levels of H_2O_2 production and increased carbonyl generation.[83] Clearly, normal testicular function is highly dependent on a functional thyroid system.

Diabetes

Experimental induction of diabetes in animal models has been shown to impair testicular function and decrease male fertility. Thus, diabetogens such as streptozotocin, enhance ROS generation and induce both lipid peroxidation and protein carbonyl expression in the testes. Moreover the oxidative stress associated with the diabetic condition is associated with DNA damage in the male germ line and high rates of embryonic loss in mated females (dominant lethal effect). These effects could be attenuated by the administration of antioxidants such as ascorbic acid, melatonin, taurine or an herbal mixture containing extracts from *Musa paradisiaca, Tamarindus indica, Eugenia jambolana* and *Coccinia indica*.[84-86] In light of recent data showing an increased level of DNA damage in the spermatozoa of diabetic patients compared with non-diabetic controls,[87] causative links between diabetes, oxidative stress in the male germ line and DNA damage appears both likely and clinically, extremely important.

Infection

Another factor that may cause oxidative stress in the testes is infection. Experimental models of infection, involving the intraperitoneal injection of bacterial lipopolysaccharide (LPS), induced lipid peroxidation in the testes and rapidly depleted this tissue of antioxidant enzyme activity in the form of SOD, catalase and the glutathione peroxidase-reductase couple. This oxidative stress was associated with the transient generation of pro-inflammatory mediators such as interleukin 1β, inducible nitric oxide synthase and cyclo-oxygenase-2.[88] The same experimental infection model has also been used to demonstrate the particular sensitivity of Leydig cell steroidogenesis to oxidative stress induced by bacterial LPS. In these studies, the oxidative stress induced by LPS stimulated lipid peroxidation in Leydig cell membranes as well as significant reductions in steroidogenic acute regulatory protein (StAR) and 3β-hydroxysteroid dehydrogenase isomerase (3β-HSD) activity. Moreover, these effects were associated with the disruption of Leydig cell mitochondrial function and, specifically, the inhibition of StAR-mediated cholesterol transfer activity.[89]

Physical Exertion

Physical exercise has been shown to up-regulate antioxidant activities in the testes of aging rats and may represent a practical way in which the detrimental effects of age on testicular function can be ameliorated.[90] A similar case could be argued for the ability of moderate exercise to ameliorate the degree of oxidative damage inflicted on the testes by chronic ethanol ingestion.[91] However, excess exercise can have the opposite effect, causing oxidative stress in the testes and generating high levels of lipid peroxidation in association with significant declines in the activities of key antioxidant enzymes including SOD, catalase, GST and GPx.[92] Such stress has a significant inhibitory effect on the both steroidogenesis and germ cell differentiation within the testes. The fact that these effects can be reversed by the administration of an antioxidant, α-tocopherol succinate, confirms the importance of oxidative stress in the aetiology of such exercise-dependent testicular dysfunction.[40]

Reproductive Hormone Imbalance

The immediate endocrine environment of the testes has a major impact on the antioxidant status of this organ. Treatments including exposure to cyclophosphamide or dimethane sulfonate that diminish the intratesticular concentration of testosterone, inhibit the testicular expression of antioxidant enzymes such as GPx, SOD and catalase.[93,94] Furthermore, these suppressive effects on antioxidant expression, as well as the disruption of spermatogenesis, can be reversed by the administration of exogenous gonadotrophin to artificially elevate intratesticular testosterone levels.[94,95] Suppression of intratesticular testosterone with exogenous steroids, including both androgens and estrogens, similarly results in the suppression of antioxidant enzyme expression, a concomitant increase in peroxidative damage, the disruption of spermatogenesis and an increase in germ cell apoptosis.[95-97] Intriguingly, the suppression of antioxidant activity in response to exogenous steroid treatment largely affects the Leydig cells that contain most of the catalase and GPx activities. Testicular SOD activities that are largely confined to the seminiferous tubules did not change dramatically under these circumstances.[95] It is therefore possible that the site of free radical generation in response to gonadotrophin withdrawal involves electron leakage from the inhibited steroidogenic pathway of the Leydig cells. These free radicals then attack the germ cells within the seminiferous tubules leading to extensive apoptosis and the disruption of spermatogenesis. The fact that aminoglutethimide, an inhibitor of the P450 cholesterol side-chain cleavage, induces extensive lipid peroxidation in the testis supports this contention.[95] Interestingly, over-stimulation of the Leydig cells by chronic exposure to hCG (100 IU/day for 30 days in rats) also stimulates high levels of ROS production from these cells, that in turn stimulate lipid peroxidation, reduction in antioxidant enzyme activities, germ cell apoptosis and the consequential disruption of spermatogenesis.[98] Thus, as we saw with the involvement of the thyroid gland in the control of testicular function,

Table 1. Impact of antioxidants on testicular damage caused by testicular torsion/detorsion

Antioxidant	Outcome	Ref.	Antioxidant	Outcome	Ref.
Garlic extract	⇓MDA ⇓XO ⇑histopathology	57	Pentoxifylline	⇓MDA ⇓ Germ cell apoptosis	159
Caffeic acid phenethyl ester	⇓MDA ⇑histopathology ⇑GPx	186	Erdostein	⇓MDA ⇑GPx ⇑Catalase ⇑histopathology	160
Caffeic acid phenethyl ester	⇓MDA ⇓MPO ⇓iNOS ⇑histopathology	60	Resveratrol	⇓Germ cell apoptosis	58
N-acetylcysteine	⇓MDA ⇑GPx	158	Dexpathenol	⇑histopathology	161
Morphine	⇓MDA ⇑GPx ⇑SOD ⇑ Catalase	187	L-carnitine	⇓MDA ⇑histopathology	59
			Propofol	⇑histopathology	162

MDA = malondialdehyde; XO = xanthine oxidase; GPx = glutathione peroxidase; MPO = myeloperoxidase; iNOS = inducible nitric oxide synthase.

a stable redox environment depends on an appropriately balanced gonadotrophic support, either hyper- or hypo- gonadotrophism will induce a state of oxidative stress in the testis.

Retinoids

While fluctuations in Leydig cell steroidogenesis may be one source of free radical generation in the testes, another is the Sertoli cell population. The latter has been shown to generate ROS following stimulation with all trans-retinoic acid (RA), a vital cofactor for spermatogenesis. Exposure of rat Sertoli cells to RA led to activation of ROS generation, lipid peroxidation and, ultimately, a loss of cell viability.[99] There is also some evidence to suggest that retinol might stimulate ROS generation in rat Sertoli cells[99,100] and that this effect is accompanied by an up-regulation of testicular antioxidant enzymes including SOD, GPx and catalase.[101] There may be nothing particularly specific about this effect since retinoids have been shown to stimulate ROS generation in a variety of other cellular systems.[102] Nevertheless, the free radical generation triggered by retinoids in the testes may explain the testicular degeneration induced by hypervitaminosis A in the rat[103] and the association between excess beta carotene intake and infertility in human males.[104]

Impact of Xenobiotics

A wide variety of different xenobiotics have also been shown to induce oxidative stress in the testes in concert with the suppression of antioxidant mechanisms. A summary of these testicular toxicants is provided in Table 2. Heavy paternal smoking, for example, is known to

Table 2. List of compounds capable of inducing oxidative stress in the testes

Compound	Ref.	Compound	Ref.
Smoking	2, 105-107	Nonylphenol	132-134
Alcohol	108-111	Adriamycin	135
Chromic acid	34, 113	Cisplatin	136-137
Iron	114,115	Cyclophosphamide	138-140
Lead	35	Hexachlorocyclohexane	141-142
Cadmium	116	Trinitrotoluene	143
Uranium	118	Aflatoxin	144
Arsenic	119	Lindane	145
Vanadate	120	Quinalphos	146
Phthalate esters	121,122	Endosulfan	147
Sulfur dioxide	123	Diethyl maleate	148
Sodium fluoride	124	Monensin	149
PCB/PCN	2,39, 125-127	Formaldehyde	150
Methoxychlor	128,129	Alloxan	151,152
Bisphenol A	1,130,131	Streptozotocin	86
		Acrylamide	153
		Ozone	154

MDA = malondialdehyde; XO = xanthine oxidase; GPx = glutathione peroxidase; MPO = myeloperoxidase; iNOS = inducible nitric oxide synthase.

generate oxidative DNA damage in the male germ line in association with a 32% reduction in the α-tocopherol content of the seminal plasma.[105] The role of oxidative stress in the genesis of this DNA damage is supported by the observation that in individuals subjected to an ascorbate depleted diet, the seminal plasma ascorbate levels decreased by a half, while DNA damage levels in the spermatozoa increased by 91%. Repletion of the ascorbate levels in the diet had the reverse effect and decreased DNA damage by 36%.[106] Experimental exposure of rats to cigarette smoke also induces lipid peroxidation in the testes in association with disturbances in testicular antioxidant enzyme activity.[2] The testicular damage induced by cigarette smoke exposure in rats is certainly oxidative in nature because it can be reversed by concomitant exposure to an antioxidant (caffeic acid phenethyl ester).[107]

In addition to smoking, excessive alcohol consumption also has a negative effect of testicular function through the induction of oxidative stress and the concomitant disruption of testicular antioxidant status.[108,109] Furthermore, the ability of antioxidants such as vitamin C or lecithin to ameliorate this pathology, confirms the importance of oxidative stress in this context.[110-111] In addition to inducing low sperm counts and poor sperm motility, it also appears that the oxidative stress created in the Leydig cells as a consequence of chronic alcohol exposure diminishes the steroidogenic capacity of the testes, lowering circulating testosterone levels.[112]

Table 2 also highlights a number of metals that are known to induce oxidative stress in the testes and compromise male infertility. Chromium, for example, is a testicular toxicant that stimulates lipid peroxidation and suppresses antioxidant enzyme activities as well as ascorbate levels in the testes.[113] Additional studies in monkeys have also shown that chromium administration decreases not only inhibit the classical array of antioxidant enzymes in the testes but also diminishes the testicular content of GSH as well as vitamins A,E and C, while H_2O_2 production and hydroxyl radical formation are increased.[34] Additional transition metals such as iron also induce lipid peroxidation, protein carbonyl expression and lipid soluble antioxidant depletion in testicular tissue with the consequent disruption of spermatogenesis.[114,115] Significantly, iron intoxication of male mice also induces a dominant lethal effect characterized by high levels of embryonic loss in females mated to iron-exposed males. In this situation, the oxidative stress induced in the testes by acute iron overload must have so damaged the DNA in the spermatozoa that the resulting embryos were non-viable.

Heavy metals such as lead, cadmium and uranium have a similar effect on the testes disrupting spermatogenesis via mechanisms that involved the induction of lipid peroxidation, depletion of ROS scavengers and disruption of testicular antioxidant enzyme activity.[35,116-118] Arsenic has also been shown to induce peroxidative damage in the testes elevating protein carbonyl expression and decreasing tissue GSH content and inhibiting 3β- and 17β-hydroxysteroid dehydrogenase activities. The importance of oxidative stress in the testicular toxicity associated with arsenic was emphasised by the ability of ascorbate to reverse these changes.[119] Similarly, vanadate is a testicular toxicant that induces lipid peroxidation in the testes along with significant suppression of testicular SOD and catalase and the disruption of 3β- and 17β- hydroxysteroid dehydrogenase activities.[120]

In addition to the above, Table 2 lists a wide variety of different industrial and environmental toxicants that are all capable of compromising male fertility by inducing a state of oxidative stress in the testes. These compounds include phthalate esters,[121,122] sulfur dioxide,[123] sodium fluoride,[124] a range of environmental estrogens (e.g., PCBs,[2,39,125-127] methoxychlor,[128,129] bisphenol A[130,131] nonylphenol[132]), chemotherapeutic agents (e.g., adriamycin,[135] cisplatin[136,137] cyclophosphamide[138-140]) hexachlorocyclohexane,[141-142] 2,4,6-trinitrotoluene,[143] aflatoxin,[144] lindane,[145] quinalphos[146] endosulfan,[147] diethyl maleate,[148] monensin,[149] formaldehyde,[150] alloxan,[151,152] streptozotocin,[86] acrylamide[153] and ozone.[154] In addition to this list of xenobiotic chemicals that can induce oxidative stress in the testes, physical factors such as static magnetic fields[155] and electromagnetic radiation in its various forms from heat[12,156] to X-ray[157] irradiation, can also trigger a state of oxidative stress in testicular tissue. Given the variety and prevalence of chemical and physical factors that can generate oxidative stress in the male gonad, there is an urgent need to identify antioxidants that can supplement the tissue's own antioxidant strategies to rescue the testes from the consequences of ROS attack.

Antioxidant Therapy

In order to determine the relative potential of different antioxidants to address oxidative stress in the testes, the testicular torsion-detorsion model has been repeatedly used. Typically this model involves the application of antioxidant therapy prior to the creation of a brief period of oxidative stress and subsequent comparison of various testicular attributes (lipid peroxidation, histopathology, DNA damage or antioxidant enzyme status) with sham operated controls (Table 1). Such analyses have recorded significant protection against oxidative stress for factors as garlic extract,[57] caffeic acid phenethyl ester (CAPE),[60] N-acetyl cysteine,[158] pentoxifylline,[159] erdostein,[160] resveratrol,[58] dexpathenol,[161] L-carnitine,[59] and propofol anaesthetic.[162]

A variety of antioxidants have also been assessed for their ability to counteract oxidative stress in the testes created by alternative mechanisms. For example: (1) CAPE has been shown to protect the testes from the oxidative stress created by exposure to dizocilpine (MK-801), a drug that is commonly used to induce schizophrenia,[163] and cigarette smoke[107] (2) lycopene, the red plant antioxidant that is a major constituent of tomatoes, is capable of reversing the oxidative damage induced in rat testes following exposure to cyclosporin A[164] or cisplatin[137] (3) extracts from the herb *Lycium barbarum*, effectively protect the testes from the oxidative damage induced by heat stress and significantly suppress the oxidative DNA damage induced in mouse testicular cells by H_2O_2[165] (4) MTEC (an aqueous-methanol extract of *Musa paradisiaca, Tamarindus indica, Eugenia jambolana* and *Coccinia indica*) protects against the oxidative testicular damage resulting from induced diabetes[84] (5) lecithin administration protects the testes from the oxidative stress induced by chronic ethanol exposure[111](6) lipoic acid has been shown to inhibit the oxidative damage resulting from exposure to cyclophosphamide,[140] adriamycin[135] and X-irradiation[157] (7) complex feruloyl oligosaccharides released from wheat bran have also been shown to protect the testes from the oxidative stress associated with alloxan-induced diabetes in rats[152] and (8) β-carotene ameliorates cadmium induced oxidative stress in the testes, suppressing lipid peroxidation and restoring SOD, GST and GSH to normal physiological levels.[166]

One of the most effective antioxidants for the protection of testicular function is melatonin. This evolutionarily conserved compound has been shown to reduce oxidative stress in the testes induced by ethanol,[167] indomethacin,[168] X- irradiation,[169] streptozotocin-induced diabetes,[86] and cisplatin.[136] In vitro studies have also shown that melatonin and its immediate precursor N-acetyl-serotonin could inhibit ascorbate-Fe (II) induced lipid peroxidation in rat testicular microsomes and mitochondria.[170,171]

The administration of antioxidants such as resveratrol, ascorbate or cocoa rich in flavanols to normal animals, not suffering from induced oxidative stress, also appears to improve testicular function, suggesting that oxidative stress is a consistent feature of testicular physiology.[172,173] In light of such results, antioxidants have frequently been administered to infertile men in the hope of improving the quality of the semen profile. Very few properly controlled double blind crossover trials have been conducted in this context. However where these conditions have been met, the results have been extremely promising.[174,175]

Conclusions

Oxidative stress is a major factor in the aetiology of male infertility. At the level of the isolated spermatozoon, ROS attack can induce lipid peroxidation and DNA fragmentation disrupting both the motility of these cells and their ability to support normal embryonic development.[176-182] At the level of the testes, oxidative stress is capable of disrupting the steroidogenic capacity of Leydig cells[183] as well as the capacity of the germinal epithelium to differentiate normal spermatozoa.[184] A large number of independent clinical studies have demonstrated a correlative relationship between male infertility and evidence of oxidative stress in the ejaculate.[180,185] Moreover the literature reviewed in this chapter reveals an abundance of experimental data in animal models demonstrating a causal relationship between the induction of oxidative stress in the testes and the impairment of male reproductive function. However these two lines of evidence have not yet come together. Although oxidative stress is clearly a dominant feature in the aetiology of male infertility, the underlying causative mechanisms remain unresolved. The plethora of physical, chemical, and pathological factors that can apparently contribute to the induction of oxidative stress in the testes is impressive and suggests that the clinical picture will be extremely complex, with each individual being subject to a unique range of causative factors as a result of differences in occupational and environmental exposures, the presence of other pathological factors such as infection or diabetes, and genetic factors that could influence everything from the way in which specific xenobiotics are metabolised to the endocrine environment in which the testes have to function.

That there are so many factors capable of inducing oxidative stress in the testes strongly suggests that this is a vulnerable tissue that is both highly dependent on oxygen to drive spermatogenesis and yet highly susceptible to the toxic effects of reactive oxygen metabolites; in this context, the testis is very like the brain. While the testes clearly do possess highly specialized antioxidant defence enzymes such as extracellular SOD, PHGPx etc, there are clear benefits to be gained by treating susceptible individuals with exogenous antioxidants. Despite the evident clinical market for an antioxidant preparation specifically designed to support male reproductive health, it is remarkable how little effort has gone into the development of such a preparation and how poor most of the clinical trials in this area have been. In animal models an impressive range of antioxidant preparations has been examined and compounds identified that are clearly capable of crossing the blood testes barrier and protecting the germinal epithelium and Leydig cells from oxidative stress. The future imperatives for this area are to go beyond the superficial phenomenology that characterizes most of the clinical research in this area in an attempt to (i) gain insights into the underlying causes of oxidative stress in the male reproductive tract and (ii) develop optimized antioxidant preparations to treat pathologies arising from an imbalance in the redox status of these tissues. The journey will be long and difficult but ultimately more rewarding than the empirical approach that characterizes the current approach to treating the infertile male.

References

1. Free MJ, Schluntz GA, Jaffe RA. Respiratory gas tensions in tissues and fluids of the male rat reproductive tract. Biol Reprod 1976; 14:481-488.
2. Peltola V, Mantyla E, Huhtaniemi I et al. Lipid peroxidation and antioxidant enzyme activities in the rat testis after cigarette smoke inhalation or administration of polychlorinated biphenyls or polychlorinated naphthalenes. J Androl 1994; 15:353-361.
3. Quinn PG, Payne AH. Oxygen-mediated damage of microsomal cytochrome P-450 enzymes in cultured leydig cells: Role in steroidogenic desensitization. J Biol Chem 1984; 259:4130-4135.
4. Chen H, Liu J, Luo L et al. Vitamin E, aging and Leydig cell steroidogenesis. Exp Gerontol 2005; 40:728-736.
5. Banfi B, Molnar G, Maturana A et al. A Ca(2+)-activated NADPH oxidase in testis, spleen, and lymph nodes. J Biol Chem 2001; 276:37594-37601.
6. Kumagai A, Kodama H, Kumagai J et al. Xanthine oxidase inhibitors suppress testicular germ cell apoptosis induced by experimental cryptorchidism. Mol Hum Reprod. 2002; 8:118-123.
7. Zangar RC, Davydov DR, Verma S. Mechanisms that regulate production of reactive oxygen species by cytochrome P450. Toxicol Appl Pharmacol 2004; 199:316-331.
8. Kaur P, Kaur G, Bansal MP. Tertiary-butyl hydroperoxide induced oxidative stress and male reproductive activity in mice: Role of transcription factor NF-kappaB and testicular antioxidant enzymes. Reprod Toxicol 2006; 22:479-484.
9. Zini A, Schlegel PN. Catalase mRNA expression in the male rat reproductive tract. J Androl 1996; 17:473-480.
10. Peltola V, Huhtaniemi I, Ahotupa M. Antioxidant enzyme activity in the maturing rat testis. J Androl 1992; 13:450-455.
11. Mruk DD, Silvestrini B, Mo MY et al. Antioxidant superoxide dismutase—A review: Its function, regulation in the testis, and role in male fertility. Contraception 2002; 65:305-311.
12. Ishii T, Matsuki S, Iuchi Y et al. Accelerated impairment of spermatogenic cells in SOD1-knockout mice under heat stress. Free Radic Res 2005; 39:697-705.
13. Gu W, Hecht NB. Developmental expression of glutathione peroxidase, catalase, and manganese superoxide dismutase mRNAs during spermatogenesis in the mouse. J Androl 1996; 17:256-262.
14. Vaisberg CN, Jelezarsky LV, Dishlianova B et al. Activity, substrate detection and immunolocalization of glutathione peroxidase (GPx) in bovine reproductive organs and semen. Theriogenology 2005; 64:416-428.
15. Baek IJ, Seo DS, Yon JM et al. Tissue expression and cellular localization of phospholipid hydroperoxide glutathione peroxidase (PHGPx) mRNA in male mice. J Mol Histol 2007; 38:237-244.
16. Kaur P, Bansal MP. Influence of selenium induced oxidative stress on spermatogenesis and lactate dehydrogenase-X in mice testis. Asian J Androl 2004; 6:227-232.
17. Avlan D, Erdougan K, Cimen B et al. The protective effect of selenium on ipsilateral and contralateral testes in testicular reperfusion injury. Pediatr Surg Int 2005; 21:274-278.
18. Bray TM, Bettger WJ. The physiological role of zinc as an antioxidant. Free Radic Biol Med 1990; 8:281-291.
19. Nair N, Bedwal S, Prasad S et al. Short-term zinc deficiency in diet induces increased oxidative stress in testes and epididymis of rats. Indian J Exp Biol 2005; 43:786-794.
20. Khan S, Khan MA, Bhatnagar D et al. Zinc protection against lipid peroxidation from cadmium. Indian J Exp Biol 1991; 29:823-825.
21. Batra N, Nehru B, Bansal MP. The effect of zinc supplementation on the effects of lead on the rat testis. Reprod Toxicol 1998; 12:535-540.
22. Ozkan KKU, Boran C, Kilinc M et al. The effect of zinc aspartate pretreatment on ischemia-reperfusion injury and early changes of blood and tissue antioxidant enzyme activities after unilateral testicular torsion-detorsion. J Pediatr Surg 2004; 39:91-95.
23. Amara S, Abdelmelek H, Garrel C et al. Preventive Effect of zinc against cadmium-induced oxidative stress in the rat testis. J Reprod Dev 2007, [Epub ahead of print].
24. Johnson FC. The antioxidant vitamins CRC. Crit Rev Food Sci Nutr 1979; 11:217-309.
25. Yoganathan T, Eskild W, Hansson V. Investigation of detoxification capacity of rat testicular germ cells and Sertoli cells. Free Radic Biol Med 1989; 7:355-359.
26. Paolicchi A, Pezzini A, Saviozzi M et al. Localization of a GSH-dependent dehydroascorbate reductase in rat tissues and subcellular fractions. Arch Biochem Biophys 1996; 333:489-495.

27. Sonmez M, Turk G, Yuce A. The effect of ascorbic acid supplementation on sperm quality, lipid peroxidation and testosterone levels of male Wistar rats. Theriogenology 2005; 63:2063-2072.
28. Senthil kumar J, Banudevi S, Sharmila M et al. Effects of Vitamin C and E on PCB (Aroclor 1254) induced oxidative stress, androgen binding protein and lactate in rat Sertoli cells. Reprod Toxicol 2004; 19:201-208.
29. Maneesh M, Jayalakshmi H, Dutta S et al. Experimental therapeutic intervention with ascorbic acid in ethanol induced testicular injuries in rats. Indian J Exp Biol 2005; 43:172-176.
30. Rao M, Narayana K, Benjamin S et al. L-ascorbic acid ameliorates postnatal endosulfan induced testicular damage in rats. Indian J Physiol Pharmacol 2005; 49:331-336.
31. Chang SI, Jin B, Youn P et al. Arsenic-induced toxicity and the protective role of ascorbic acid in mouse testis. Toxicol Appl Pharmacol 2007; 218:196-203.
32. Sen Gupta R, Sen Gupta E et al. Vitamin C and vitamin E protect the rat testes from cadmium-induced reactive oxygen species. Mol Cells 2004; 17:132-139.
33. Verma RJ, Nair A. Ameliorative effect of vitamin E on aflatoxin-induced lipid peroxidation in the testis of mice. Asian J Androl 2001; 3:217-221.
34. Aruldhas MM, Subramanian S, Sekar P et al. Chronic chromium exposure-induced changes in testicular histoarchitecture are associated with oxidative stress: Study in a non-human primate (Macaca radiata Geoffroy). Hum Reprod 2005; 20:2801-2813.
35. Marchlewicz M, Wiszniewska B, Gonet B et al. Increased lipid peroxidation and ascorbic acid utilization in testis and epididymis of rats chronically exposed to lead. Biometals 2007; 20:13-19.
36. Lucesoli F, Fraga CG. Oxidative stress in testes of rats subjected to chronic iron intoxication and alpha-tocopherol supplementation. Toxicology 1999; 132:179-186.
37. Gavazza MB, Catala A. The effect of alpha-tocopherol on lipid peroxidation of microsomes and mitochondria from rat testis. Prostaglandins Leukot Essent Fatty Acids 2006; 74:247-254.
38. Ghosh D, Das UB, Misro M. Protective role of alpha-tocopherol-succinate (provitamin-E) in cyclophosphamide induced testicular gametogenic and steroidogenic disorders: A correlative approach to oxidative stress. Free Radic Res 2002; 36:1209-1218.
39. Latchoumycandane C, Mathur PP. Effects of vitamin E on reactive oxygen species-mediated 2,3,7,8-tetrachlorodi-benzo-p-dioxin toxicity in rat testis. J Appl Toxicol 2002; 22:345-351.
40. Manna I, Jana K, Samanta PK. Intensive swimming exercise-induced oxidative stress and reproductive dysfunction in male wistar rats: Protective role of alpha-tocopherol succinate. Can J Appl Physiol 2004; 29:172-185.
41. Jedlinska-Krakowska M, Bomba G et al. Impact of oxidative stress and supplementation with vitamins E and C on testes morphology in rats. J Reprod Dev 2006; 52:203-209.
42. Zhou DX, Qiu SD, Zhang J et al. The protective effect of vitamin E against oxidative damage caused by formaldehyde in the testes of adult rats. Asian J Androl 2006; 8:584-588.
43. Mogulkoc R, Baltaci AK, Aydin L et al. Pinealectomy increases oxidant damage in kidney and testis caused by hyperthyroidism in rats. Cell Biochem Funct 2006; 24:449-453.
44. Awad H, Halawa F, Mostafa T et al. Melatonin hormone profile in infertile males. Int J Androl 2006; 29:409-413.
45. Semercioz A, Onur R, Ogras S et al. Effects of melatonin on testicular tissue nitric oxide level and antioxidant enzyme activities in experimentally induced left varicocele. Neuro Endocrinol Lett 2003; 24:86-90.
46. Liu Z, Lin H, Ye S et al. Remarkably high activities of testicular cytochrome c in destroying reactive oxygen species and in triggering apoptosis. Proc Natl Acad Sci USA 2006; 103:8965-8970.
47. Ahotupa M, Huhtaniemi I. Impaired detoxification of reactive oxygen and consequent oxidative stress in experimentally cryptorchid rat testis. Biol Reprod 1992; 46:1114-1118.
48. Ikeda M, Kodama H, Fukuda J et al. Role of radical oxygen species in rat testicular germ cell apoptosis induced by heat stress. Biol Reprod 1999; 61:393-399.
49. Ishii T, Matsuki S, Iuchi Y et al. Accelerated impairment of spermatogenic cells in SOD1-knockout mice under heat stress. Free Radic Res 2005; 39:697-705.
50. Smith GR, Kaune GH, Parodi ChD et al. Extent of sperm DNA damage in spermatozoa from men examined for infertility: Relationship with oxidative stress. Rev Med Chil 2007; 135:279-286.
51. Chaki SP, Ghosh D, Misro MM. Simultaneous increase in germ cell apoptosis and oxidative stress under acute unilateral testicular ischaemia in rats. Int J Androl 2003; 26:319-328.
52. Taneli F, Vatansever S, Ulman C et al. The effect of spermatic vessel ligation on testicular nitric oxide levels and germ cell-specific apoptosis in rat testis. Acta Histochem 2005; 106:459-466.
53. Lysiak JJ, Zheng S, Woodson R et al. Caspase-9-dependent pathway to murine germ cell apoptosis: Mediation by oxidative stress, BAX, and caspase 2. Cell Tissue Res 2007; 328:411-49.
54. Guimaraes SB, Aragao AA, Santos JM et al. Oxidative stress induced by torsion of the spermatic cord in young rats. Acta Cir Bras 2007; 22:30-33.

55. Anim JT, Kehinde EO, Prasad A et al. Morphological responses of the rabbit testis to ischemic/reperfusion injury due to torsion. Urol Int 2005; 75:258-263.
56. Kehinde EO, Anim JT, Mojiminiyi OA et al. Allopurinol provides long-term protection for experimentally induced testicular torsion in a rabbit model. BJU Int 2005; 96:686-687.
57. Unsal A, Eroglu M, Avci A et al. Protective role of natural antioxidant supplementation on testicular tissue after testicular torsion and detorsion. Scand J Urol Nephrol 2006; 40:17-22.
58. Uguralp S, Usta U, Mizrak B. Resveratrol may reduce apoptosis of rat testicular germ cells after experimental testicular torsion. Eur J Pediatr Surg 2005; 15:333-336.
59. Dokmeci D, Inan M, Basaran UN et al. Protective effect of L-carnitine on testicular ischaemia-reperfusion injury in rats. Cell Biochem Funct 2007, 25(6):611-8.
60. Atik E, Gorur S, Kiper AN. The effect of caffeic acid phenethyl ester (CAPE) on histopathological changes in testicular ischemia-reperfusion injury. Pharmacol Res 2006; 54:293-297.
61. Turner TT, Bang HJ, Lysiak JL. The molecular pathology of experimental testicular torsion suggests adjunct therapy to surgical repair. J Urol 2004; 172:2574-2578.
62. Sarica K, Kupeli B, Budak M et al. Influence of experimental spermatic cord torsion on the contralateral testis in rats: Evaluation of tissue free oxygen radical scavenger enzyme levels. Urol Int 1997; 58:208-212.
63. Saba M, Morales CR, De Lamirande E et al. Morphological and biochemical changes following acute unilateral testicular torsion in prepubertal rats. J Urol 1997; 157:1149-1154.
64. Filho DW, Torres MA, Bordin AL et al. Spermatic cord torsion, reactive oxygen and nitrogen species and ischemia-reperfusion injury. Mol Aspects Med 2004; 25:199-210.
65. Hendin BN, Kolettis PN, Sharma RK et al. Varicocele is associated with elevated spermatozoal reactive oxygen species production and diminished seminal plasma antioxidant capacity. J Urol 1999; 161:1831-1834.
66. Agarwal A, Prabakaran S, Allamaneni SS. Relationship between oxidative stress, varicocele and infertility: A meta-analysis. Reprod Biomed Online 2006; 12:630-633.
67. Smith R, Kaune H, Parodi D et al. Increased sperm DNA damage in patients with varicocele: Relationship with seminal oxidative stress. Hum Reprod 2006; 21:986-993.
68. Hurtado de Catalfo GE, Ranieri-Casilla A, Marra FA et al. Oxidative stress biomarkers and hormonal profile in human patients undergoing varicocelectomy. Int J Androl 2007, 30(6):519-30.
69. Shiraishi K, Naito K. Generation of 4-hydroxy-2-nonenal modified proteins in testes predicts improvement in spermatogenesis after varicocelectomy. Fertil Steril 2006; 86:233-235.
70. Ishikawa T, Fujioka H, Ishimura T et al. Increased testicular 8-hydroxy-2'-deoxyguanosine in patients with varicocele. BJU Int 2007, 100(4):863-6.
71. Ozdamar AS, Soylu AG, Culha M et al. Testicular oxidative stress: Effects of experimental varicocele in adolescent rats. Urol Int 2004; 73:343-347.
72. Saleh RA, Agarwal A, Sharma RK et al. Evaluation of nuclear DNA damage in spermatozoa from infertile men with varicocele. Fertil Steril 2003; 80:1431-1436.
73. Pasqualotto FF, Sharma RK, Nelson DR et al. Relationship between oxidative stress, semen characteristics, and clinical diagnosis in men undergoing infertility investigation. Fertil Steril 2000; 73:459-464.
74. Mitropoulos D, Deliconstantinos G, Zervas A et al. Nitric oxide synthase and xanthine oxidase activities in the spermatic vein of patients with varicocele: A potential role for nitric oxide and peroxynitrite in sperm dysfunction. J Urol 1996; 156(6):1952-1958.
75. Gomez E, Buckingham DW, Brindle J et al. Development of an image analysis system to monitor the retention of residual cytoplasm by human spermatozoa: Correlation with biochemical markers of the cytoplasmic space, oxidative stress, and sperm function. J Androl 1996; 17:276-287.
76. Baker MA, Reeves G, Hetherington L et al. Proteomic analysis of human spermatozoa. Proteomics Clin Appl 2007; 1:524-532.
77. Williams AC, Ford WC. Functional significance of the pentose phosphate pathway and glutathione reductase in the antioxidant defences of human sperm. Biol Reprod 2004; 71:1309-1316.
78. Zini A, Defreitas G, Freeman M et al. Varicocele is associated with abnormal retention of cytoplasmic droplets by human spermatozoa. Fertil Steril 2000; 74:461-464.
79. Zini A, Buckspan M, Jamal M et al. Effect of varicocelectomy on the abnormal retention of residual cytoplasm by human spermatozoa. Hum Reprod 1999; 14:1791-1793.
80. Sahoo DK, Roy A, Chattopadhyay S et al. Effect of T3 treatment on glutathione redox pool and its metabolizing enzymes in mitochondrial and post-mitochondrial fractions of adult rat testes. Indian J Exp Biol 2007; 45:338-346.
81. Zamoner A, Barreto KP, Filho DW et al. Hyperthyroidism in the developing rat testis is associated with oxidative stress and hyperphosphorylated vimentin accumulation. Mol Cell Endocrinol 2007; 267:116-126.

82. Krassas GE, Pontikides N, Deligianni V et al. A prospective controlled study of the impact of hyperthyroidism on reproductive function in males. J Clin Endocrinol Metab 2002; 87:3667-3671.
83. Choudhury S, Chainy GB, Mishro MM. Experimentally induced hypo- and hyper-thyroidism influence on the antioxidant defence system in adult rat testis. Andrologia 2003; 35:131-140.
84. Mallick C, Mandal S, Barik B et al. Protection of testicular dysfunctions by MTEC, a formulated herbal drug, in streptozotocin induced diabetic rat. Biol Pharm Bull 2007; 30:84-90.
85. Shrilatha B, Muralidhara. Early oxidative stress in testis and epididymal sperm in streptozotocin-induced diabetic mice: Its progression and genotoxic consequences. Reprod Toxicol 2007; 23:578-587.
86. Armagan A, Uz E, Yilmaz HR et al. Effects of melatonin on lipid peroxidation and antioxidant enzymes in streptozotocin-induced diabetic rat testis. Asian J Androl 2006; 8:595-600.
87. Agbaje IM, Rogers DA, McVicar CM et al. Insulin dependent diabetes mellitus: Implications for male reproductive function. Hum Reprod 2007, 22(7):1871-7.
88. Reddy MM, Mahipal SV, Subhashini J et al. Bacterial lipopolysaccharide-induced oxidative stress in the impairment of steroidogenesis and spermatogenesis in rats. Reprod Toxicol 2006; 22:493-500.
89. Allen JA, Diemer T, Janus P et al. Bacterial endotoxin lipopolysaccharide and reactive oxygen species inhibit Leydig cell steroidogenesis via perturbation of mitochondria. Endocrine 2004; 25:265-275.
90. Somani SM, Husain K. Exercise training alters kinetics of antioxidant enzymes in rat tissues. Biochem Mol Biol Int 1996; 38:587-595.
91. Husain K, Somani SM. Interaction of exercise training and chronic ethanol ingestion on testicular antioxidant system in rat. J Appl Toxicol 1998; 18:421-429.
92. Manna I, Jana K, Samanta PK. Effect of intensive exercise-induced testicular gametogenic and steroidogenic disorders in mature male Wistar strain rats: A correlative approach to oxidative stress. Acta Physiol Scand 2003; 178:33-40.
93. Zini A, Schlegel PN. Effect of hormonal manipulation on mRNA expression of antioxidant enzymes in the rat testis. J Urol 2003; 169:767-771.
94. Ghosh D, Das UB, Ghosh S et al. Testicular gametogenic and steroidogenic activities in cyclophosphamide treated rat: A correlative study with testicular oxidative stress. Drug Chem Toxicol 2002; 25:281-292.
95. Peltola V, Huhtaniemi I, Metsa-Ketela T et al. Induction of lipid peroxidation during steroidogenesis in the rat testis. Endocrinology 1996; 137:105-112.
96. Chainy GB, Samantaray S, Samanta L. Testosterone-induced changes in testicular antioxidant system. Andrologia 1997; 29:343-349.
97. Chaki SP, Misro MM, Gautam DK et al. Estradiol treatment induces testicular oxidative stress and germ cell apoptosis in rats. Apoptosis 2006; 11:1427-1437.
98. Gautam DK, Misro MM, Chaki SP et al. hCG treatment raises H_2O_2 levels and induces germ cell apoptosis in rat testis. Apoptosis 2007; 12(7):1173-82.
99. Conte da Frota Jr ML, Gomes da Silva E, Behr GA et al. All-trans retinoic acid induces free radical generation and modulate antioxidant enzyme activities in rat Sertoli cells. Mol Cell Biochem 2006; 285:173-179.
100. Klamt F, Dal-Pizzol F, Ribeiro NC et al. Retinol-induced elevation of ornithine decarboxylase activity in cultured rat Sertoli cells is attenuated by free radical scavenger and by iron chelator. Mol Cell Biochem 2000; 208:71-76.
101. Dal-Pizzol F, Klamt F, Benfato MS et al. Retinol supplementation induces oxidative stress and modulates antioxidant enzyme activities in rat sertoli cells. Free Radic Res 2001; 34:395-404.
102. Murata M, Kawanishi S. Oxidative DNA damage by vitamin A and its derivative via superoxide generation. J Biol Chem 2000; 275:2003-2008.
103. Biswas NM, Deb C. Testicular degeneration in rats during hypervitaminosis A. Endokrinologie 1965; 49:64-69.
104. Adamopoulos D, Venaki E, Koukkou E et al. Association of carotene rich diet with hypogonadism in a male athlete. Asian J Androl 2006; 8:488-492.
105. Fraga CG, Motchnik PA, Wyrobek AJ et al. Smoking and low antioxidant levels increase oxidative damage to sperm DNA. Mutat Res 1996; 351:199-203.
106. Fraga CG, Motchnik PA, Shigenaga MK et al. Ascorbic acid protects against endogenous oxidative DNA damage in human sperm. Proc Natl Acad Sci USA 1991; 88:11003-11006.
107. Ozyurt H, Pekmez H, Parlaktas BS et al. Oxidative stress in testicular tissues of rats exposed to cigarette smoke and protective effects of caffeic acid phenethyl ester. Asian J Androl 2006; 8:189-193.
108. Nordmann R, Ribiere C, Rouach H. Ethanol-induced lipid peroxidation and oxidative stress in extrahepatic tissues. Alcohol Alcohol 1990; 25:231-237.

109. Schlorff EC, Husain K, Somani SM. Dose and time dependent effects of ethanol on antioxidant system in rat testes. Alcohol 1999; 18:203-214.
110. Amanvermez R, Demir S, Tuncel OK et al. Alcohol-induced oxidative stress and reduction in oxidation by ascorbate/L-cys/ L-met in the testis, ovary, kidney, and lung of rat. Adv Ther 2005; 22:548-558.
111. Maneesh M, Jayalekshmi H, Dutta S et al. Effect of exogenous lecithin on ethanol-induced testicular injuries in Wistar rats. Indian J Physiol Pharmacol 2005; 49:297-304.
112. Maneesh M, Dutta S, Chakrabarti A et al. Alcohol abuse-duration dependent decrease in plasma testosterone and antioxidants in males. Indian J Physiol Pharmacol 2006; 50:291-296.
113. Acharya UR, Mishra M, Tripathy RR et al. Testicular dysfunction and antioxidative defense system of Swiss mice after chromic acid exposure. Reprod Toxicol 2006; 22:87-91.
114. Lucesoli F, Caligiuri M, Roberti MF et al. Dose-dependent increase of oxidative damage in the testes of rats subjected to acute iron overload. Arch Biochem Biophys 1999; 372:37-43.
115. Doreswamy K, Muralidhara. Genotoxic consequences associated with oxidative damage in testis of mice subjected to iron intoxication. Toxicology 2005; 206:169-178.
116. Santos FW, Oro T, Zeni G et al. Cadmium induced testicular damage and its response to administration of succimer and diphenyl diselenide in mice. Toxicol Lett 2004; 152:255-263.
117. Koizumi T, Li ZG. Role of oxidative stress in single-dose, cadmium-induced testicular cancer. J Toxicol Environ Health 1992; 37:25-36.
118. Linares V, Belles M, Albina ML et al. Assessment of the pro-oxidant activity of uranium in kidney and testis of rats. Toxicol Lett 2006; 167:152-161.
119. Chang SI, Jin B, Youn P et al. Arsenic-induced toxicity and the protective role of ascorbic acid in mouse testis. Toxicol Appl Pharmacol 2007; 218:196-203.
120. Chandra AK, Ghosh R, Chatterjee A et al. Effects of vanadate on male rat reproductive tract histology, oxidative stress markers and androgenic enzyme activities. J Inorg Biochem 2007, [Epub ahead of print].
121. Kasahara E, Sato EF, Miyoshi M et al. Role of oxidative stress in germ cell apoptosis induced by di(2-ethylhexyl)phthalate. Biochem J 2002; 365:849-856.
122. Lee E, Ahn MY, Kim HJ et al. Effect of di(n-butyl) phthalate on testicular oxidative damage and antioxidant enzymes in hyperthyroid rats. Environ Toxicol 2007; 22:245-255.
123. Meng Z, Bai W. Oxidation damage of sulfur dioxide on testicles of mice. Environ Res 2004; 96:298-304.
124. Ghosh D, Das Sarkar S, Maiti R et al. Testicular toxicity in sodium fluoride treated rats: Association with oxidative stress. Reprod Toxicol 2002; 16:385-390.
125. Murugesan P, Balaganesh M, Balasubramanian K et al. Effects of polychlorinated biphenyl (Aroclor 1254) on steroidogenesis and antioxidant system in cultured adult rat Leydig cells. J Endocrinol 2007; 192:325-338.
126. al-Bayati ZA, Wahba ZZ, Stohs SJ. 2,3,7,8-Tetrachlorodibenzo-p-dioxin (TCDD)-induced alterations in lipid peroxidation, enzymes, and divalent cations in rat testis. Xenobiotica 1988; 18:1281-128.
127. Latchoumycandane C, Chitra KC, Mathur PP. The effect of 2,3,7,8-tetrachlorodibenzo-p-dioxin on the antioxidant system in mitochondrial and microsomal fractions of rat testis. Toxicology 2002; 171:127-135.
128. Latchoumycandane C, Mathur PP. Effect of methoxychlor on the antioxidant system in mitochondrial and microsome-rich fractions of rat testis. Toxicology 2002; 176:67-75.
129. Latchoumycandane C, Mathur PP. Induction of oxidative stress in the rat testis after short-term exposure to the organochlorine pesticide methoxychlor. Arch Toxicol 2002; 76:692-698.
130. Kabuto H, Hasuike S, Minagawa N et al. Effects of bisphenol A on the metabolisms of active oxygen species in mouse tissues. Environ Res 2003; 93:31-35.
131. Chitra KC, Latchoumycandane C, Mathur PP. Induction of oxidative stress by bisphenol A in the epididymal sperm of rats. Toxicology 2003; 185:119-127.
132. Chitra KC, Latchoumycandane C, Mathur PP. Effect of nonylphenol on the antioxidant system in epididymal sperm of rats. Arch Toxicol 2002; 76:545-551.
133. Gong Y, Han XD. Nonylphenol-induced oxidative stress and cytotoxicity in testicular Sertoli cells. Toxicol 2006; 22:623-630.
134. Chitra KC, Mathur PP. Vitamin E prevents nonylphenol-induced oxidative stress in testis of rats. Indian J Exp Biol 2004; 42:220-223.
135. Prahalathan C, Selvakumar E, Varalakshmi P. Lipoic acid ameliorates adriamycin-induced testicular mitochondriopathy. Reprod Toxicol 2005; 20:111-116.
136. Atessahin A, Sahna E, Turk G et al. Chemoprotective effect of melatonin against cisplatin-induced testicular toxicity in rats. J Pineal Res 2006; 41:21-27.

137. Atessahin A, Karahan I, Turk G et al. Protective role of lycopene on cisplatin-induced changes in sperm characteristics, testicular damage and oxidative stress in rats. Reprod Toxicol 2006; 21:42-47.
138. Ghosh D, Das UB, Misro M. Protective role of alpha-tocopherol-succinate (provitamin-E) in cyclophosphamide induced testicular gametogenic and steroidogenic disorders: A correlative approach to oxidative stress. Free Radic Res 2002; 36:1209-1218.
139. Ghosh D, Das UB, Ghosh S et al. Testicular gametogenic and steroidogenic activities in cyclophosphamide treated rat: A correlative study with testicular oxidative stress. Drug Chem Toxicol 2002; 5:281-292.
140. Selvakumar E, Prahalathan C, Mythili Y et al. Protective effect of DL-alpha-lipoic acid in cyclophosphamide induced oxidative injury in rat testis. Reprod Toxicol 2004; 19:163-167.
141. Samanta L, Roy A, Chainy GB. Changes in rat testicular antioxidant defence profile as a function of age and its impairment by hexachlorocyclohexane during critical stages of maturation. Andrologia 1999; 31:83-90.
142. Samanta L, Sahoo A, Chainy GB. Age-related changes in rat testicular oxidative stress parameters by hexachlorocyclohexane. Arch Toxicol 1999; 73:96-107.
143. Homma-Takeda S, Hiraku Y, Ohkuma Y et al. 2,4,6-trinitrotoluene-induced reproductive toxicity via oxidative DNA damage by its metabolite. Free Radic Res 2002; 36:555-566.
144. Verma RJ, Nair A. Ameliorative effect of vitamin E on aflatoxin-induced lipid peroxidation in the testis of mice. Asian J Androl 2001; 3:217-221.
145. Sujatha R, Chitra KC, Latchoumycandane C et al. Effect of lindane on testicular antioxidant system and steroidogenic enzymes in adult rats. Asian J Androl 2001; 3:135-138.
146. Debnath D, Mandal TK. Study of quinalphos (an environmental oestrogenic insecticide) formulation (Ekalux 25 E.C.)-induced damage of the testicular tissues and antioxidant defence systems in Sprague-Dawley albino rats. J Appl Toxicol 2000; 20:197-204.
147. Rao M, Narayana K, Benjamin S et al. L-ascorbic acid ameliorates postnatal endosulfan induced testicular damage in rats. Indian J Physiol Pharmacol 2005; 49:331-336.
148. Kaur P, Kalia S, Bansal MP. Effect of diethyl maleate induced oxidative stress on male reproductive activity in mice: Redox active enzymes and transcription factors expression. Mol Cell Biochem 2006; 291:55-61.
149. Singh M, Kalla NR, Sanyal SN. Effect of monensin on the enzymes of oxidative stress, thiamine pyrophosphatase and DNA integrity in rat testicular cells in vitro. Exp Toxicol Pathol 2006; 58:203-208.
150. Zhou DX, Qiu SD, Zhang J et al. The protective effect of vitamin E against oxidative damage caused by formaldehyde in the testes of adult rats. Asian J Androl 2006; 8:584-588.
151. El-Missiry MA. Enhanced testicular antioxidant system by ascorbic acid in alloxan diabetic rats. Comp Biochem Physiol C Pharmacol Toxicol Endocrinol 1999; 124:233-237.
152. Ou SY, Jackson GM, Jiao X et al. Protection against oxidative stress in diabetic rats by wheat bran feruloyl oligosaccharides. J Agric Food Chem 2007; 55:3191-3195.
153. Yousef MI, El-Demerdash FM. Acrylamide-induced oxidative stress and biochemical perturbations in rats. Toxicology 2006; 219:133-141.
154. Jedlinska-Krakowska M, Bomba G, Jakubowski K et al. Impact of oxidative stress and supplementation with vitamins E and C on testes morphology in rats. J Reprod Dev 2006; 52:203-209.
155. Amara S, Abdelmelek H, Garrel C et al. Effects of subchronic exposure to static magnetic field on testicular function in rats. Arch Med Res 2006; 37:947-952.
156. Ikeda M, Kodama H, Fukuda J et al. Role of radical oxygen species in rat testicular germ cell apoptosis induced by heat stress. Biol Reprod 1999; 61:393-399.
157. Manda K, Ueno M, Moritake T et al. Alpha-lipoic acid attenuates x-irradiation-induced oxidative stress in mice. Cell Biol Toxicol 2007; 23:129-137.
158. Cay A, Alver A, Kucuk M et al. The effects of N-acetylcysteine on antioxidant enzyme activities in experimental testicular torsion. J Surg Res 2006; 131:199-203.
159. Liu ZM, Zheng XM, Yang ZW et al. Protective effect of pentoxifylline on spermatogenesis following testicular torsion/detorsion in rats. Zhonghua Nan Ke Xue 2006; 12:323-325.
160. Koc A, Narci A, Duru M et al. The protective role of erdosteine on testicular tissue after testicular torsion and detorsion. Mol Cell Biochem 2005; 280:193-199.
161. Etensel B, Ozkisacik S, Ozkara E et al. The protective effect of dexpanthenol on testicular atrophy at 60th day following experimental testicular torsion. Pediatr Surg Int 2007; 23:271-275.
162. Yagmurdur H, Ayyildiz A, Karaguzel E et al. The preventive effects of thiopental and propofol on testicular ischemia-reperfusion injury. Acta Anaesthesiol Scand 2006; 50:1238-1243.
163. Ozyurt B, Parlaktas BS, Ozyurt H et al. A preliminary study of the levels of testis oxidative stress parameters after MK-801-induced experimental psychosis model: Protective effects of CAPE. Toxicology 2007; 230:83-89.

164. Turk G, Atessahin A, Sonmez M et al. Lycopene protects against cyclosporine A-induced testicular toxicity in rats. Theriogenology 2007; 67:778-785.
165. Luo Q, Li Z, Huang X et al. Lycium barbarum polysaccharides: Protective effects against heat-induced damage of rat testes and H_2O_2-induced DNA damage in mouse testicular cells and beneficial effect on sexual behavior and reproductive function of hemicastrated rats. Life Sci 2006; 79:613-621.
166. El-Missiry MA, Shalaby F. Role of beta-carotene in ameliorating the cadmium-induced oxidative stress in rat brain and testis. J Biochem Mol Toxicol 2000; 14:238-243.
167. Oner-Iyidogan Y, Gurdol F, Oner P. The effects of acute melatonin and ethanol treatment on antioxidant enzyme activities in rat testes. Pharmacol Res 2001; 44:89-93.
168. Othman AI, El-Missiry MA, Amer MA. The protective action of melatonin on indomethacin-induced gastric and testicular oxidative stress in rats. Redox Rep 2001; 6:173-177.
169. Hussein MR, Abu-Dief EE, Abou El-Ghait AT et al. Melatonin and roentgen irradiation of the testis. Fertil Steril 2006; 86:750-752.
170. Gavazza M, Catala A. Melatonin preserves arachidonic and docosapentaenoic acids during ascorbate-Fe2+ peroxidation of rat testis microsomes and mitochondria. Int J Biochem Cell Biol 2003; 35:359-366.
171. Gavazza MB, Catala A. Protective effect of N-acetyl-serotonin on the non-enzymatic lipid peroxidation in rat testicular microsomes and mitochondria. J Pineal Res 2004; 37:153-160.
172. Juan ME, Gonzalez-Pons E, Munuera T et al. Trans-resveratrol, a natural antioxidant from grapes, increases sperm output in healthy rats. J Nutr 2005; 135:757-760.
173. Orozco TJ, Wang JF, Keen CL. Chronic consumption of a flavanol- and procyanindin-rich diet is associated with reduced levels of 8-hydroxy-2'-deoxyguanosine in rat testes. J Nutr Biochem 2003; 14:104-110.
174. Suleiman SA, Ali ME, Zaki ZM et al. Lipid peroxidation and human sperm motility: Protective role of vitamin E. J Androl 1996; 17:530-537.
175. Keskes-Ammar L, Feki-Chakroun N, Rebai T et al. Sperm oxidative stress and the effect of an oral vitamin E and selenium supplement on semen quality in infertile men. Arch Androl 2003; 49:83-94.
176. Aitken RJ, De Iuliis GN. Origins and consequences of DNA damage in male germ cells. Reprod Biomed Online 2007; 14:727-733.
177. Aitken RJ, Baker MA. Oxidative stress, sperm survival and fertility control. Mol Cell Endocrinol 2006; 250:66-69.
178. Aitken RJ. Founders' Lecture: Human spermatozoa: Fruits of creation, seeds of doubt. Reprod Fertil Dev 2004; 16:655-664.
179. Aitken RJ. The Amoroso Lecture: The human spermatozoon—A cell in crisis? J Reprod Fertil 1999; 115:1-7.
180. Sikka SC. Relative impact of oxidative stress on male reproductive function. Curr Med Chem 2001; 8:851-862.
181. Agarwal A, Gupta S, Sikka S. The role of free radicals and antioxidants in reproduction. Curr Opin Obstet Gynecol 2006; 18:325-332.
182. Kumar TR, Muralidhara. Male-mediated dominant lethal mutations in mice following prooxidant treatment. Mutat Res 1999; 444:145-149.
183. Hales DB, Allen JA, Shankara T et al. Mitochondrial function in Leydig cell steroidogenesis. Ann N Y Acad Sci 2005; 1061:120-134.
184. Naughton CK, Nangia AK, Agarwal A. Pathophysiology of varicoceles in male infertility. Hum Reprod Update 2001; 7:473-481.
185. Agarwal A, Gupta S, Sikka S. The role of free radicals and antioxidants in reproduction. Curr Opin Obstet Gynecol 2006; 18:325-332.
186. Uz E, Sogut S, Sahin S et al. The protective role of caffeic acid phenethyl ester (CAPE) on testicular tissue after testicular torsion and detorsion. World J Urol 2002; 20:264-270.
187. Salmasi AH, Beheshtian A, Payabvash S et al. Effect of morphine on ischemia-reperfusion injury: Experimental study in testicular torsion rat model. Urology 2005; 66:1338-1342.

Chapter 10

Nitric Oxide and Cyclic Nucleotides:
Their Roles in Junction Dynamics and Spermatogenesis

Nikki P.Y. Lee* and C. Yan Cheng

Abstract

Spermatogenesis is a highly complicated process in which functional spermatozoa (haploid, 1n) are generated from primitive mitotic spermatogonia (diploid, 2n). This process involves the differentiation and transformation of several types of germ cells as spermatocytes and spermatids undergo meiosis and differentiation. Due to its sophistication and complexity, testis possesses intrinsic mechanisms to modulate and regulate different stages of germ cell development under the intimate and indirect cooperation with Sertoli and Leydig cells, respectively. Furthermore, developing germ cells must translocate from the basal to the apical (adluminal) compartment of the seminiferous epithelium. Thus, extensive junction restructuring must occur to assist germ cell movement. Within the seminiferous tubules, three principal types of junctions are found namely anchoring junctions, tight junctions, and gap junctions. Other less studied junctions are desmosome-like junctions and hemidesmosome junctions. With these varieties of junction types, testes are using different regulators to monitor junction turnover. Among the uncountable junction modulators, nitric oxide (NO) is a prominent candidate due to its versatility and extensive downstream network. NO is synthesized by nitric oxide synthase (NOS). Three traditional NOS, specified as endothelial NOS (eNOS), inducible NOS (iNOS), and neuronal NOS (nNOS), and one testis-specific nNOS (TnNOS) are found in the testis. For these, eNOS and iNOS were recently shown to have putative junction regulation properties. More important, these two NOSs likely rely on the downstream soluble guanylyl cyclase/cGMP/protein kinase G signaling pathway to regulate the structural components at the tight junctions and adherens junctions in the testes. Apart from the involvement in junction regulation, NOS/NO also participates in controlling the levels of cytokines and hormones in the testes. On the other hand, NO is playing a unique role in modulating germ cell viability and development, and indirectly acting on some aspects of male infertility and testicular pathological conditions. Thus, NOS/NO bears an irreplaceable role in maintaining the homeostasis of the microenvironment in the seminiferous epithelium via its different downstream signaling pathways.

Introduction

Among the organs in the mammalian body, testis is one of the exceptional organs having complex cellular structures and organization. After puberty, testis functions as a sperm producing factory, generating up to millions of spermatozoa on a daily basis through the entire adulthood.[1] In order to fulfill its reproductive function, testis is compartmentalized into two broad partitions, the seminiferous tubules and the inter-tubular areas (Fig. 1).[2,3] In the seminiferous tubules, the

*Corresponding Author: Nikki P.Y. Lee—Departments of Medicine and Surgery, University of Hong Kong, Queen Mary Hospital, Hong Kong, China. Email: nikkilee@hkucc.hku.hk

Molecular Mechanisms in Spermatogenesis, edited by C. Yan Cheng. ©2008 Landes Bioscience and Springer Science+Business Media.

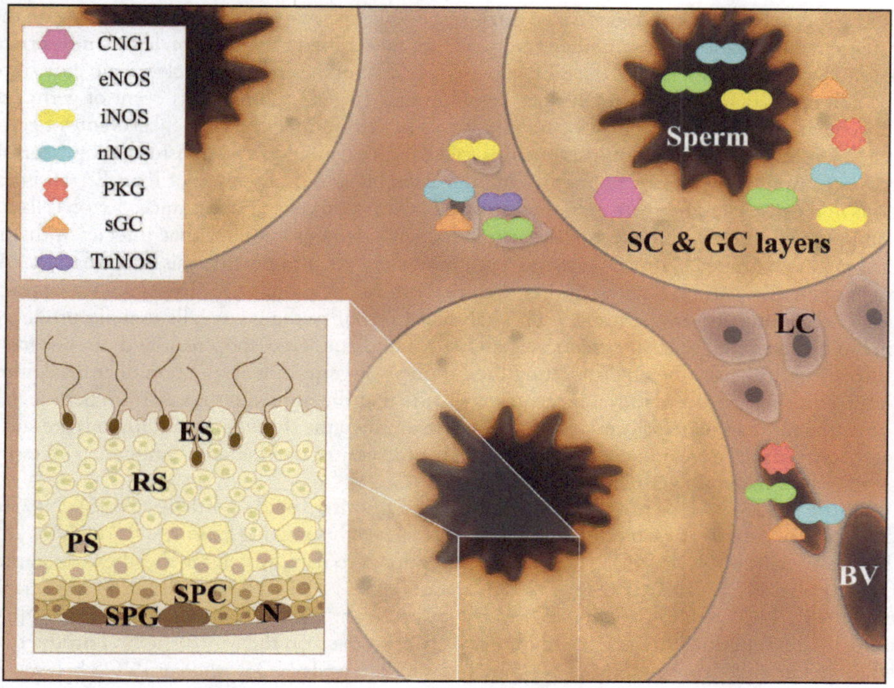

Figure 1. Cellular localization of different NOS/NO signaling pathway components in the testes. Schematic drawing depicting the gross morphology of a testis cross-section. Seminiferous tubules are prominent structures found in the testes. Area surrounding the seminiferous tubules is termed interstitial area, which harbors Leydig cells and blood vessels. The inset diagram illustrates different germ cell layers of a seminiferous tubule. During spermatogenesis, spermatogonium migrates from the basal compartment to the adluminal compartment, during which spermatogonium differentiates into advanced germ cell types, namely preleptotene/leptotene spermatocytes, pachytene spermatocytes, round spermatids, and elongated spermatids, before spermatozoa are released into the tubule lumen. Components of the NOS/NO pathway, such as CNG1, eNOS, iNOS, nNOS, PKG, sGC, and TnNOS, are represented by the symbols tabulated. They are localized in specific locations within the testes, such as in the Sertoli cell and germ cell layers (SC & GC layers), sperm, Leydig cells (LC), and blood vessel (BV). Abbreviations used: BV, blood vessel; CNG1, cyclic nucleotide-gated channel 1; eNOS, endothelial NOS; ES, elongated spermatid; GC, germ cell; iNOS, inducible NOS; LC, Leydig cells; N, Sertoli cell nucleus; nNOS, neuronal NOS; PKG, protein kinase G; PS, pachytene spermatocyte; RS, round spermatid; N, Sertoli cell nucleus; sGC, soluble guanylyl cyclase; SC, Sertoli cells; SPC, preleptotene/leptotene spermatocyte; SPG, spermatogonium; TnNOS, testis-specific nNOS.

epithelium is physically divided into the adluminal compartment and basal compartment by the blood-testis barrier (BTB) which is constituted by adjacent Sertoli cells near the basement membrane.[4,5] Different cell types situate in specialized testicular locations. Sertoli cells and assorted germ cell types namely spermatogonia, spermatocytes, and spermatids are found in the seminiferous epithelium.[6] Myoid cells locate adjacent to the tubules and Leydig cells reside in the inter-tubular space known as the interstitium.[2] Each cell type performs different function, however they are communicating with each other to share the core role in sperm production during spermatogenesis. Apart from that, the male sex hormone level namely testosterone in the systemic circulation is also produced and regulated by the Leydig cells in the testis via steroidogenesis. These processes cannot be fully executed, if they are not equipped with precisely regulated interactive mechanisms during spermatogenesis. In rodents, the germ-line lineage spermatogonia, initially residing on the basement membrane of the seminiferous epithelium must differentiate into preleptotene spermatocytes, which in turn, traverse the BTB at stages VII-VIII of the epithelial cycle to gain entry into the adluminal compartment for further development[7] (Fig. 1). During this event of germ cell movement, Sertoli cells also play a paramount role in determining the molecular events of germ cell development, including mitosis, meiosis, cellular differentiation and transformation.[8] Sertoli cells accomplish this in part by monitoring the assembly and disassembly of inter-Sertoli junctions in the testes and partly by initiating cross-talk with germ cells.[9] For instance, Sertoli cells are equipped with certain architectural machineries, such as microtubules, that interact with the movement-associated germ cell proteins (e.g., motor proteins) to provide this coordination.[9] As such, premature germ cell release from the epithelium will be prohibitive. To sustain the optimal germ cell population in the testis, more than half (~75%) of the germ cells that are produced including spermatogonia, spermatocytes and spermatids undergo apoptosis, and are phagocytosed by Sertoli cells, thereby restricting the numbers of germ cells in the seminiferous epithelium. This spontaneous removal mechanism ensures that the limited resources from Sertoli cells (note: the number of Sertoli cells in adult rats remain the same throughout adulthood) are sufficient for germ cell development, and are within the capacity of the testes, by eliminating excessive germ cells to maintain germ cell quality.

Nitric oxide (NO) is a free radical synthesized by nitric oxide synthase (NOS). NOS is composed of two identical monomers with molecular weights ranging from 130 to 160 kDa.[10,11] Three isoforms of NOS, NOS I, II, and III, are known to date, which are the alternate names for neuronal NOS (nNOS) (Mr, ~320 kDa), inducible NOS (iNOS) (Mr, ~260 kDa), and endothelial NOS (eNOS) (Mr, ~270 kDa), respectively.[12] On the other hand, these NOS isoforms are functionally categorized into two groups, based on their intrinsic NO production efficacy. The constitutive group of NOS includes nNOS and eNOS, whereas iNOS belongs to the inducible form. Despite of these differences, all of them execute the same enzymatic reaction by converting L-arginine into NO and L-citrulline, using the cosubstrates of O_2 and nicotinamide adenine dinucleotide phosphate (NADPH). In addition, tetrahydrobiopterin (BH_4), flavin adenine dinucleotide (FAD), flavin mononucleotide (FMN), heme, calcium ions, and zinc ions are other necessary cofactors of this reaction.[11,13] nNOS and eNOS usually synthesize NO in nanomole range, unlike the micromole range of NO generated by iNOS. Excessive level of NO, at >1 μM, has a direct detrimental effect on the physiological system, via the production of peroxynitrile, after interacting with oxygen or superoxide.[14] In contrast, low concentration of NO, at <1 μM, works as an upstream regulatory molecule, goading the downstream signaling proteins, such as soluble guanylyl cyclase (sGC) that sequentially produces cGMP and activates protein kinase G (PKG).[15,16] An inimitable form of nNOS is being documented as testis-specific nNOS (TnNOS).[17] In short, the multifarious effects exhibited by NO are paramount in the general body metabolism. With the identification of a unique isoform of NOS, TnNOS, in the testis, an interest to examine the role of NOS and NO in spermatogenesis and steroidogenesis is expanding. As a complement to the earlier data regarding to the localization studies of NOS/NO and their related proteins and molecules, the functions of NOS/NO in spermatogenesis and steroidogenesis are being unfolded due to the establishment of several in vivo models or in clinical situations. Results derived from these studies advance the knowledge of NOS/NO in the testes and open the gate for the diagnosis and treatment of male reproductive dysfunctions.

NOS/NO in Junction Dynamics

Germ cells undergo various stages of differentiation during spermatogenesis, and these cells must also migrate from the basal compartment to adluminal compartment during maturation in the testis. To facilitate the course of germ cell movement, coordinated junction restructuring takes place between Sertoli and germ cells, resulting in the luminal release of spermatozoa. This phenomenon seems to be simple superficially; however, the mechanism(s) underneath is perhaps one of the most complicated procedures in the mammalian body. Unlike other endothelia and epithelia with assorted junction zones, seminiferous epithelium contains hybrid junctions instead.[18-20] The most imperative exposition of this heterogeneity is the BTB, which encompasses a minimal of three junction types: the tight junction (TJ), the gap junction (GJ), and the adherens junction (AJ).[20] As such, the passage of preleptotene spermatocytes through the BTB depends on the dynamic changes of the junction structures at the BTB. In the testes, junctions are broadly classified into three types, the anchoring junctions, the TJ, and the GJ. The former junction is further divided into two sub-groups, the actin cytoskeleton-based AJ, known alternatively as the ectoplasmic specialization (ES),[3,9] and the intermediate filament-based. Fundamental structure of junction complex consists of integral membrane or transmembrane proteins, which are indirectly linked to the underlying cytoskeletons via adaptors. In addition, peripheral regulatory proteins, such as kinases or phosphatases, are also found in the vicinity or in direct contact with these junction complexes. Thus, controlling the spatial and physical distributions of these junctions and their status are one of the important tasks for the successful generation of spermatozoa in a timely manner. Among numerous signaling molecules, NOS/NO is one of the important regulators of the junction integrity in the seminiferous epithelium.[21] The roles of NOS/NO in the junction dynamics are also implicated in other endothelia and epithelia. Below are discussions of the pertinent studies of these structural components in the testes and how NOS/NO alters the junction stability and integrity by affecting integral membrane proteins, adaptors, cytoskeletons, and regulatory proteins.

Integral Membrane Proteins

Three types of transmembrane proteins in the testis have been extensively studied in recent years. First, occludins, claudins, and junctional adhesion molecules (JAM) are restricted to TJ at the BTB.[4,21] Second, connexins are the known GJ proteins in the testes, with their distributions from the basal to the adluminal compartment in the seminiferous epithelium.[20,22] Third, different assortment of proteins in anchoring junctions.[9] Anchoring junctions are further divided according to their cytoplasmic associated cytoskeletons that serve as their attachment sites. Cadherins are the prominent proteins located between cells at the sites of actin-based AJ, such as basal ES at the BTB;[9] whereas integrins are found between cells and extracellular matrix at the sites of focal adhesion as well as at the Sertoli-germ cell interface at the apical ES. The structures and the components of these testicular junctions are resemblance of other epithelia in mammals. However, their relative locations are unique in the testes. For instance, ES is a testis-specific AJ type, but it is also a hybrid anchoring junction having the properties of both AJ and focal adhesion.[18,19] The physiological basis of these unusual features are currently unknown but recent studies have illustrated that there are cross-talk between different junction types in the seminiferous epithelium, which is mediated by the associated adaptors and/or the underlying cytoskeletons.[19,20]

Adaptors

Adaptors are proteins that originally thought to have a restricted function by maintaining junction integrity in which they link the transmembrane proteins to the underlying cytoskeletons, such as actin, microtubule, or intermediate filament. Subsequent studies in recent years have shown that adaptors are functionally much more diversified than initially conceived, such as by recruiting signaling molecules (e.g., kinases, phosphatases) to the junction site and by mediating cross-talk between different junctional protein complexes in the testes.[19] These expanded functionalities of adaptors are not entirely unexpected in view of their widespread occurrence in different junctional complexes. Amidst all the currently known adaptors, ZO-1 is known for its ability to conjoin occludin and connexin and it is found in both TJ and GJ.[19] As such, one junction type (e.g., TJ) can impose indirect influence to other junctions (e.g., GJ) via a common adaptor (e.g., ZO-1). This view has been validated in at least two other studies in the testis. When rats were treated with a blocking connexin peptide, disruption of connexin functions using pan-connexin peptide renders the disruption of occludin-based TJ, but not N-cadherin-based AJ in the testes.[23] This proves the vulnerability of the occludin-associated complex following a dysfunction of connexin-based GJ, since pan-connexin peptide with sequence conserved among all connexins virtually blocks all connexin-associated functions in the testes.[23] In addition, the structural association of γ-catenin, an AJ adaptor, and ZO-1, a TJ adaptor, is weakened after treatment of rats using adjudin, which is shown to have a role in disturbing the AJ without compromising the TJ in the testes.[3,24] These findings substantiate the significance of adaptors that mediate cross-talk between different junction types in the testes. Apart from that, other functions are recently uncovered for adaptors, including their participation in cytokine signaling in the testes and immune-related activities[25,26] Based on this emerging evidence, adaptors are proteins with diversified physiological functions in maintaining spermatogenesis, in particular the events of junction restructuring.

Cytoskeletons

Actin filaments, intermediate filaments, and microtubules are the three cytoskeletons found in mammalian cells including testes.[8] Actin filaments are assembled by the polymerization of the actin monomers, whereas microtubules are largely composed of α- and β-tubulins, which form the heterodimers as the basic constituents.[8,27] In spite of the identification of at least five categories of intermediate filament elements in the testes, vimentin is one of the most studied intermediate filament components in the testis.[8,28] Recently, the physiological roles ascribed to cytoskeletons are rapidly expanding. In addition to their roles that provide the cellular structural support and cell motility,[29] they are proven to participate in other signaling mechanisms, such as in the transcriptional regulation of genes in the nucleus.[30] Remarkably, nuclear actin and myosin are among two of the vital elements.[31] Other functional activities include the organization of chromosomes, and their allocation and segregation during mitosis.[32] In the seminiferous epithelium, actin is intimately involved in the development of acrosomes.[33] On the other hand, tubulin-based microtubules are known to serve as the track, which works in concert with motor proteins to direct the trans-epithelial movement of spermatids from basal to the apical compartment or vice versa.[9] Cytoskeletons have specific locations within the seminiferous epithelium. Due to the multiplexing nature of the junctions in the testes, the underlying junctions are intimately lying in the proximity of each other or even exhibiting an overlapping position. This further implicates the possible interaction among different cytoskeletons. Studies in other epithelia have illustrated that cytoskeletons mediate cross-talk between junctions.[34,35] Interestingly, there are accumulating evidence regarding the signal transduction properties of different cytoskeletal elements, such as the intermediate filament.[36] Due to the coherent complex nature of junctions in the testes, much work is needed in this area to decipher the functional roles of different cytoskeletons and their interactions during spermatogenesis.

Studies of NOS/NO in the Testes

Many proteins and/or molecules are known modulators of the junction integrity and functionality in the testes[25,37] including NO. NO is highly efficient in these processes due to its small molecular size and diffusible nature, making its sites of action distance away from its production sites. The major source of NO in the testes derives from macrophages found in the microvessels and in the inter-tubular compartment in the interstitium, making Leydig cells as one of the most immediate responders to NO (Fig. 1).[38,39] This effect inevitably alters the metabolic activities in Leydig cells, modulating their testosterone output during steroidogenesis (see below). Indeed, testicular macrophages are prominent cellular regulators in Leydig cell physiology, due to their proximal location with Leydig cells and that they are also the cellular source of growth factors and/or cytokines.[39] Apart from that, NO also influences the activity of Sertoli and germ cells within the seminiferous tubules. However, the effects exhibited are not as remarkable as those observed in Leydig cells due to the intrinsic physical distance between the interstitium and the seminiferous epithelium. However, NO released from the different forms of NOS found in the seminiferous epithelium is the major regulator of the spermatogenetic process. Several NOSs are found in different testicular cells. Three major forms of NOS and their defined locations in the testes are known to date (Table 1 and Fig. 1). Germ cells express eNOS, whereas Leydig cells produce iNOS abundantly.[21] On the other hand, minor amounts of nNOS are produced by Sertoli cells. In spite of the presence of these classic NOSs, a testis-specific NOS variant has been identified and entitled as the truncated form of nNOS (TnNOS).[17] Its expression is limited to Leydig cells, strongly implicating its role in steroidogenesis.[40] This testicular forms of NOS seems to be an appropriate subject of an intensive investigation, however, its functions are not fully deciphered due to the lack of knockout mouse model.

In order to fully appreciate the physiological effects of NOS/NO, recent studies have extended to their effectors, which are the executioners of the NOS/NO signaling pathway. The components of the sGC/cGMP/PKG pathway are expressed in a cyclic manner during the seminiferous epithelial cycle in the testes[41-43] (Table 1 and Fig. 1). Spatially, iNOS is depicted to exist in coherent locations with their associated proteins, such as sGC and PKG., as demonstrated by immunohistochemistry and immunofluorescent microscopy.[41,42,44] These observations emphasize the close association of components of NOS/NO pathways in the seminiferous epithelium. A panel of junction proteins has been shown to be putative NOS-binding proteins using the techniques of coimmunoprecipitation and immunoblottings. For instance,

Table 1. Cellular localization of NOS signaling pathway components and their putative associated proteins in mammalian testes

	Cellular Localization*								
Proteins	**SC**	**GC**	**AC**	**LC**	**MC**	**MF**	**EC**	**SP**	**Putative Associated Proteins†**
CNG 1	+	+	-	-	-	-	-	-	n.k.
eNOS	+	+	/	+	/	+	+	+	actin, β-catenin, eNOS, iNOS, N-cadherin, occludin, sGC, α-tubulin, vimentin
iNOS	+	+	/	+	+	/	-	+	actin, β-catenin, eNOS, iNOS, N-cadherin, occludin, sGC, α-tubulin, vimentin
nNOS	+	-	+	+	/	+	+	+	sGC, cGMP
PKG	+	+	+	-	-	+	+	-	β-catenin, sGC
sGC	+	+	+	+	+	+	+	-	actin, afadin, cadherin, catenin, connexins, eNOS, espin, iNOS, JAM, nectin, nNOS, occludin, PKC, PKG, ponsin, sGC, tubulin, vimentin, ZO-1
TnNOS	-	-	-	+	-	-	-	-	n.k.

*Cellular localization was revealed by RT-PCR, IB, IHC, and/or IF. †Putative associated proteins were assessed by co-IP, IHC, and/or IF. This table was prepared based on the following research articles and reviews.[40-44,59,60,67-75] *Abbreviations used:* +, presence; -, absence; /, not positively identified; AC, acrosome; CNG 1, cyclic nucleotide-gated channel 1; co-IP, coimmunoprecipitation; EC, endothelial cells in blood vessels; eNOS, endothelial NOS; IB, immunoblot; IF, immunofluorescent microscopy; IHC, immunohistochemistry; GC, germ cells; iNOS, inducible NOS; JAM, junctional adhesion molecule; LC, Leydig cells; MC, myoid cells; MF, myofibroblasts; n.k., not known; nNOS, neuronal NOS; NOS, nitric oxide synthase; PKG, protein kinase G; SC, Sertoli cells; sGC, soluble guanylyl cyclase; RT-PCR, reverse transcription polymerase chain reaction; SP, spermatozoa; TnNOS, testis-specific nNOS; ZO-1, zonula occludens-1.

iNOS and eNOS were shown to associate with occludin-based TJ complexes in the testes.[44] Besides, these two NOS isoforms also link to the N-cadherin-based junction network.[42] Additionally, sGC, the downstream effector of the NOS pathway, is structurally associated with both AJ and TJ protein complexes in the testes.[43] In this context, NOS/NO is a putative regulator of junction restructuring in the testes as illustrated in other functional studies. Zinc (II) protoporphyrin-IX, a broad spectrum NOS inhibitor and a sGC inhibitor, was shown to perturb the TJ integrity in Sertoli cell cultures.[44] This event also accompanied by a down-regulation in the amount of intracellular cGMP and the occludin protein steady-state levels.[44] iNOS and eNOS were also shown to dissociate from the N-cadherin/β-catenin protein complexes during the Adjudin-induced AJ restructuring in the rat testes that led to germ cell depletion from the epithelium.[42] Apart from that, the administration of KT-5823, a PKG inhibitor, delayed the actions of Adjudin in mediating germ cell loss from the seminiferous epithelium.[42] Significantly, a tighter association of sGC with cadherin-based protein complex was observed during Adjudin-induced junction restructuring in vivo, whilst a weakened interaction was found between sGC and TJ protein complexes[43] (Table 2 and Fig. 2). Based on these findings, the significance of the NOS/NO/sGC/PKG pathway in AJ dynamics in the testes is increasingly clear. In short, the NOS/NO pathway is one of the versatile mechanisms utilized by the testes to regulate junction dynamics.

Studies of NOS/NO in Other Systems That Can Be the Basis of Future Studies in the Testes

As described above, NOS/NO is a novel pathway to regulate AJ and TJ dynamics in the testes. However, information regarding the ability of NOS/NO in regulating other junction types, such as gap junctions and other anchoring junctions (e.g., desmosome-like junctions), are lacking. Recent studies have shown that NO regulates connexin 35-associated gap junction coupling in neurons.[45] However, it remains to be determined if there is any interaction between NO and connexins in the testes. Also, NO has a negative role in modulating integrin-linked kinase, a protein kinase related to the integrin-associated protein complex, in rat kidneys[46] (Table 2). However, these results still need to be validated in the testes.

NOS/NO and Spermatogenesis

NOS/NO and the Hormone/Cytokine/Paracrine/Autocrine System in the Testis

Hormones and cytokines are known to have versatile functions ranging from the modulation of endocrine systems to the fine-tuning of immune systems. Within the microenvironment in the testis, testosterone, the major male sex hormone, dominates the processes of spermatogenesis. The synthesis of testosterone by Leydig cells is under the control of luteinizing hormone (LH) released from the pituitary gland. For cytokines, they are mostly derived from the immune cells (e.g., macrophages) in the circulation and diffuse into the testicles via the blood vessels.[39] Importantly, large part of the NO produced in the testes is derived from activated testicular macrophages, which are having high levels of iNOS.[47] These exogenous and endogenous sources of hormones and cytokines are involved in constraining the expression of different forms of NOS in the testes, and as such, indirectly affecting the testicular NO steady-state level.[21]

On the other side, NO coordinates the testicular production of hormones and cytokines. Exposure of Leydig cell cultures to an NO donor, S-nitrosoglutathione can elicite an inhibition of testosterone production in vitro.[47] Other studies have demonstrated that the activated macrophage-produced NO is associated with a reduction in the testosterone producing activity in Leydig cells.[48] Notably, this inhibition is at least in part involved with the blockade of the P450 steroidogenic enzymes.[48]

Table 2. Participation of NOS/NO in the regulation of junctions in testes and other epithelia

Organ or Tissue/ Junction Type	NOS	Target Junction Proteins	Regulation	Selected References
Testis/TJ	eNOS, iNOS	n.k.	-	44
Testis/AJ	iNOS	N-Cadherin, β-Catenin	-	42
Hepatobiliary duct/GJ	iNOS	Occludin, ZO-1, ZO-2, ZO-3	-	76
Brain/TJ	gNOS	Occludin	+	77
Vascular/GJ	gNOS	Connexin 37	-	78
Muscular/GJ	gNOS	Connexin 43	-	79
Neuronal/GJ	gNOS	n.k.	+	80

This table only contains selected examples of NOS and the role of NO in junctions including the testes and other nongonadal tissues. Other important studies are not cited due to the page limit. *Abbreviations and symbols used:* +, positive regulation; -, negative regulation; nk, information not known; AJ, adherens junction; eNOS, endothelial NOS; iNOS, inducible NOS; GJ, gap junction; gNOS, studies involved the activation of general NOS activity in the systems; NO, nitric oxide; NOS, nitric oxide synthase; TJ, tight junction; ZO, zonula occludens.

In short, the bi-directional relationship manifested by NOS/NO and the hormone/cytokine level is crucial in maintaining the physiological function of the testes.

NOS/NO in Germ Cell Development and Differentiation

Germ Cell Apoptosis and Germ Cell Output in the Seminiferous Epithelium

The number of total germ cells produced by the testes is tightly regulated in order to secure the production of viable and fertile germ cells within the supporting capacity of the Sertoli cells in the testes. In the rat, Sertoli cells begin to proliferate at day 16 post-coitus, and at birth, the number of Sertoli cells is about 1 million per testis; and by day 15 post-natal, the number of Sertoli cells rises to ~40 million, however, proliferation ceases to occur thereafter.[49] The Sertoli cell number remains relatively constant throughout adulthood.[50] Thus, this fixed number of Sertoli cells cannot nurture unlimited number of germ cells generated from the primordial spermatogonia. To remove redundant and abnormal perhaps unhealthy germ cells, an elimination mechanism involving germ cell apoptosis is being utilized by the testes. More than half of the germ cells, perhaps ~75%, particular spermatogonia and spermatocytes, undergo spontaneous apoptosis during normal spermatogenesis. Besides estrogens (e.g., 17β-estradiol) that regulate the germ cell number via apoptosis (see below) (for a review, see ref. 51), another mechanism via phagocytosis is also used by the testis. In brief, apoptotic germ cells destined to be phagocytosed by Sertoli cells are recognized via an externalized phosphatidylserine on the apoptotic germ cell surface, which, in turn, coheres the class B scavenger receptor type I (SR-BI) on Sertoli cell surface[52] since Sertoli cells also serve as the scavenger in the epithelium. If the SR-BI on the Sertoli cell surface is inactivated by a monoclonal anti-SR-BI antibody, this causes an increase in residual apoptotic germ cells in the epithelium.[52] Using these mechanisms, the sperm output by the testis can be finely maintained without overwhelming the Sertoli cells.

Notwithstanding, uncontrolled apoptosis would disintegrate the harmonized microenvironment and the Sertoli:germ cell ratios in the seminiferous epithelium during spermatogenesis. As such, these apoptotic events can also be triggered by external stimuli or artificially induced, such

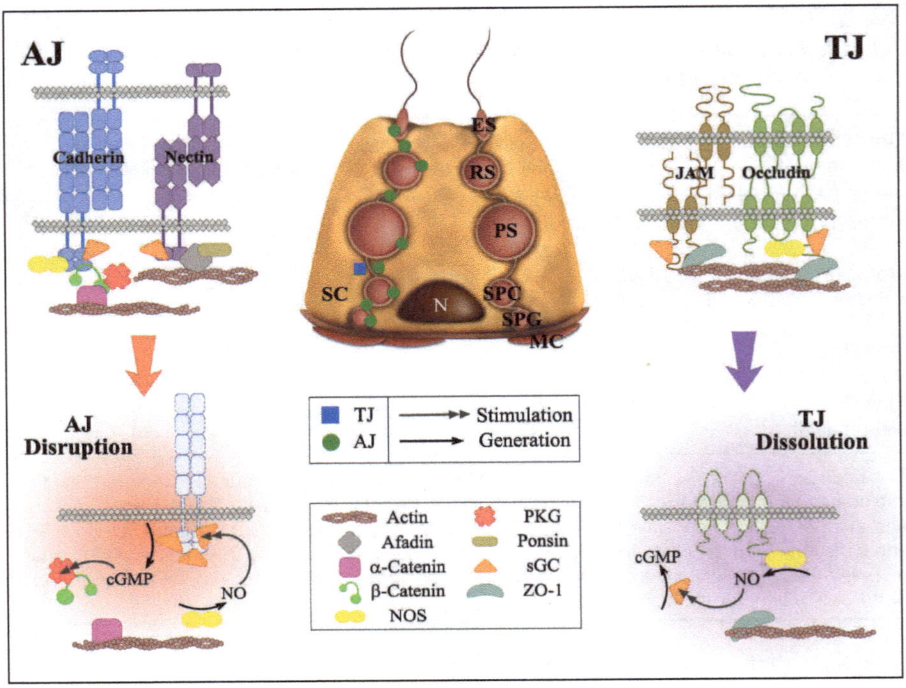

Figure 2. The NOS/NO signaling pathways that regulate AJ and TJ dynamics in the testes. This is a simplified schematic diagram summarizing recent studies regarding the role of the NOS/NO signaling pathway that regulates junction dynamics in the testis using the Adjudin model.[42-44] Abbreviations used: AJ, adherens junction; ES, elongated spermatid; JAM, junctional adhesion molecule; MC, myoid cells; N, Sertoli cell nucleus; NO, nitric oxide; NOS, nitric oxide synthase; PKG, protein kinase G; PS, pachytene spermatocyte; RS, round spermatid; SC, Sertoli cell; sGC, soluble guanylyl cyclase; SPC, preleptotene/leptotene spermatocyte; SPG, spermatogonium; TJ, tight junction; ZO-1, zonula occludens-1.

as testosterone deprivation and local testicular heating,[53] which are detrimental to spermatogenesis. Based on these other models, several germ cell apoptotic pathways have also been identified. At the molecular levels, caspases, especially caspase 3,[53] and Fas/Fas ligand (Fas L)[54] are the main regulatory molecules. These pathways are probably inter-connected and mediated by junction proteins, such as connexins, during apoptosis in the testes.[23] There are reports in the literature illustrating an excessive NO level can directly trigger massive germ cell apoptosis in the testes. These are clearly depicted in the artificial spermatic vessel ligation model[55] and in the mouse model of congenital cryptorchidism,[56] both of which were shown to elevate NO testicular levels and uncontrolled germ cell apoptosis. The role of NO in germ cell apoptosis has been further strengthened by the observation that treatment of Hoxa 11 knockout mice having congenital cryptorchidism using L-NAME, an NOS inhibitor, to block the NO-mediated effects can grossly attenuate germ cell apoptosis.[56] Normal aging process also illustrates the association of NO and apoptosis.[57] In aged testes, aggravated NOS activity and an induced iNOS level were shown to accompany with high incidence of germ cell apoptosis.[57] iNOS and eNOS are also postulated to participate in germ cell apoptosis in the testes.[21] Specifically, eNOS has been known to be highly expressed in degenerating germ cells in comparison with other germ cell types.[58,59] In addition, iNOS plays a determining role in restricting the germ cell numbers in the testes, since testes from $iNOS^{-/-}$ mice are heavier on average when compared to normal testes,[60] and a marked reduction

Table 3. Correlation of testis function and NOS/NO in human diseases and mouse models

NOS Type	Testicular Dysfunction/Model	Correlaetion/ Observation	Selected References
Human diseases			
eNOS	Obstructive azoospermia	Insignificant expression change	63
	Varicocele	Insignificant expression change	63
	Idiopathic azoospermia	Reduces eNOS level	63
iNOS	Sertoli cell only syndrome	Induces iNOS level	81
Mouse models			
eNOS	Congenital cryptorchidism	Induces eNOS level associated with apoptosis	56
	Ischemia-reperfusion	Induces eNOS level associated with apoptosis	58
iNOS	Aging	Induces iNOS level associated with apoptosis	57

This table only includes selected examples and references, many important studies in the field were not included since we did not intend to be exhaustive because of the page limit.

on germ cell apoptosis, in particular pachytene spermatocytes and round spermatids, is noted.[60] These observations thus clearly illustrate the unequivocal role of NO in triggering germ cell apoptosis in the testes. Nonetheless, the downstream NO pathway(s) that regulates germ cell apoptosis is presently not known.

NOS/NO in Fertility and Pathogenesis

Male fertility has always been a primary concern in human reproduction. At the molecular level, fertility partly refers to the successful fusion of male and female gametes, which depends on several factors for its completion. The quality and quantity of sperm and sperm concentrations are several of the key issues directly affecting fertilization. As mentioned earlier, apoptosis is one of the key processes that maintains the quality and quantity of germ cells in the testes.[61] Thus, if apoptosis fails to control these variables, a lack of viable and fertile germ cells will be the consequence. If testes fail to produce sufficient number of healthy spermatozoa without defects, infertility is unavoidable. Several etiologies are known to goad infertility, such as varicocele, tumors, and azoospermia. Also, DNA integrity in sperm is another major determinant.[62] It is known that an unbalanced levels of NO or dysregulation of NOS in the testes contribute to some of these defects (Table 3). For instance, a reduced testicular eNOS protein level was observed in patients with idiopathic azoospermia versus patients with obstructive azoospermia or varicocele and healthy individual.[63] Besides, excess NO in human varicocele conditions was demonstrated to be harmful to the sperm motility.[64] Despite all this, a physiological level of NO is required for successful fertilization.[65] Apart from that, NO is also known to participate in sperm transport from the rete testis to the epididymis. The propelling force that transports spermatozoa to the epididymis via the rete testis is generated by the contraction and relaxation of the tunica albuginea in the testis, which, in turn, is regualted by PKG, a downstream effector of NOS/NO.[66] In short, NOS/NO has diversified roles in testis pathogenesis.

Concluding Remarks and Future Perspectives

NO is a versatile molecule with diversified functions ranging from coordinating cell and blood vessel permeability to junction regulation. It is produced by four isoforms of NOS, namely eNOS, iNOS, nNOS, and TnNOS. NOS/NO is depicted to regulate disparate junction dynamics, at AJ and TJ, in the testes. However, the significance of NOS/NO in the regulation of other junction types, such as gap junctions and desmosomes, are not fully deciphered and much effort is needed to uncover the associated mechanisms and identify the proteins that are involved. Apart from that, NOS/NO is illustrated to have roles in monitoring the levels of hormones and cytokines, indirectly controlling the processes of spermatogenesis and steroidogenesis. Importantly, NOS/NO also takes part in the regulation of germ cell development and differentiation, partially via the coordination of germ cell apoptosis and maintaining the correct ratio of Sertoli:germ cells in the epithelium, securing the efficacy in the production of viable and fertile spermatozoa. As such, NOS/NO is crucial to maintain male fertility and pathogenesis. An expanded research in this area can form the foundation of identifying candidate molecules for male contraception and to understand male reproductive pathogenesis.

Acknowledgements

This work was supported in part by grants from the National Institutes of Health (NICHD U01 HD045908, and U54 HD29990 Project 3) and the CONRAD Program (CICCR CIG 01-72).

References

1. Johnson AD, Gomes WR, Vandemark NL. The Testis Volume 1: Development, Anatomy, and Physiology. New York: Academic Press, 1970.
2. Russell L, Ettlin RA, Sinha Hikim AP et al. Histological and Histopathological Evaluation of the Testis. Clearwater: Cache River, 1990:1-52.
3. Mruk DD, Cheng CY. Cell-cell interactions at the ectoplasmic specialization in the testis. Trends Endocrinol Metab 2004; 15:439-447.
4. Wong CH, Cheng CY. The blood-testis barrier: Its biology, regulation, and physiological role in spermatogenesis. Curr Top Dev Biol 2005; 71:263-296.
5. Parreira GG, Melo RCN, Russell L. Relationship of Sertoli-Sertoli tight junctions to ectoplasmic specialization in conventional and en face views. Biol Reprod 2002; 67:1232-1241.
6. Russell LD. Sertoli-germ cell interrelations: A review. Gamete Res 1980; 3:179-202.
7. Russell L. Movement of spermatocytes from the basal to the adluminal compartment of the rat testis. Amer J Anat 1977; 148:313-328.
8. Mruk DD, Cheng CY. Sertoli-Sertoli and Sertoli-germ cell interactions and their significance in germ cell movement in the seminiferous epithelium during spermatogenesis. Endocr Rev 2004; 25:747-806.
9. Lee NPY, Cheng CY. Ectoplasmic specialization, a testis-specific cell-cell actin-based adherens junction type: Is this a potential target for male contraceptive development? Human Reprod Update 2004; 10:349-369.
10. Stuehr DJ. Structure-function aspects in the nitric oxide synthases. Annu Rev Pharmacol Toxicol 1997; 37:339-359.
11. Bogdan C. Nitric oxide and the regulation of gene expression. Trends Cell Biol 2001; 11:66-75.
12. Forstermann U, Gath I, Schwarz P et al. Isoforms of nitric oxide synthase: Properties, cellular distribution and expressional control. Biochem Pharmacol 1995; 50:1321-1332.
13. Alderton WK, Cooper CE, Knowles RG. Nitric oxide synthases: Structure, function and inhibition. Biochem J 2001; 357:593-615.
14. Davis KL, Martin E, Turko IV et al. Novel effects of nitric oxide. Annu Rev Pharmacol Toxicol 2001; 41:203-236.
15. Hanafy KA, Krumenacker JS, Murad F. NO, nitrotyrosine, and cyclic GMP in signal transduction. Medical Science Monitor 2001; 7:801-819.
16. Hofmann F, Ammendola A, Schlossmann J. Rising behind NO: cGMP-dependent protein kinases. J Cell Sc 2000; 113:1671-1676.
17. Wang Y, Goligorsky MS, Lin M et al. A novel, testis-specific mRNA transcript encoding an NH_2-terminal truncated nitric oxide synthase. J Biol Chem 1997; 272:11392-11401.
18. Schneeberger EE, Lynch RD. The tight junction: A multifunctional complex. Am J Physiol Cell Physiol 2004; 286:C1213-C1228.
19. Lee NPY, Cheng CY. Mini-review: Adaptors, junction dynamics, and spermatogenesis. Biol Reprod 2004; 71:392-404.
20. Lee NPY, Yeung WSB, Luk JM. Junction interaction in the seminiferous epithelium: Regulatory roles of connexin-based gap junction. Front Biosci 2007; 12:1552-1562.

21. Lee NPY, Cheng CY. Nitric oxide/nitric oxide synthase, spermatogenesis, and tight junction dynamics. Biol Reprod 2004; 70:267-276.
22. Pointis G, Segretain D. Role of connexin-based gap junction channels in testis. Trends Endocrinol Metab 2005; 16:300-306.
23. Lee NPY, Leung KW, Wo JY et al. Blockage of testicular connexins induced apoptosis in rat seminiferous epithelium. Apoptosis 2006; 11:1215-1229.
24. Yan HH, Cheng CY. Blood-testis barrier dynamics are regulated by an engagement/disengagement mechanism between tight and adherens junctions via peripheral adaptors. Proc Natl Acad Sci USA 2005; 102:11722-11727.
25. Xia W, Mruk DD, Lee WM et al. Cytokines and junction restructuring during spermatogenesis-a lession to learn from the testis. Cytokine Growth Factor Rev 2005; 16:469-493.
26. Togni M, Lindquist J, Gerber A et al. The role of adaptor proteins in lymphocyte activation. Mol Immunol 2004; 41:615-630.
27. Nogales E. Structural insights into microtubule function. Annu Rev Biophys Biomol Struct 2001; 30:397-420.
28. Helfand BT, Chang L, Goldman RD. The dynamic and motile properties of intermediate filaments. Annu Rev Cell Dev Biol 2003; 19:445-467.
29. Small JV, Resch GP. The comings and goings of actin: Coupling protrusion and retraction in cell motility. Curr Opin Cell Biol 2005; 17:517-523.
30. Pederson T, Aebi U. Nuclear actin extends, with no contraction in sight. Mol Biol Cell 2005; 16:5055-5060.
31. de Lanerolle P, Johnson T, Hofmann WA. Actin and myosin I in the nucleus: What next? Nat Struct Mol Biol 2005; 12:742-746.
32. McIntosh JR, Grishchuk EL, West RR. Chromosome-microtubule interactions during mitosis. Annu Rev Cell Dev Biol 2002; 18:193-219.
33. Breitbart H, Cohen G, Rubinstein S. Role of actin cytoskeleton in mammalian sperm capacitation and the acrosome reaction. Reproduction 2005; 129:263-268.
34. Chou YH, Helfand BT, Goldman RD. New horizons in cytoskeletal dynamics: Transport of intermediate filaments along microtubule tracks. Curr Opin Cell Biol 2001; 13:106-109.
35. Chang L, Goldman RD. Intermediate filaments mediate cytoskeletal crosstalk. Nat Rev Mol Cell Biol 2004; 5:601-613.
36. Helfand BT, Chou YH, Shumaker DK et al. Intermediate filament proteins participate in signal transduction. Trends Cell Biol 2005; 15:568-570.
37. Wong CH, Cheng CY. Mitogen-activated protein kinases, adherens junction dynamics, and spermatogenesis: A review of recent data. Dev Biol 2005; 286:1-15.
38. Hutson JC. Physiologic interactions between macrophages and Leydig cells. Exp Biol Med 2006; 231:1-7.
39. Hales DB. Testicular macrophage modulation of Leydig cell steroidogenesis. J Reprod Immunol 2002; 57:3-18.
40. Wang Y, Newton DC, Miller TL et al. An alternative promoter of the human neuronal nitric oxide synthase gene is expressed specifically in Leydig cells. Am J Pathol 2002; 160:369-380.
41. Shi F, Wang T. Stage- and cell-specific expression of soluble guanylyl cyclase alpha and beta subunits, cGMP-dependent protein kinase I alpha and beta, and cyclic nucleotide-gated channel subunit 1 in the rat testis. J Androl 2005; 26:258-263.
42. Lee NPY, Mruk DD, Wong CH et al. Regulation of Sertoli-germ cell adherens junction dynamics in the testis via the nitric oxide synthase (NOS)/cGMP/protein kinase G (PRKG)/β-catenin (CATNB) signaling pathway: An in vitro and in vivo study. Biol Reprod 2005; 73:458-471.
43. Sarkar O, Xia W, Mruk DD. Adjudin-mediated junction restructuring in the seminiferous epithelium leads to displacement of soluble guanylate cyclase from adherens junctions. J Cell Physiol 2006; 208:175-187.
44. Lee NPY, Cheng CY. Regulation of Sertoli cell tight junction in the rat testis via the nitric oxide synthase/soluble guanylate cyclase/cGMP/protein kinase G signaling pathway: An in vitro study. Endocrinology 2003; 144:3114-3129.
45. Patel LS, Mitchell CK, Dubinsky WP et al. Regulation of gap junction coupling through the neuronal connexin Cx35 by nitric oxide and cGMP. Cell Commun Adhes 2006; 13:41-54.
46. Beck KF, Walpen S, Eberhardt W, Pfeilschifter J. Downregulation of integrin-linked kinase mRNA expression by nitric oxide in rat glomerular mesangial cells. Life Sci 2001; 69:2945-2955.
47. Weissman BA, Niu E, Ge R et al. Paracrine modulation of androgen synthesis in rat Leydig cells by nitric oxide. J Androl 2005; 26:369-378.
48. Pomerantz DK, Pitelka V. Nitric oxide is a mediator of the inhibitory effect of activated macrophages on production of androgen by the Leydig cell of the mouse. Endocrinology 1998; 139:922-931.

49. Orth JM. Proliferation of Sertoli cells in fetal and postnatal rats: A quantitative autoradiographic study. Anat Rec 1982; 203:485-492.
50. Wang ZX, Wreford NG, de Kretser DM. Determination of Sertoli cell numbers in the developing rat testis by stereological methods. Int J Androl 1989; 12:58-64.
51. Shaha C. Estrogen and spermatogenesis. In: Cheng CY, ed. Molecular Mechanisms in Spermatogenesis. Austin: Landes Bioscience, 2007, (in press).
52. Nakanishi Y, Shiratsuchi A. Phagocytic removal of apoptotic spermatogenic cells by Sertoli cells: Mechanisms and consequences. Biol Pharm Bull 2004; 27:13-16.
53. Sinha Hikim AP, Lue Y, Diaz-Romero M et al. Deciphering the pathways of germ cell apoptosis in the testis. J Steroid Biochem Mol Biol 2003; 85:175-182.
54. Koji T. Male germ cell death in mouse testes: Possible involvement of Fas and Fas ligand. Med Electron Microsc 2001; 34:213-222.
55. Taneli F, Vatansever S, Ulman C et al. The effect of spermatic vessel ligation on testicular nitric oxide levels and germ cell-specific apoptosis in rat testis. Acta Histochem 2005; 106:459-466.
56. DeFoor WR, Kuan CY, Pinkerton M et al. Modulation of germ cell apoptosis with a nitric oxide synthase inhibitor in a murine model of congenital cryptorchidism. J Urol 2004; 172:1731-1735.
57. Sinha Hikim AP, Vera Y, Vernet D et al. Involvement of nitric oxide-mediated intrinsic pathway signaling in age-related increase in germ cell apoptosis in male Brown-Norway rats. J Gerontol A Biol Sci Med Sci 2005; 60:702-708.
58. Zini A, Abitbol J, Girardi SK et al. Germ cell apoptosis and endothelial nitric oxide synthase (eNOS) expression following ischemia-reperfusion injury to testis. Arch Androl 1998; 41:57-65.
59. Zini A, O'Bryan MK, Magid MS et al. Immunohistochemical localization of endothelial nitric oxide synthase in human testis, epididymis, and vas deferens suggests a possible role for nitric oxide in spermatogenesis, sperm maturation, and programmed cell death. Biol Reprod 1996; 55:935-941.
60. Lue Y, Hikim APS, Wang C et al. Functional role of inducible nitric oxide synthase in the induction of male germ cell apoptosis, regulation of sperm number, and determination of testes size: Evidence from null mutant mice. Endocrinology 2003; 144:3092-3100.
61. Sakkas D, Seli E, Manicardi GC et al. The presence of abnormal spermatozoa in the ejaculate: Did apoptosis fail? Hum Fertil 2004; 7:99-103.
62. O'Brien J, Zini A. Sperm DNA integrity and male infertility. Urology 2005; 65:16-22.
63. Fujisawa M, Yamanaka K, Tanaka H et al. Expression of endothelial nitric oxide synthase in the Sertoli cells of men with infertility of various causes. BJU Int 2001; 87:85-88.
64. Kisa U, Basar MM, Ferhat M et al. Testicular tissue nitric oxide and thiobarbituric acid reactive substance levels: Evaluation with respect to the pathogenesis of varicocele. Urol Res 2004; 32:196-199.
65. Kim BH, Kim CH, Jung KY et al. Involvement of nitric oxide during in vitro fertilization and early embryonic development in mice. Arch Pharm Res 2004; 27:86-93.
66. Middendorff R, Muller D, Mewe M et al. The tunica albuginea of the human testis is characterized by complex contraction and relaxation activities regulated by cyclic GMP. J Clin Endocrinol Metab 2002; 87:3486-3499.
67. Meroni SB, Suburo AM, Cigorraga SB. Interleukin-1β regulates nitric oxide production and γ-glutamyl transpeptidase activity in Sertoli cells. J Androl 2000; 21:855-861.
68. Burnett AL, Ricker DD, Chamness SL et al. Localization of nitric oxide synthase in the reproductive organs of the male rat. Biol Reprod 1995; 52:1-7.
69. Herrero MB, Perez Martinez S, Viggiano JM et al. Localization by indirect immunofluorescence of nitric oxide synthase in mouse and human spermatozoa. Reprod Fertil Dev 1996; 8:931-934.
70. Middendorff R, Muller D, Wichers S et al. Evidence for production and functional activity of nitric oxide in seminiferous tubules and blood vessels of the human testis. J Clin Endocrinol Metabol 1997; 82:4154-4161.
71. Davidoff MS, Middendorff R, Mayer B et al. Nitric oxide synthase (NOS-I) in Leydig cells of the human testis. Arch Histol Cytol 1995; 58:17-30.
72. Herrero MB, Goin JC, Boquet M et al. The nitric oxide synthase of mouse spermatozoa. FEBS Letts 1997; 411:39-42.
73. O'Bryan MK, Schlatt S, Gerdprasert O et al. Inducible nitric oxide synthase in the rat testis: Evidence for potential roles in both normal function and inflammation-mediated infertility. Biol Reprod 2000; 63:1285-1293.
74. O'Bryan MK, Zini A, Cheng CY et al. Human sperm endothelial nitric oxide synthase expression: Correlation with sperm motility. Fertil Steril 1998; 70:1143-1147.
75. Davidoff MS, Middendorff R, Mayer B et al. Nitric oxide/cGMP pathway components in the Leydig cells of the human testis. Cell Tissue Res 1997; 287:161-170.

76. Han X, Fink MP, Uchiyama T et al. Increased iNOS activity is essential for hepatic epithelial tight junction dysfunction in endotoxemic mice. Am J Physiol Gastrointest Liver Physiol 2004; 286:G126-G136.
77. Yamagata K, Tagami M, Takenaga F et al. Hypoxia-induced changes in tight junction permeability of brain capillary endothelial cells are associated with IL-1beta and nitric oxide. Neurobiol Dis 2004; 17:491-499.
78. Kameritsch P, Khandoga N, Nagel W et al. Nitric oxide specifically reduces the permeability of Cx37-containing gap junctions to small molecules. J Cell Physiol 2005; 203:233-242.
79. Roh CR, Heo JH, Yang SH et al. Regulation of connexin 43 by nitric oxide in primary uterine myocytes from term pregnant women. Am J Obstet Gynecol 2002; 187:434-440.
80. O'Donnell P, Grace AA. Cortical afferents modulate striatal gap junction permeability via nitric oxide. Neuroscience 1997; 76:1-5.
81. Sezer C, Koksal IT, Usta MF et al. Relationship between mast cell and iNOS expression in testicular tissue associated with infertility. Arch Androl 2005; 51:149-158.

CHAPTER 11

The Sertoli Cell Cytoskeleton

A. Wayne Vogl,* Kuljeet S. Vaid and Julian A. Guttman

Abstract

The cytoskeleton of terminally differentiated mammalian Sertoli cells is one of the most elaborate of those that have been described for cells in tissues. Actin filaments, intermediate filaments and microtubules have distinct patterns of distribution that change during the cyclic process of spermatogenesis. Each of the three major cytoskeletal elements is either concentrated at or related in part to intercellular junctions. Actin filaments are concentrated in unique structures termed ectoplasmic specializations that function in intercellular adhesion, and at tubulobulbar complexes that are thought to be involved with junction internalization during sperm release and movement of spermatocytes through basal junctions between neighboring Sertoi cells. Intermediate filaments occur in a perinuclear network which has peripheral extensions to desmosome-like junctions with adjacent cells and to small hemidesmosome-like attachments to the basal lamina. Unlike in most other epithelia where the intermediate filaments are of the keratin type, intermediate filaments in mature Sertoli cells are of the vimentin type. The function of intermediate filaments in Sertoli cells is not entirely clear; however, the pattern of filament distribution and the limited experimental data available are consistent with a role in maintaining tissue integrity when the epithelium is mechanically stressed. Microtubules are abundant in Sertoli cells and are predominantly oriented parallel to the long axis of the cell. Microtubules are involved with maintaining the columnar shape of Sertoli cells, with transporting and positioning organelles in the cytoplasm, and with secreting seminiferous tubule fluid. In addition, microtubule-based transport machinery is coupled to intercellular junctions to translocate and position adjacent spermatids in the epithelium. Although the cytoskeleton of Sertoli cells has structural and functional properties common to cells generally, there are a number of properties that are unique and that appear related to processes fundamental to spermatogenesis and to interfacing somatic cells both with similar neighboring somatic cells and with differentiating cells of the germ cell line.

Introduction

The cytoskeleton in animal cells consists of actin filaments, intermediate filaments and microtubules. These filamentous polymers are associated with a plethora of associated molecules that determine the balance between soluble subunits and polymers, the way in which the polymers are linked to others of the same and different types, and the way in which various molecules, protein complexes and organelles are transported and positioned in cells. The cytoskeleton not only is a determinant of cell shape, but also plays significant roles in cell division, intracellular transport and cell movement, and in establishing and maintaining tissue organization and integrity.

*Corresponding Author: A. Wayne Vogl—Department of Cellular and Physiological Sciences, Division of Anatomy and Cell Biology, Faculty of Medicine, Life Sciences Centre, The University of British Columbia, 2350 Health Sciences Mall, Vancouver, British Columbia, Canada, V6T 1Z3. Email: vogl@interchange.ubc.ca

Molecular Mechanisms in Spermatogenesis, edited by C. Yan Cheng. ©2008 Landes Bioscience and Springer Science+Business Media.

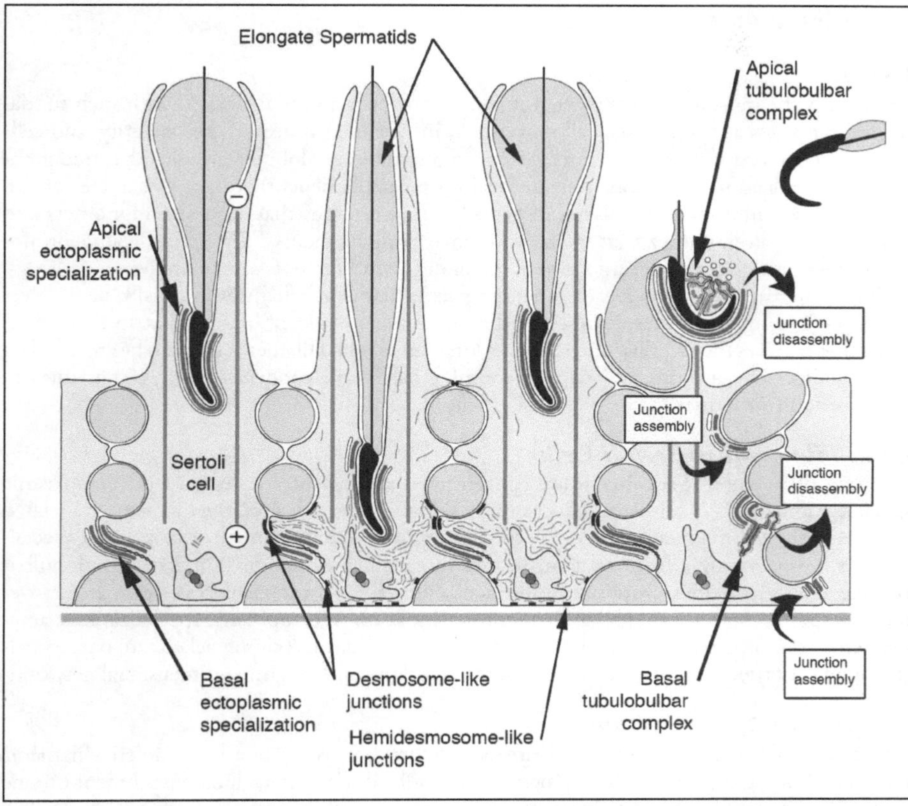

Figure 1. Schematic diagram showing the distribution of major elements of the Sertoli cell cytoskeleton at progressive stages of spermatogenesis in the rat seminiferous epithelium. Actin filaments are shown in red, intermediate filaments are in blue, and microtubules are in green. Actin filaments are concentrated in ectoplasmic specializations and tubulobulbar complexes. Intermediate filaments are concentrated around the nucleus and extend to desmosome-like attachments with adjacent Sertoli and spermatogenic cells and to hemidesmosome-like attachments with the basal lamina. Microtubules are predominantly oriented parallel to the long axis of the cell.

In Sertoli cells, actin filaments, intermediate filaments and microtubules are abundant and are concentrated in specific regions (Fig. 1). They also are dynamic; that is, their patterns of organization change during spermatogenesis.[1] Interestingly, all three elements of the cytoskeleton are related, at least in part, to sites of intercellular attachment and may play significant roles in translocating, positioning, and anchoring spermatogenic cells in the seminiferous epithelium and in establishing and maintaining epithelial organization. This association with intercellular junctions and with specialized structures related to junction turnover indicates that the cytoskeleton also may participate in the mechanism of sperm release and in the process by which spermatocytes move through basal inter-Sertoli junction complexes as these cells move from basal to adluminal compartments of the epithelium.

Actin Filaments

General

Actin is the most abundant protein in eukaryotic cells and is associated with such fundamental processes as cytokinesis, cell movement, intracellular transport, cell polarity, and cell/cell and cell/substratum attachment.[2-5] Actin monomers are globular proteins that under appropriate nucleation conditions polymerize into polar filaments that have a diameter of 5-8 nm. There are more than 60 classes of actin binding proteins that sequester monomers and nucleate, cap, sever, stabilize, cross-link and move along filaments.[6] The actin-dependent motor proteins associated with cargo movement along actin filaments are the myosins.[7]

There are two major models of generating actin filament structures in cells. One involves the Arp2/3 complex that results in three-dimensional networks of branched actin filaments.[8] The other involves the formins[3] and results in long unbranched filaments that can be cross-linked into bundles. The formins and Arp2/3 complex may work cooperatively at certain sites to generate actin structures.[9]

Actin Filaments in Sertoli Cells

Actin filaments in Sertoli cells are concentrated in two specific regions: (1) ectoplasmic specializations, and (2) tubulobulbar complexes (Fig. 1). At both sites, the filaments are related to areas of the plasma membrane involved with intercellular attachment. Ectoplasmic specializations are primarily a form of actin-related intercellular adhesion junction. Tubulobulbar complexes are structures proposed to internalize junctions prior to sperm release and movement of spermatocytes through basal junction complexes. At ectoplasmic specializations, actin filaments occur in bundles in which the filaments are unipolar and close-packed into paracrystals (hexagonal arrays). At tubulobulbar complexes, the filaments form three-dimensional networks.

Ectoplasmic Specializations

Ectoplasmic specializations are tripartite structures consisting of a layer of actin filaments together with regions of the plasma membrane involved with intercellular attachment on one side of the filament layer and a cistern of endoplasmic reticulum on the other[10-19] (Fig. 1). The intercellular gap between cells at ectoplasmic specializations narrows to about 90 angstroms.[10]

Ectoplasmic specializations occur at two locations in Sertoli cells (Fig. 2): (1) At heterotypic sites of attachment between Sertoli cells and spermatids in apical regions of the seminiferous epithelium; (2) As part of the homotypic junction complex between neighboring Sertoli cells near the base of the seminiferous epithelium.

At apical sites, ectoplasmic specializations assemble as spermatids polarize and become situated in apical Sertoli cell crypts. Ectoplasmic specializations develop in Sertoli cell regions of the crypts juxtaposed to acrosomal regions of spermatid heads. No structures similar to ectoplasmic specializations develop in the spermatid heads. At certain stages of spermatogenesis, notably stage V in the rat, intermediate filament associated junctions (desmosome-like) appear to intercalate themselves into ectoplasmic specializations in regions adjacent to the dorsal curvature of spermatid heads,[1,20] and then later disappear. When spermatids are mechanically separated from the seminiferous epithelium, intact ectoplasmic specializations remain attached to the surfaces of the cells, indicating that the three components of the junction (plasma membrane, actin filaments and endoplasmic reticulum of the Sertoli cell) are a structural unit.[21]

At basal sites of attachment between Sertoli cells, ectoplasmic specializations occur in each of the adjacent cells and therefore the junctions are bilateral. Ectoplasmic specializations appear to overlap with and incorporate other junction types such as tight and gap junctions into their structure[10,22,23] (Fig. 3). Together with desmosome-like junctions and the other junction types, ectoplasmic specializations form large junction complexes. Tight junctions in these complexes form the "blood-testis" or "blood-Sertoli" barrier.

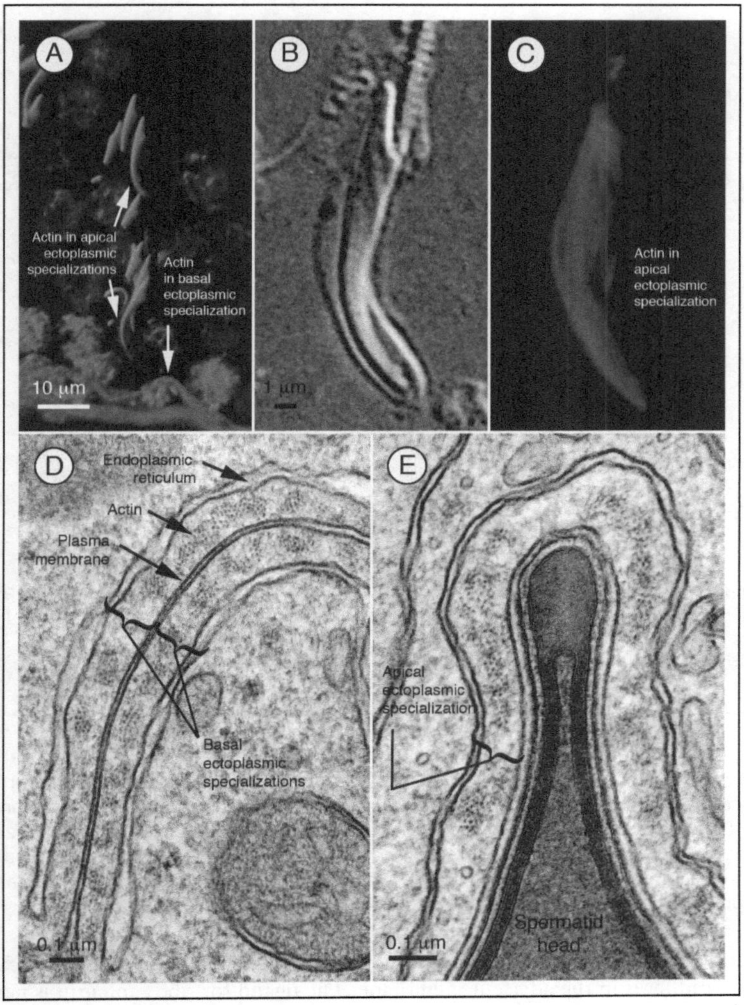

Figure 2. Apical and basal ectoplasmic specializations (rat). A) Confocal projection of a section of rat seminiferous epithelium at approximately stage V of spermatogenesis. Actin is red and nuclei are blue. Apical ectoplasmic specializations are associated with elongate spermatids in this image, and basal ectoplasmic specializations occur as part of the junction complex between adjacent Sertoli cells. B,C) Paired DIC (differential interference contrast) and fluorescence images of an elongate spermatid with attached ectoplasmic specialization that has been mechanically dissociated from the seminiferous epithelium. Actin staining mainly is present in the ectoplasmic specialization attached to the spermatid head. D) Electron micrograph of basal ectoplasmic specializations at a site of inter-Sertoli cell attachment. E) Electron micrograph of apical ectoplasmic specialization at a site of attachment to a mature spermatid.

Most available evidence, from studies where localization clearly occurs both at apical and at basal sites and/or where codistribution with actin filaments has been determined, is consistent with the conclusion that the integral membrane adhesion molecules present at mature ectoplasmic specializations in vivo are mainly $\alpha6\beta1$ integrin,[24,25] nectin-2,[26] and JAMs.[27]

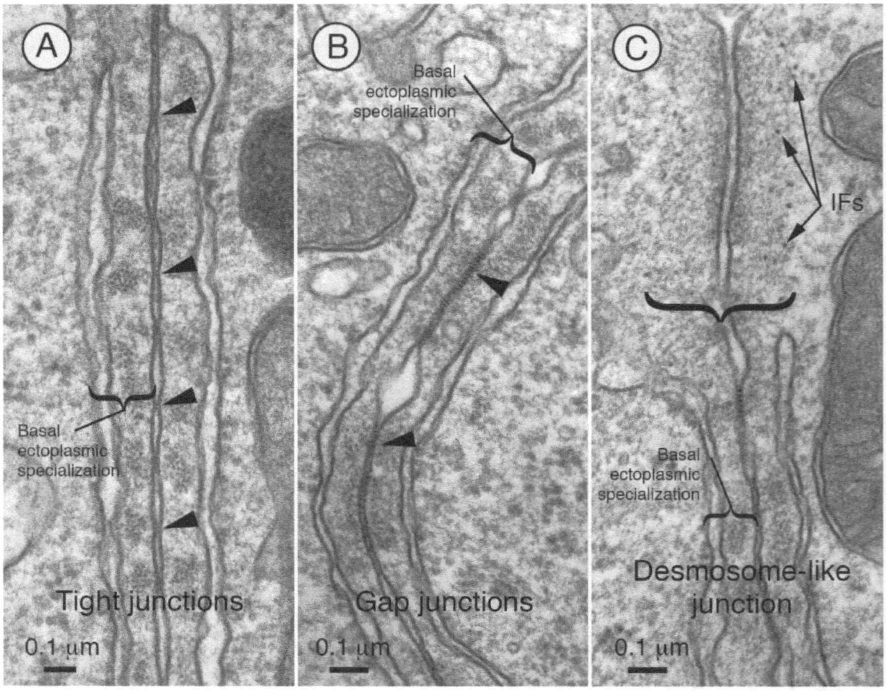

Figure 3. Electron micrographs of basal ectoplasmic specializations (rat). In basal junction complexes between adjacent Sertoli cells, other junction types overlap with, occur within or are intercalated amongst ectoplasmic specializations. A) In this image, tight junctions (arrowheads) are incorporated into the structure of the two opposing ectoplasmic specializations. B) Gap junctions (arrowheads) occur within the adhesion complex in this image. C) A desmosome-like junction, enclosed by the bracket, is closely related to an ectoplasmic specialization situated in the lower half of the image. IFs, intermediate filaments.

N-cadherin also is reported present at the sites.[28-30] Presumably the ligand for N-cadherin is another N-cadherin in the adjacent membrane. The ligand for $\alpha6\beta1$ integrin is not entirely clear, although laminin $\gamma3$ recently has been identified as a candidate at apical sites.[31] The ligand for nectin-2 is nectin-3 in spermatid membranes at apical sites and another nectin-2 on the neighboring Sertoli cell at basal sites.[26] Nectin-2 knockout male mice are infertile and show loss of actin filaments and intercellular adhesion at ectoplasmic specializations—a result that highlights the importance of this type of adhesion junction to spermatogenesis.[26]

In addition to integral membrane adhesion proteins and actin filaments, other elements present at ectoplasmic specializations include the adaptor proteins vinculin[32] and afadin,[26] that facilitate the relationship between integral membrane adhesion elements and the underlying actin cytoskeleton. The catenins also are reported as present.[33] Actin binding proteins concentrated at the sites include α-actinin,[34] fimbrin,[35] espin,[36] Keap 1,[37] and cortactin.[38] Although myosin VIIa is present in the structures,[39] myosin II is not[40] and the actin bundles are not considered to have contractile potential. Nonmuscle cofilin is not localized at the sites.[41] Paxillin is not concentrated at the sites but is generally expressed in the cytoplasm of Sertoli cells.[42]

Regulation of Actin Filament Dynamics at Ectoplasmic Specializations

The regulation of ectoplasmic specializations recently has received a great deal of attention because they are thought to contain potential molecular targets for male contraceptives.[18,29,33,43-45] It is proposed that intercellular attachment at ectoplasmic specializations is regulated directly by TGF-β3 through the Ras/MEK/ERK signaling pathway.[33] Attachment also may be influenced at a higher order level by hormones.[46-50]

The mechanisms of actin polymerization and depolymerization at ectoplasmic specializations have not been studied in detail, although changes in actin dynamics are suspected to be linked to changes in the status of adhesion elements in the plasma membrane. The unipolar, hexagonally packed and un-branched arrangement of actin filaments in ectoplasmic specializations indicates that predominantly a formin-based mechanism of polymerization rather than an Arp 2/3-based mechanism may be involved. Although not yet localized to ectoplasmic specializations, the formins have been implicated in actin polymerization at adherens junctions generally in epithelia and a model involving activation by Rho GTPases has been proposed.[51] Once filaments are formed at ectoplasmic specializations, espin, fimbrin and α-actinin are likely involved with cross-linking the filaments into bundles and inter-relating the bundles to each other.

It has long been suspected that the endoplasmic reticulum component of ectoplasmic specializations may function to regulate calcium within the micro-environment of the junction plaque[52] and thereby influence junction dynamics, possibly through effects on regulating calcium dependent actin-severing proteins such as gelsolin/scinderin.[53,54] This class of proteins also binds to phosphatidylinositol 4,5-bisphosphate (PtdIns(4,5)*P*2) in the plasma membrane and is released when PtdIns(4,5)*P*2 is converted to inositol (1,4,5)-trisphosphate (Ins(1,4,5)*P*3) and diacylglycerol by phosphoinositide-specific phospholipase C. The Ins(1,4,5)*P*3, which is released from the plasma membrane, acts to release calcium from the endoplasmic reticulum, which in turn stimulates the actin severing activity of the free actin-binding proteins. The hypothesis that actin filament dynamics, particularly disassembly, is regulated in part by calcium dependent actin-binding proteins that also bind to PtdIns(4,5)*P*2 in the plasma membrane is attractive because it ties together the three structural elements of ectoplasmic specializations—the endoplasmic reticulum, the actin layer, and the plasma membrane.

We have reevaluated our original experiments in which we demonstrated the presence of gelsolin at the sites and feel our initial findings may largely have been due to secondary binding to the sites of exogenous gelsolin present both in serum used in our antibody blocking buffers and in serum contaminants in our spermatid/ectoplasmic specialization isolates.[55] Although the calcium dependent actin-binding protein/phosphoinositide hypothesis generally is still viable, we now believe that gelsolin may not be a significant player. This conclusion is consistent with the observation that the reproductive capacity of gelsolin knock-out animals is not impaired.[56] The roles of the endoplasmic reticulum and of calcium-dependent actin-binding proteins at ectoplasmic specializations remains to be clarified.

Function of Actin filaments in Ectoplasmic Specializations

The arrangement of actin bundles in mammalian ectoplasmic specializations, and the hexagonal packing of actin filaments within the bundles, may function structurally to reinforce and stabilize large intercellular adhesion domains in an epithelium where cells progressively change position and shape during spermatogenesis and in areas where the plasma membrane has an irregular contour. This is particularly true at apical sites where Sertoli cells are attached to spermatid heads. The observation that the patterns of actin bundles in ectoplasmic specializations change to conform to the maturing shape of spermatid heads during spermatogenesis is consistent with this function. The loss of adhesion between Sertoli cells and early elongate spermatids[57] and the disruption of the structural and functional integrity of basal junction complexes[58] after intratesticular injection of cytochalasin D are consistent with the argument that actin filaments stabilized adhesion domains in the plasma membrane.

Tubulobulbar Complexes

Tubulobulbar complexes are elaborate structures that develop at apical and basal sites of intercellular attachment in the seminiferous epithelium (Fig. 1). They are most pronounced at apical sites of adhesion between Sertoli cells and spermatids (Figs. 4 and 5)[59] where the formation of multiple generations of these structures precedes sperm release. In this apical location, the structures consist of a number of tubular extensions from the plasma membrane of spermatid heads that protrude into corresponding plasma membrane invaginations of the adjacent Sertoli cell. The structures have swollen or "bulbar" ends that often have small tubular extensions with "coated pits" at their termini. A network of actin filaments cuffs the long tubular invaginations of the Sertoli cell and the bulbar regions are closely related to cisternae of endoplasmic reticulum. The terminal parts of the complexes are associated with numerous vesicles, some of which have been identified as lysosomes.[59-61] The large bulbar regions of the complexes are thought to "bud" from the structures and be degraded.

A number of functions have been attributed to tubulobulbar complexes. They have been suggested to anchor spermatids to the epithelium based on the observation that they are the last structures to disengage at sperm release.[59,60] They also are considered to function as a route by which Sertoli cells can eliminate cytoplasm from spermatids.[62] Support for this argument comes from the observation that the development of tubulobulbar complexes correlates with the time during which cytoplasmic volume of spermatids dramatically decreases,[62] and spermatids are much larger when tubulobulbar complexes do not develop in association with them.[63] Another suggested function is that they facilitate the shaping of spermatid

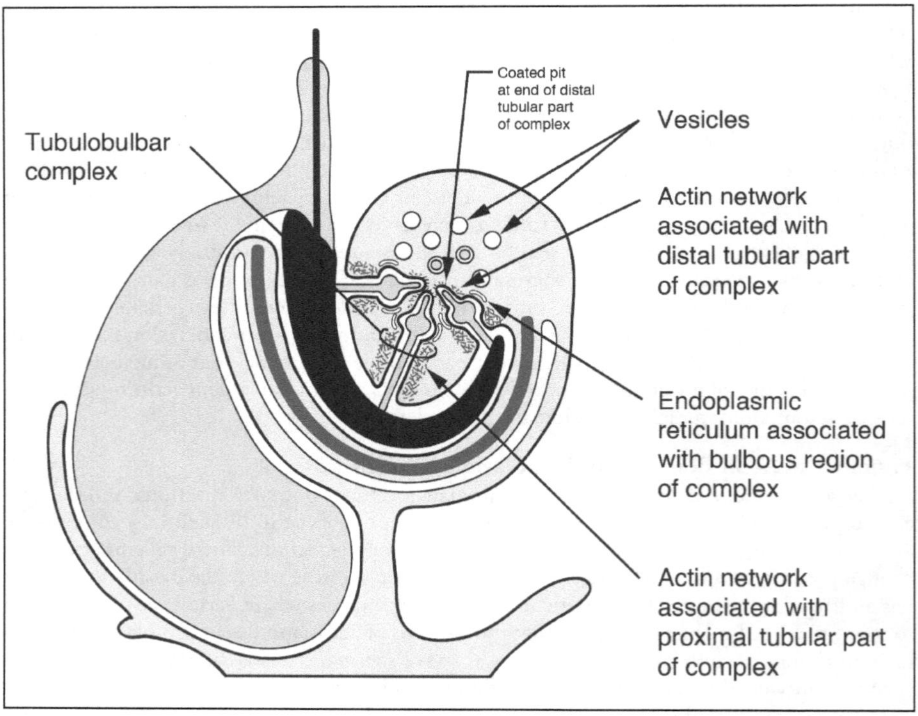

Figure 4. Schematic diagram of tubulobulbar complexes. Shown here is a magnified view of the apical region of a Sertoli cell that is related to a mature spermatid (rat). Three tubulobulbar complexes and their parts are illustrated.

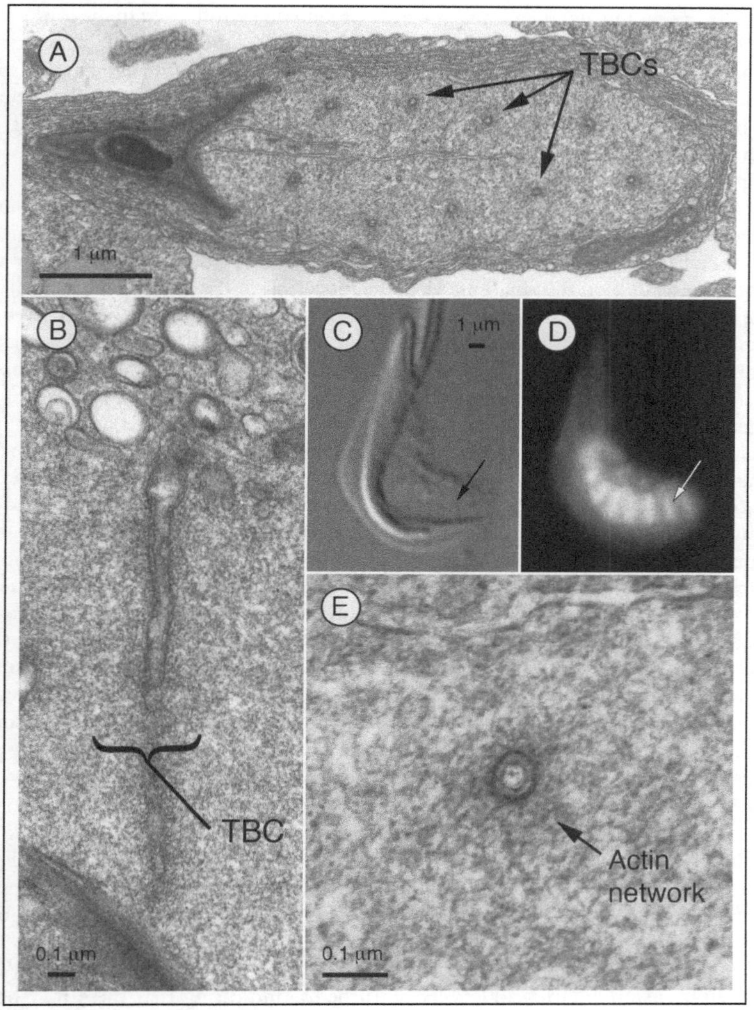

Figure 5. Apical tubulobulbar complexes (rat). A) Electron micrograph of a section through a late spermatid head and associated tubulobulbar complexes (TBCs). Multiple tubulobulbar complexes are shown in cross section. B) Electron micrograph of a longitudinal section through a tubulobulbar complex (TBC). C,D) Paired DIC and fluorescence images of tubulobulbar complexes (arrows) associated with the head of a late spermatid. The filamentous actin in (D) is labeled with fluorescent phallotoxin and appears as an elongate cuff around the tubular membrane components of each complex. E) Electron micrograph a cross section through a single tubulobulbar complex. The actin filaments of the complex form a network surrounding the membrane components. This organization of actin filaments into a network is clearly different from the hexagonally packed bundles of filaments seen in ectoplasmic specializations (see Fig. 2D).

heads.[64] An additional function, and the one that we favor, is that tubulobulbar complexes internalize integral membrane junction proteins during junction disassembly,[61] a hypothesis initially put forward by Russell[57,60] and later by Pelletier.[22]

Generally in cells integral membrane junction proteins are synthesized in the rough endoplasmic reticulum where they are inserted into the membrane. They generally pass through the Golgi, and then "junction vesicles" are transported to and inserted into the basolateral plasma membrane. Here the proteins are mobile in the plane of the membrane and eventually may become incorporated into junctions. There is recent evidence that the trajectory of junction vesicles from Golgi to plasma membrane may not be as direct as initially thought. E-Cadherin, for example, may pass through a recycling endosome prior to delivery to the plasma membrane.[65] During constitutive or induced junction turnover, the junction proteins in the membrane are internalized by endocytosis and may either be degraded or recycled. The emerging mechanism for the internalization of adherens and tight junction components appears to be one of disengagement from ligands on the adjacent cell and endocytosis of the proteins in each adjacent cell as part of either clathrin- or a caveolin-mediated pathways[66-70] or by clathrin and caveolin independent mechanisms such as macropinocytosis[71] depending on cell context and regulation.[72]

Interestingly, intact gap junctions, consisting of connexons in the plasma membranes of both adjacent cells, are typically removed from the surface and internalized by one of the cells and targeted to lysosomes.[73,74] A similar mechanism recently has been observed for "moving" epithelial cells internalizing intercellular tight junctions.[75] In this experimental system (MDCK and mouse Eph4 cells), adjacent junction membranes do not detach from one another. Rather, they are coendocytosed as double membrane vesicles into one of the adjacent cells and targeted for degradation. This type of mechanism also has been observed in colon and ovarian adenocarcinoma cell lines.[76,77] We propose that this mechanism may be the normal method of junction internalization by tubulobulbar complexes in the seminiferous epithelium of the testis.

The model we propose is one in which Sertoli cells internalize junction proteins by the "budding-off" of large double membrane vesicles, from tubulobulbar complexes, that then either fuse with lysosomes and are degraded or are selectively recycled to the plasma membrane. In other words, junction proteins in one cell together with the attached junction proteins in the membrane of the adjacent cell are internalized together at tubulobulbar complexes. Although this mechanism would basically be a caveolin- and clathrin-independent pathway, our model also includes the possibility that some sorting by clathrin- and caveolin-mediated pathways of proteins may occur prior to and/or after budding of double membrane vesicles from the complexes, and that some of these junction molecules may eventually be recycled back to the plasma membrane. The observation that there are small vesicles, "coated pits" and multivesicular bodies associated with tubulobulbar complexes is consistent with this possibility.

Pertinent to the junction internalization hypothesis are a number of key observations made by Russell and coworkers[57,59,60,78] in their now classic ultrastructural descriptions. First, the structures develop in areas occupied by ectoplasmic specializations or in areas where ectoplasmic specializations are pharmacologically perturbed,[57] indicating that there may be a functional relationship between junctions and tubulobulbar complexes. Second, tubulobulbar complexes not only develop at apical junctions between Sertoli cells and spermatids, but also develop at basal junction complexes between adjacent Sertoli cells (Fig. 6), indicating that the primary function of tubulobulbar complexes is not related only to spermatid maturation. Finally, ultrastructurally identifiable gap and tight junctions occur in the bulbous regions of basal tubulobulbar complexes,[78] indicating that junction elements do occur in these structures.

We recently have confirmed that tubulobulbar complexes at apical junctions with spermatids develop in regions previously occupied by ectoplasmic specializations. We also have found that double membrane vesicles occur at the ends of the complexes and that lysosomal and endosomal markers are associated with vesicles in similar locations.[61] In addition, protein kinase Cα, a signaling molecule known to regulate endocytosis of junction proteins in other systems[66,79,80] is concentrated in regions containing tubulobulbar complexes. Significantly, immunological probes for nectin-2 (Sertoli cell) and nectin-3 (spermatid) react in a vesicular pattern with the ends of tubulobulbar complexes in fluorescence experiments, indicating that the two molecules each from different cells may be internalized together by Sertoli cells.

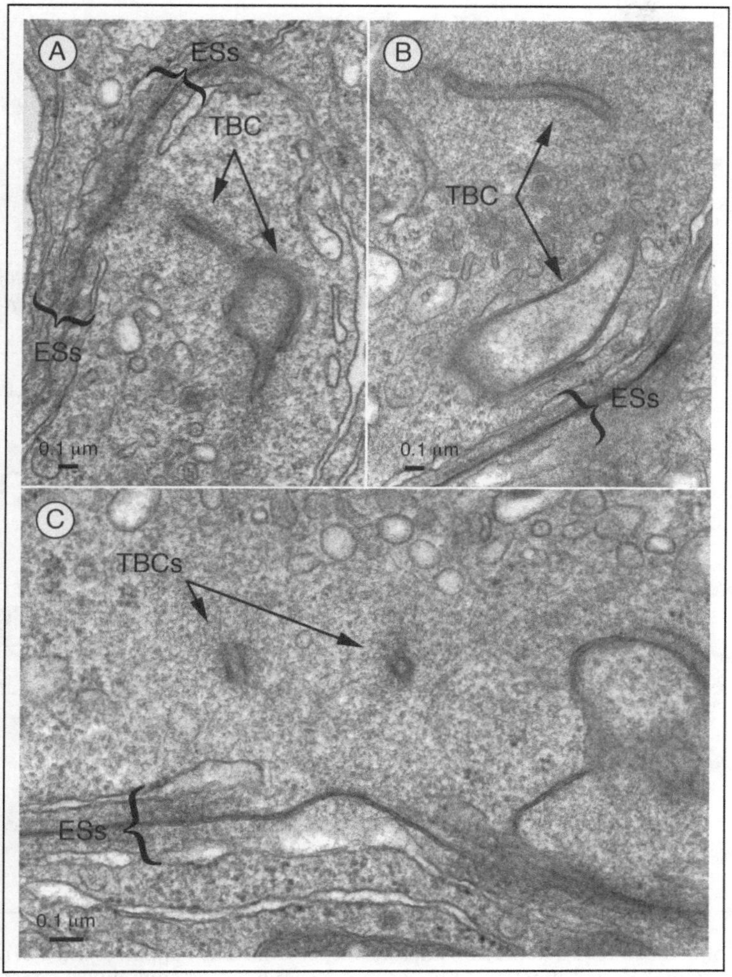

Figure 6. Electron micrographs of tubulobulbar complexes (TBC) associated with basal junction complexes between adjacent Sertoli cells. A,B) Longitudinal sections through the 'tubular' and 'bulbar' regions of tubulobulbar complexes. C) Cross section through two tubulobulbar complexes (TBCs). In all three images, the tubulobulbar complexes occur in regions associated with ectoplasmic specializations (ESs).

The junction internalization hypothesis of tubulobulbar function does not rule out the possibility that other processes may be involved in junction turnover, particularly at basal sites where junctions must disassemble above and assemble below spermatocytes as these cells translocate between basal and adluminal compartments of the epithelium (Fig. 7). At basal sites, tubulobulbar complexes are smaller than at apical sites and are much less numerous than might be predicted if they were the sole means for junction turnover. One alternative possibility is that junction components separate from those in the adjacent Sertoli cell and are endocytosed directly from the plasma membrane as occurs in other epithelia, and then are either degraded or recycled. Another is that some junction molecules dissociate from their ligands and move within the plane of the membrane around translocating spermatocytes to reattach to their partner ligands below.

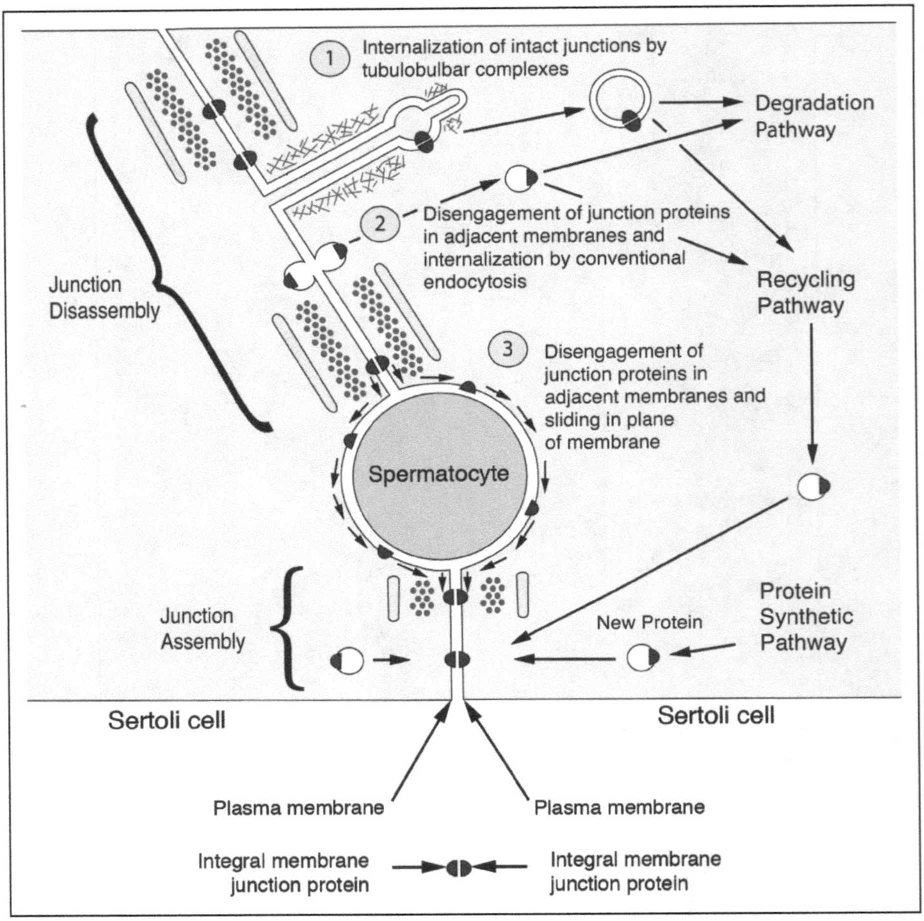

Figure 7. Shown here are a number of alternatives for what may happen to integral membrane junction proteins during junction turnover in the seminiferous epithelium. Intact junctions may be internalized by tubulobulbar complexes and then either be recycled to newly assembling junctions or be degraded. Alternatively, junction proteins may disengage from their ligands in adjacent membranes and then be internalized by standard endocytic pathways in each cell, and then degraded or recycled. Another possibility is that junction proteins disengage from their ligands, move within the plane of the membrane, and then are recruited into newly assembling junctions elsewhere in the cell. Newly assembling junctions incorporate new protein from synthetic pathways and 'old' protein from recycling compartments. Although a basal junction complex between two Sertoli cells is illustrated here, a similar model could be proposed for junctions that disassemble during sperm release and that assemble in association with early elongate spermatids. It is likely that the Sertoli cell cytoskeleton, particularly actin filaments and microtubules, are involved in the proposed pathways.

At both basal and apical sites, the contributions from reused (recycled or moved in the plane of the membrane) and of newly synthesized junction proteins to the formation of junction complexes below spermatocytes and to newly formed ectoplasmic specializations at sites of attachment to early elongating spermatids needs to be investigated further.

Actin Filament Dynamics at Tubulobulbar Complexes

Little is known about the actin filaments associated with tubulobulbar complexes. What is known is that the actin filaments appear arranged into a three dimensional cuff that surrounds the length of each tubular component of the complexes. The arrangement of filaments into a network is consistent with the possibility that the Arp2/3 complex is involved in formation of the structures, although this remains to be verified.

The fact that tubulobulbar complexes originate from areas previously occupied by ectoplasmic specializations raises the possibility that the actin network might result partly from a remodeling of preexisting actin filaments in the junction plaques. Support for this possibility is that tubulobulbar complexes contain some of the same protein components that are found in ectoplasmic specializations.[61]

Among actin-related components known to be associated with tubulobulbar complexes are paxillin,[42] espin, myosin VIIa, and Keap 1.[61] One component found associated with tubulobulbar complexes that does not appear to be concentrated at ectoplasmic specializations is the calcium-independent actin-depolymerizing protein nonmuscle cofilin,[41] a protein that is regulated by phosphorylation. The presence of cofilin at tubulobulbar complexes fits nicely with an Arp2/3 model of actin network formation at these sites.

The Function of Actin at Tubulobulbar Complexes

The function of the actin filament networks at tubulobulbar complexes is not known; however one obvious possibility is that the filaments facilitate the formation and maintenance of the elongate tubular shape of the complexes. This conclusion is consistent with the observation that tubular parts of the complexes do not form after intratesticular injection of cytochalasin D.[81] During normal spermatogenesis, disassembly of the filament networks near the ends of the complexes may lead to the formation of the bulbs and to the eventual budding of large double membrane vesicles from the complexes. The biological function of having numerous elongate tubes associated with junction disassembly may be related to increasing the surface area for the internalization of the huge amounts of junctional membrane during sperm release and during the movement of spermatocytes through basal junction complexes.

Intermediate Filaments

General

Intermediate filaments generally are classified into five Types (I - V) on the basis of gene substructure and sequence homology in a specific region of the proteins.[82] Type I to IV form 8-12 nm diameter cytoplasmic filaments while type V consists of the lamins that form part of a meshwork on the inner aspect of the nuclear membrane. Unlike actin filaments and microtubules, intermediate filaments are formed from filamentous rather than globular subunits and the resulting polymers lack polarity. There are no intermediate filament dependent motor proteins. Also, filament dynamics are not dependent on nucleotide binding and hydrolysis by subunits and there is only a small pool of soluble subunits in vivo.[82] Importantly for their function, and unlike actin filaments and microtubules, there is growing evidence that cytoplasmic intermediate filaments are flexible, extensible and tough.[83,84]

Generally in epithelial cells, intermediate filaments form perinuclear networks that extend peripherally to attach to cell/cell and cell/substratum adhesion junctions.[85] Through this relationship of strong yet elastic cytoskeletal elements with adhesion sites, a significant function of intermediate filaments is to provide tissues, particularly epithelia, with mechanical support and the ability to maintain tissue integrity and be resilient to mechanical deformation.[85]

Other functions of cytoplasmic intermediate filaments include establishing the positions of organelles, providing scaffolds for signaling and other protein complexes, facilitating resistance to metabolic stress, and determining cytoarchitecture.[82,86-88] The nuclear lamins have been implicated in determining nuclear shape and providing structural support for the nuclear membrane. They also may play roles in positioning nuclear pores and anchoring chromatin to the nuclear envelope, and in the biogenesis of nuclear membranes.[89]

Intermediate Filaments in Sertoli Cells

In Sertoli cells, cytoplasmic intermediate filaments are major components of the cytoskeleton. The filaments mainly consist of vimentin (Type III),[90] although keratins (Type I and II) are expressed during development,[91] and in certain other situations.[92,93] Nestin (Type IV) also is expressed in Sertoli cells during development.[94] Nuclear lamins are present in Sertoli cells,[95,96] but have not been extensively studied.

Intermediate filaments in terminally differentiated Sertoli cells form a network around the nucleus with peripheral extensions to desmosome-like junctions with adjacent Sertoli and spermatogenic cells and to hemidesmosome-like structures that connect the cell to the basal lamina (Figs. 1, 8, 9 and10).[1,97] When spermatids are embedded deep within Sertoli cell apical crypts, transient demosome-like junctions are intercalated into the ectoplasmic specializations in regions along the dorsal curvature of the spermatid heads (Figs. 1, 8 and 11).[1] At these locations, intermediate filaments appear to pass through a defect in the ectoplasmic specialization and associate with a density on the plasma membrane. Desmosome-like junctions are dynamic during spermatogenesis[11] so it is not surprising that the intermediate filament patterns also change during spermatogenesis.[1]

Generally in cells, desmosomes consist of the desmosomal cadherins (desmogleins and desmocollins) that are the integral membrane adhesion molecules, the armadillo proteins (plakoglobin and plakophilins) that link the desmosomal cadherins to the intermediate filament cytoskeleton and/or function as signaling or regulatory molecules, and the plakins (desmoplakin, plectin, envoplakin and periplakin) that regulate the linkage between the membrane complexes and underlying intermediate filaments.[98] Hemidesmosomes consist of the integral membrane proteins integrin ($\alpha6\beta4$) and type XVII collagen (also called bullous pemphigoid antigen-2) that links the membrane to the basal lamina, and the plakins (bullous pemphigoid antigen-1 and plectin) that link the integral membrane proteins to intermediate filaments.[99,100]

Remarkably little is known about desmosome-like and hemidesmosome-like junctions in the seminiferous epithelium. Desmosome-like junctions with spermatogenic cells are macular or spot-like in appearance. They are characterized by sub-plasma membrane densities on both the Sertoli and spermatogenic cell sides of the junctions (Fig. 10)[101] and by a discontinuous and poorly defined intermediate dense line between adjacent plasma membranes. Intermediate filaments are related only to the Sertoli cell side of the junctions. Desmosome-like junctions between neighboring Sertoli cells are similar to those formed with spermatogenic cells except that intermediate filaments are related to both sides of the junctions.[11] The junctions are most apparent in basal regions where they form part of, and are intercalated into, the junction complexes between Sertoli cells (Fig. 10A)[15,102] and appear to form discontinuous belts around the cells. Desmosome-like junctions between Sertoli cells also are present in apical regions.[11]

The presence of desmosomal cadherins and desmosome related armadillo proteins at desmosome-like junctions in the seminiferous epithelium has not been confirmed; however, there exists the possibility that members of the classical cadherins and related catenins may be incorporated into these junctions.[42,102,103] If true, the presence of classical cadherins at these sites, in addition to any desmosomal cadherins that occur at the sites, would enable these desmosome-like junctions to interact with actin filaments as well as with intermediate filaments. In Sertoli cells, the interaction would be mainly with intermediate filaments, although maybe not exclusively so. In spermatogenic cells, where intermediate filaments do not associate with the plaques, the interaction might instead be with the cortical actin network. One of the plakins (plectin) has been localized to the sites (Fig. 8)[20] and presumably participates in linking the vimentin filaments to the junction plaques in Sertoli cells. Plectin also is associated with the Sertoli cell nuclear membrane where it may serve a similar function (Fig. 8).[20]

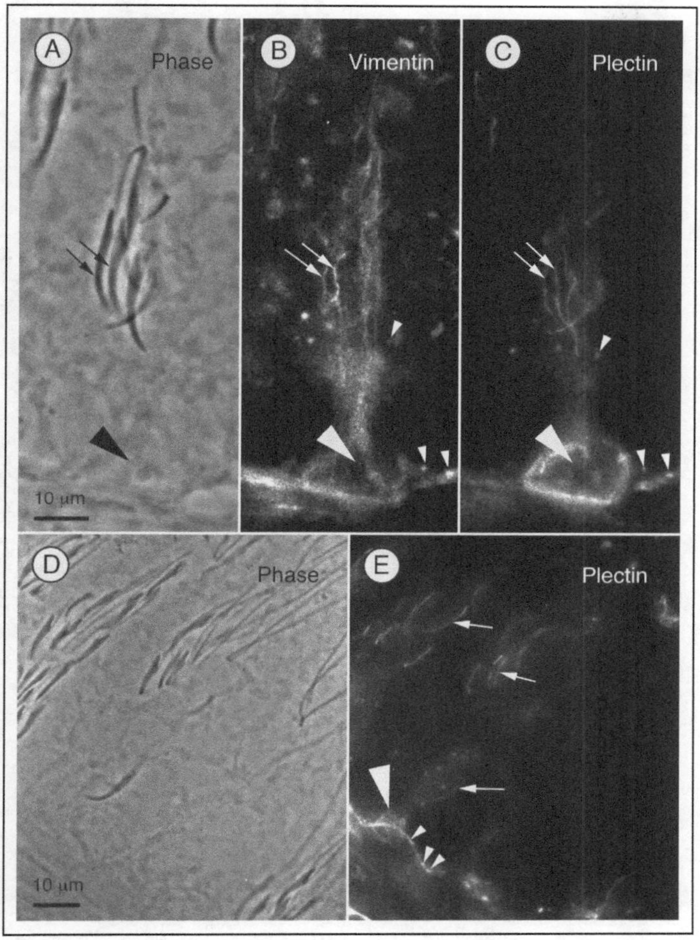

Figure 8. Distribution of vimentin intermediate filaments and plectin in Sertoli cells (rat). A,B,C) Phase and related immunofluorescence images of a section of seminiferous epithelium labeled for vimentin and plectin. Intermediate filaments are concentrated around the basally situated Sertoli cell nucleus (large arrowhead) and extend apically into regions associated with crypts or invaginations containing elongate spermatids. Plectin is concentrated around the Sertoli cell nucleus and in regions of apical crypts adjacent to the dorsal curvature of spermatid heads (arrows). Intermediate filaments and plectin also are associated with desmosome-like junctions, some of which are indicated by punctate staining in (B) and (C) (small arrowheads). D,E) Paired phase and fluorescence images of a section of seminiferous epithelium labeled for plectin. Clearly visible here is plectin associated with linear desmosome-like attachments with the dorsal aspects of elongate spermatids (arrows). In addition, plectin is associated with the Sertoli cell nucleus (large arrowhead). Also visible is plectin associated with desmosome-like junctions that are incorporated into the basal junction complex between two adjacent Sertoi cells (small arrowheads).

Virtually nothing is known about the molecular components of the small hemidesmosome-like junctions located at the base of Sertoli cells, which is surprising considering the important structural and signaling properties of these junctions in other systems.[99]

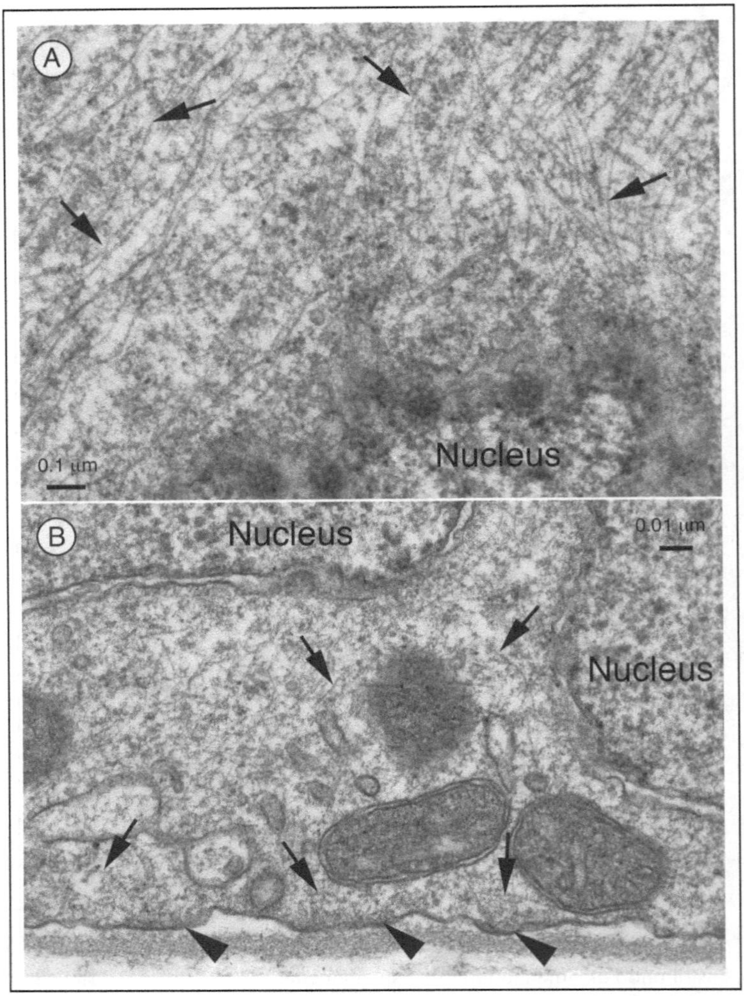

Figure 9. Electron micrographs of intermediate filaments (arrows) that surround the nucleus (A) and that also are associated with hemidesmosome-like structures at the base of the cell (arrowheads) (B).

The function of intermediate filaments in Sertoli cells has not been clearly defined. The vimentin knock-out mouse is reproductively viable[104] and the morphology of the adult seminiferous epithelium appears remarkably normal.[105] The only phenotype observed in the Sertoli cells is a complete lack of cytoplasmic intermediate filaments. Even though desmosome-like membrane associated plaques are present, there are no intermediate filaments associated with them. It is possible that intermediate filaments in Sertoli cells play a mechanical strengthening role, but they do so only when the epithelium is stressed in a particular fashion or to sufficient levels. It has long been known that desmosome-like junctions maintain seminiferous epithelial integrity when exposed to hypertonic buffers.[101] Intermediate filaments may facilitate this role in this and other[106] mechanically stressful situations.

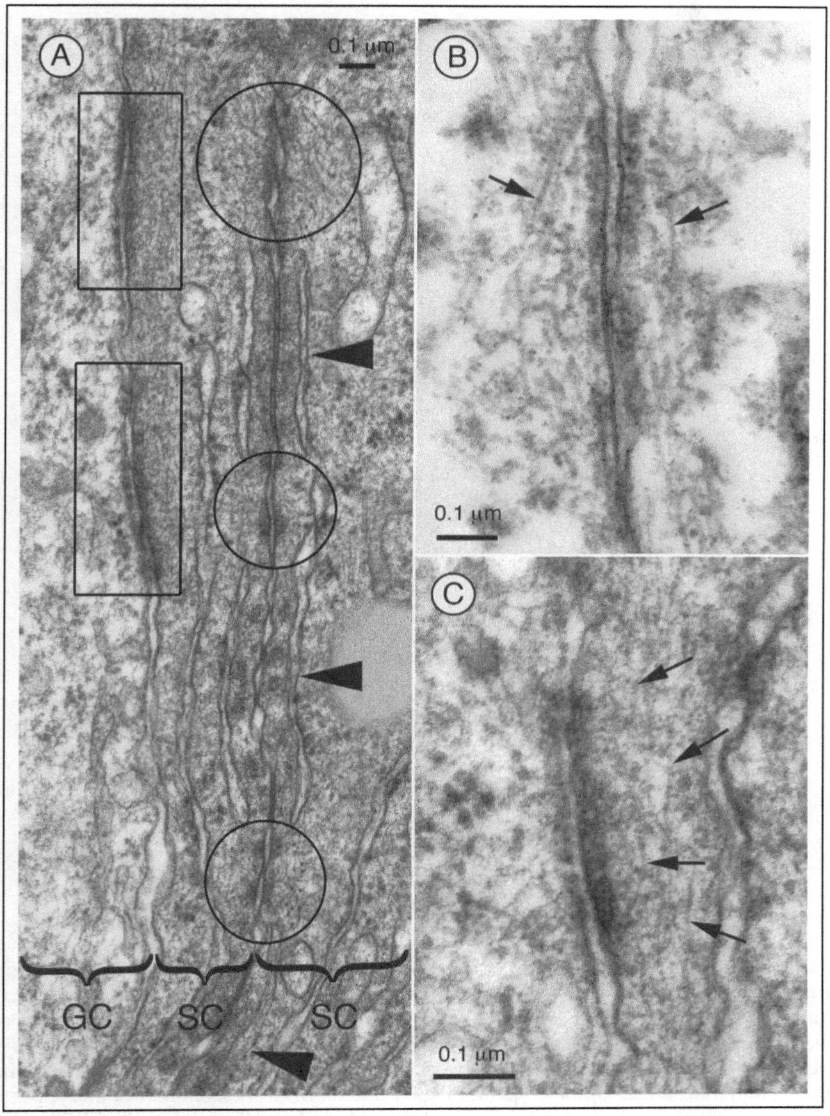

Figure 10. Electron micrographs of desmosome-like junctions. A) Shown here is a section through parts of two Sertoli cells (SC) and part of a spermatogenic cell (GC) (rat). In the seminiferous epithelium, desmosome-like junctions occur both between adjacent Sertoli cells (examples are circled in this image) and between Sertoli cells and spermatogenic cells (GC) (examples are boxed in this image). In this image, desmosome-like junctions are clearly intercalated into the basal junction complex indicated by the ectoplasmic specializations (arrowheads). B) A desmosome-like junction between two Sertoli cells (ground squirrel). The cells have been fixed, extracted with detergent and treated with tannic acid. The arrows indicate intermediate filaments. C) A desmosome-like junction between a Sertoli cell and spermatogenic cell fixed using conventional techniques (rat). Intermediate filaments (arrows) are present only on the Sertoli cell side of the junction.

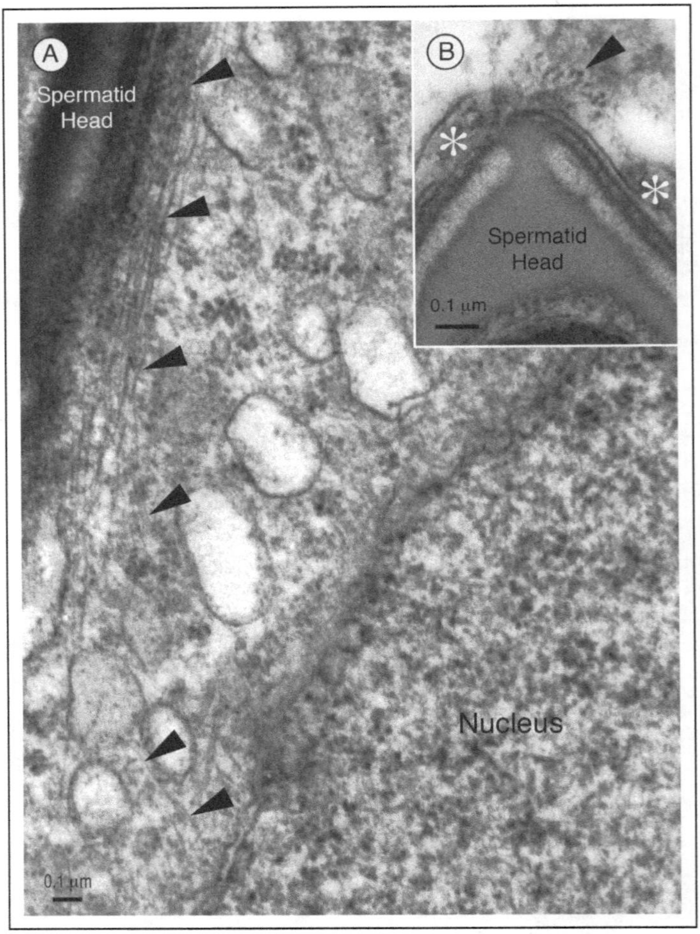

Figure 11. Filament associated desmosome-like attachment between Sertoli cell and elongate spermatids approximately at stage V of spermatogenesis in the rat. A) Longitudinal section of the perinuclear region of a Sertoli cell and a crypt containing an elongate spermatid. Intermediate filaments (arrowheads) extend from the perinuclear region to a desmosome-like plaque adjacent to the dorsal curvature of the spermatid head. This region is intercalated into the ectoplasmic specialization that surrounds the crypt (see Figs. 1 and 8). B) Cross section through the part of an apical Sertoli cell crypt adjacent the dorsal curvature of an elongate spermatid head. Intermediate filaments of a desmosome-like junction are flanked by ectoplasmic specializations (asterisks).

Microtubules

General

Microtubules are dynamic cytoskeletal components that influence cell shape and provide tracts for intracellular vesicular transport. Microtubules are long, 25 nm in diameter, tubular polymers formed by α and β tubulin heterodimers. These heterodimeric subunits confer an intrinsic polarity to microtubules providing distinct plus- (fast growing) and minus- (slow growing) ends, allowing these structures to be used as rails for directional cargo transport by the microtubule dependent kinesin and dynein motor proteins.[107-109] In most cells microtubules originate at nucleation sites called microtubule organizing centers (MTOCs), the classical center of which is the centriole containing centrosome.[110] Microtubules then radiate out to the cell periphery with their minus ends, or slow growing ends, at the MTOC. Other general patterns of microtubule distribution are common,[111] as is noncentrosomal nucleation of microtubules.[112]

Microtubules in Sertoli Cells

Sertoli cells are tall columnar epithelial cells that maintain their elongate morphology largely with the microtubule cytoskeleton. Experiments using the microtubule disrupting drugs colchicine and vinblastine in the testis result in a dramatic loss of Sertoli cell architecture as well as the sloughing of germ cells.[106,113,114]

Sertoli cell microtubules are abundant apical to the basally located nucleus where they are predominantly arranged parallel to the long axis of the cell (Fig. 12),[15] although microtubules do occur in basal regions of the cell and form elaborate arrays in apical cytoplasm associated with late spermatids.[115-117] Unlike what occurs in many other cells, microtubules are nucleated at the periphery of Sertoli cells and not in regions associated with the perinuclear centrioles. This conclusion is based on the observations that the majority of microtubules are oriented

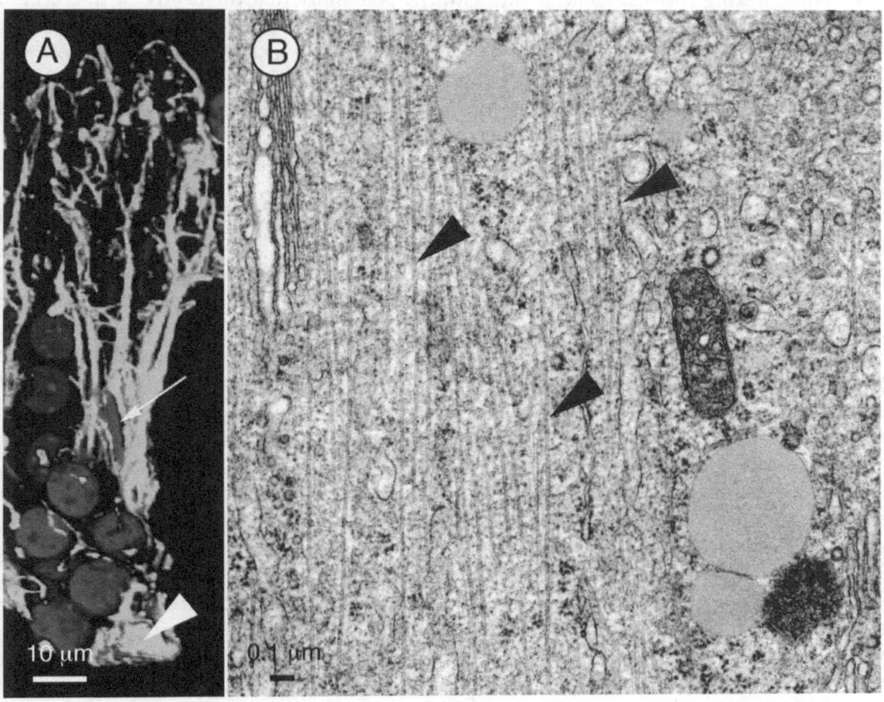

Figure 12. Sertoli cell microtubules. A) Shown here is a confocal projection of the microtubule pattern in a Sertoli cell (rat) from approximately stage V of spermatogenesis. Microtubules are in green and nuclei are in blue. The arrow indicates the head of an elongate spermatid and the arrowhead indicates the position of the Sertoli cell nucleus. Notice that the microtubules are predominantly oriented parallel to the long axis of the Sertoli cell. B) Electron micrograph of a longitudinal section through an apical stalk of a ground squirrel Sertoli cell. Microtubules (arrowheads) are uniformly aligned parallel to the axis of the stalk.

with their minus-ends at the apex and their plus-ends at the base of Sertoli cells.[118,119] Also, microtubules polymerize from the periphery or apex of Sertoli cells in the testis during recovery from nocodozole treatment.[120] Additionally, the microtubule nucleating protein, γ-tubulin, is present at peripheral sites.[121] Moreover, when γ-tubulin is over expressed in Sertoli cells it concentrates in peripheral regions associated with elongate spermatid heads.[122]

During spermatogenesis, the microtubule patterns in Sertoli cells change; in other words, the patterns are stage specific and change according to the developmental stages of spermatogenic cells with which they are associated.[1,115,117,123] In lateral processes associated with early spermatogenic cells, microtubules are scarce. However, a marked increase in microtubules is apparent in Sertoli cell projections associated with round spermatids. Later, microtubules concentrate in the cytoplasm around spermatid heads adjacent to the acrosomes, and form linear tracts of microtubules parallel to Sertoli cell crypts containing the attached elongate spermatids. Prior to sperm release, Sertoli cell microtubules often are concentrated in, or form specialized structures in, cytoplasm associated with spermatid heads. In addition, microtubules are present in projections associated with the lobe of residual spermatid cytoplasm. The findings that microtubules in Sertoli cells contain tyrosinated tubulin, which tend to be correlated with unstable populations of microtubules, and that the levels of tyrosinated tubulin change during spermatogenesis, are consistent with the observation that microtubule patterns in Sertoli cells are dynamic during spermatogenesis and with the possibility that the degree of microtubule stability may be stage specific.[117,123]

In addition to a structural function, microtubules also are essential for the directional transport of intracellular cargo generally in cells. These cytoskeletal elements use the molecular motors, kinesin and cytoplasmic dynein to transport vesicles, proteins, and other cellular elements throughout the cell. These motors convert ATP as an energy source for their motility events. The kinesins together constitute a superfamily that has recently been reorganized to contain 14 families plus an additional group of orphan kinesins.[124] Hirokawa's group[125] has identified 45 kinesin genes in mouse and human databases. These protein machines transport cargo primarily towards the plus-ends of microtubules, although an increasing number of minus-end directed motors have been discovered. Cytoplasmic dynein is generally considered a minus-end directed molecular motor, although bidirectional movements of single dynein-dynactin complexes have been reported in vitro.[126] Both of these groups of motor proteins have developed elaborate techniques for selecting cargoes, docking those cargoes to appropriate motors and targeting these cellular components to the appropriate locations.[107,127-129]

In Sertoli cells, general housekeeping and other transport events such as those that occur between different membrane compartments and those involving the transport of organelles from one position to another likely involve microtubule-based motor proteins. This conclusion is based mainly on data from cells in general, and on the correlation of organelle position with microtubules,[116,130,131] changes observed after microtubule perturbation[81,114,132] and localization of motor proteins in Sertoli cells.[133-135]

One transport event that occurs during spermiogenesis is the translocation of spermatids in the seminiferous epithelium.[136-139] This event occurs as the result of a change in position of apical crypts that contain the differentiating germ cells. When the crypts initially form in the apices of Sertoli cells, they are shallow and, together with the attached spermatids, occur in apical regions of the epithelium. At certain stages, the crypts deepen (most dramatically at stages IV-V in rat) and the attached spermatids, specifically their heads, become located near the base of the epithelium. As spermatids mature, the crypts again become shallow and spermatids are returned to the apex of the epithelium for eventual release. The biological significance of transporting spermatids deep into the epithelium is not known. What is known is that the process occurs generally in vertebrates and appears fundamental to the process of spermatogenesis. Entrenchment within the epithelium may provide increased mechanical support for elongate shaped spermatogenic cells, facilitate development of the sperm tail, provide increased surface contact for exchange of materials or signals between Sertoli cells and the developing spermatids, or have other as yet unknown functions.

Based on observations that Sertoli cell microtubules are found in close opposition to ectoplasmic specializations attached to spermatid heads[131,140] and that microtubules are oriented parallel to the direction of spermatid translocation, it has been proposed that the mechanism responsible for changes in position of elongate spermatids during spermatogenesis in mammals involves the transport of ectoplasmic specializations and the attached spermatids along microtubule tracts in Sertoli cells.[115,140] It is proposed that microtubule-based motors attached to the cytoplasmic face of the endoplasmic reticulum component of ectoplasmic specializations transport the junction/spermatid complex first basally and then apically in the epithelium.[115,118,141]

A number of lines of evidence support this hypothesis. First, pharmacological disruption (depolymerization) of microtubules in Sertoli cells alters the position of spermatids in the seminiferous epithelium.[106,114] Second, microtubules bind to isolated ectoplasmic specializations in an ATP-dependent fashion. Moreover, the binding has a profile of sensitivity to pharmacological agents that is consistent with those of some known microtubule based motors.[141] At the ultrastructural level, this nucleotide-dependent binding occurs on the cytoplasmic face of the endoplasmic reticulum component of the junction plaques.[142] Third, isolated junction plaques transport microtubules. In an in vitro motility assay, exogenous microtubules move, in an ATP-dependent fashion, on isolated spermatid/junction complexes.[143] Fourth, junction plaques transport microtubules in both directions. To account for the "down-and-up" movement in vivo, isolated junction plaques should move microtubules in plus-end and minus-end directions. This prediction has now been verified.[144] Fifth, cytoplasmic dynein is associated with the junction plaques. Antibodies to the 74 kDa intermediate chain (IC74) of cytoplasmic dynein strongly react at the light microscopic levels with Sertoli cell regions known to contain the junction plaques,[135] and react with the cytoplasmic face of the endoplasmic reticulum component of the junction plaque at the ultrastructural level.[144] Significantly, this immunoreactivity occurs during the period of spermatid translocation. This result is the first evidence, from immunolocalization studies, that a microtubule-based motor occurs in plaque regions at the appropriate time during spermatogenesis. Further support for the association of cytoplasmic dynein with the junction plaques was obtained by using gelsolin (an actin severing enzyme) to disassemble the plaques and release the endoplasmic reticulum component of the plaques into solution. When assessed by immunoblots, GRP94 (a marker for endoplasmic reticulum) and cytoplasmic dynein (indicated by IC74) were enriched in supernatants collected from low speed centrifugation of gelsolin treated spermatid/junction complexes relative to controls.[135]

Although cytoplasmic dynein has been localized to ectoplasmic specializations and is likely the motor responsible for the apical movement of spermatids in the mammalian seminiferous epithelium, the plus-end directed motor, likely a kinesin, responsible for the basal movement has yet to be identified.

Concluding Remarks

The association of the cytoskeleton with sites of intercellular attachment and with processes such as the release of sperm cells from the epithelium, the movement of spermatocytes through basal junction complexes between Sertoli cells and the translocation of spermatids in the seminiferous epithelium indicates that the cytoskeletal machinery of Sertoli cells is likely fundamental to spermatogenesis and may potentially contain molecular targets for contraception.

Although much has been learned about the organization and function of the Sertoli cell cytoskeleton over the last few years, there still is a great deal to be learned.

The mechanism of regulating actin dynamics in ectoplasmic specializations and at tubulobulbar complexes has yet to be defined. The role of the endoplasmic reticulum both at ectoplasmic specializations and at tubulobulbar complexes is completely unknown, except that at apical ectoplasmic specialization microtubule transport machinery has been coupled through the endoplasmic reticulum to the junction plaque in order to translocate and position spermatids in the epithelium. The precise role of actin at ectoplasmic specializations and tubulobulbar complexes remains to be determined.

The molecular composition of desmosome-like and hemidesmosome-like junctions in Sertoli cells, and how their linkages to the intermediate filament cytoskeleton is formed and controlled remains to be elucidated. Desmosome-like junctions are a major component of the intercellular contact machinery in the seminiferous epithelium and, like ectoplasmic specializations, their association with spermatogenic cells is cell specific and therefore dynamic. Desmosome-like junctions between neighboring Sertoli cells are part of, and are integrated into, the basal junction complex and are therefore presumably disassembled above and assembled below translocating spermatocytes. The hypothesis that intermediate filaments, together with their attachment to desmosome-like and hemidesmosome-like junctions, maintain epithelial integrity when the tissue is mechanically stressed has yet to be experimentally tested.

Although microtubule-based transport mechanisms are fundamental to intracellular motility generally in cells, the coupling of this machinery to a junction plaque to position adjacent cells in an epithelium is unique to Sertoli cells. Cytoplasmic dynein has been localized to the junction sites; however, the predicted plus-end directed motor, likely a kinesin, has not. The microtubule-based spermatid translocation hypothesis has yet to be tested in vivo, and the biological function of spermatid translocation itself remains to be determined.

References

1. Amlani S, Vogl AW. Changes in the distribution of microtubules and intermediate filaments in mammalian Sertoli cells during spermatogenesis. Anat Rec 1988; 220:143-160.
2. Winder SJ, Ayscough KR. Actin-binding proteins. J Cell Sci 2005; 118:651-654.
3. Kovar DR. Molecular details of formin-mediated actin assembly. Curr Opin Cell Biol 2006; 18:11-7.
4. Bos JL. Linking Rap to cell adhesion. Curr Opin Cell Biol 2005; 17:123-128.
5. DeMali KA, Burridge K. Coupling membrane protrusion and cell adhesion. J Cell Sci 2003; 116:2389-2397.
6. Pollard TD. Introduction to actin and actin-binding proteins. In: Kreis T, Vale R, eds. Guidebook to the Cytoskeletal and Motor Proteins. New York: Oxford University Press, 1999:3-11.
7. Mooseker MS, Cheney RE. Unconventional myosins. Annual Rev Cell Dev Biol 1995; 11:633-675.
8. Pollard TD, Borisy GG. Cellular motility driven by assembly and disassembly of actin filaments. Cell 2003; 112:453-465.
9. Zigmond S. Formin' adherens junctions. Nature Cell Biol 2004; 6:12-14.
10. Dym M, Fawcett DW. The blood-testis barrier in the rat and the physiological compartmentation of the seminiferous epithelium. Biol Reprod 1970; 3:308-326.
11. Russell LD, Peterson RN. Sertoli cell junctions: Morphological and functional correlates. Int Rev Cytol 1985; 94:177-211.
12. Vogl AW. Distribution and function of organized concentrations of actin filaments in mammalian spermatogenic cells and Sertoli cells. Int Rev Cytol 1989; 119:1-56.
13. Vogl A, Pfeiffer DC, Redenbach DM. Sertoli cell cytoskeleton: Influence on spermatogenic cells. In: Baccetti B, ed. Proceedings of the VI international congress on spermatology. Comparative Spermatology 20 years after. Italy, Serona Symposia: Raven Press, 1991:709-715.
14. Vogl AW, Pfeiffer DC, Redenbach DM. Ectoplasmic ("junctional") specializations in mammalian Sertoli cells: Influence on spermatogenic cells. Ann NY Acad Sci 1991; 637:175-202.
15. Vogl AW, Pfeiffer DC, Redenbach DM et al. Sertoli cell cytoskeleton. In: Russell LD, Griswold MD, eds. The Sertoli Cell. Clearwater: Cache River Press, 1993:39-86.
16. Vogl AW, Pfeiffer DC, Mulholland D et al. Unique and multifunctional adhesion junctions in the testis: Ectoplasmic specializations. Arch Histol Cytol 2000; 63:1-15.
17. Toyama Y, Maekawa M, Yuasa S. Ectoplasmic specializations in the Sertoli cell: New vistas based on genetic defects and testicular toxicology. Anat Sci Int 2003; 78:1-16.
18. Lee NP, Cheng CY. Ectoplasmic specialization, a testis-specific cell-cell actin-based adherens junction type: Is this a potential target for male contraceptive development? Hum Reprod Update 2004; 10:349-369.
19. Mruk DD, Cheng CY. Cell-cell interactions at the ectoplasmic specialization in the testis. Trends Endocrinol Metab 2004; 15:439-447.
20. Guttman JA, Mulholland DJ, Vogl AW. Plectin is concentrated at intercellular junctions and at the nuclear surface in morphologically differentiated rat Sertoli cells. Anat Rec 1999; 254:418-428.
21. Romrell LJ, Ross MH. Characterization of Sertoli cell-germ cell junctional specializations in dissociated testicular cells. Anat Rec 1979; 193:23-41.

22. Pelletier RM. Cyclic modulation of Sertoli cell junctional complexes in a seasonal breeder: The mink (Mustela vison). Am J Anat 1988; 183:68-102.
23. Pelletier RM, Friend DS. The Sertoli cell junctional complex: Structure and permeability to filipin in the neonatal and adult guinea pig. Am J Anat 1983; 168:213-228.
24. Palombi F, Salanova M, Tarone G et al. Distribution of β1 integrin subunit in rat seminiferous epithelium. Biol Reprod 1992; 47:1173-1182.
25. Salanova M, Stefanini M, De Curtis I et al. Integrin receptor alpha 6 beta 1 is localized at specific sites of cell-to-cell contact in rat seminiferous epithelium. Biol Reprod 1995; 52:79-87.
26. Ozaki-Kuroda K, Nakanishi H, Ohta H et al. Nectin couples cell-cell adhesion and the actin scaffold at heterotypic testicular junctions. Curr Biol 2002; 12:1145-1150.
27. Gliki G, Ebnet K, Aurrand-Lions M et al. Spermatid differentiation requires the assembly of a cell polarity complex downstream of junctional adhesion molecule-C. Nature 2004; 431:320-324.
28. Wine RN, Chapin RE. Adhesion and signaling proteins spatiotemporally associated with spermiation in the rat. J Androl 1999; 20:198-213.
29. Yan HH, Cheng CY. Blood-testis barrier dynamics are regulated by an engagement/disengagement mechanism between tight and adherens junctions via peripheral adaptors. Proc Natl Acad Sci USA 2005; 102:11722-11727.
30. Sarkar O, Xia W, Mruk DD. Adjudin-mediated junction restructuring in the seminiferous epithelium leads to displacement of soluble guanylate cyclase from adherens junctions. J Cell Physiol 2006; 208:175-187.
31. Siu MK, Cheng CY. Interactions of proteases, protease inhibitors, and the beta1 integrin/laminin gamma3 protein complex in the regulation of ectoplasmic specialization dynamics in the rat testis. Biol Reprod 2004; 70:945-964.
32. Grove BD, Pfeiffer DC, Allen S et al. Immunofluorescence localization of vinculin in ectoplasmic ("junctional") specializations of rat Sertoli cells. Am J Anat 1990; 188:44-56.
33. Xia W, Cheng CY. TGF-β3 regulates anchoring junction dynamics in the seminiferous epithelium of the rat testis via the Ras/ERK signaling pathway: An in vivo study. Dev Biol 2005; 280:321-343.
34. Franke WW, Grund C, Fink A et al. Location of actin in the microfilament bundles associated with the junctional specializations between Sertoli cells and spermatids. Biol Cell 1978; 31:7-14.
35. Grove BD, Vogl AW. Sertoli cell ectoplasmic specializations: A type of actin-associated adhesion junction? J Cell Sci 1989; 93:309-323.
36. Bartles JR, Wierda A, Zheng L. Identification and characterization of espin, an actin-binding protein localized to the F-actin-rich junctional plaques of Sertoli cell ectoplasmic specializations. J Cell Sci 1996; 109:1229-1239.
37. Velichkova M, Guttman J, Warren C et al. A human homologue of Drosophila kelch associates with myosin-VIIa in specialized adhesion junctions. Cell Motil Cytoskeleton 2002; 51:147-164.
38. Kai M, Irie M, Okutsu T et al. The novel dominant mutation Dspd leads to a severe spermiogenesis defect in mice. Biol Reprod 2004; 70:1213-1221.
39. Hasson T, Walsh J, Cable J et al. Effects of shaker-1 mutations on myosin-VIIa protein and mRNA expression. Cell Motil Cytoskeleton 1997; 37:127-138.
40. Vogl AW, Soucy LJ. Arrangement and possible function of actin filament bundles in ectoplasmic specializations of ground squirrel Sertoli cells. J Cell Biol 1985; 100:814-825.
41. Guttman JA, Obinata T, Shima J et al. Nonmuscle cofilin is a component of tubulobulbar complexes in the testis. Biol Reprod 2004; 70:805-812.
42. Mulholland DJ, Dedhar S, Vogl AW. Rat seminiferous epithelium contains a unique junction (Ectoplasmic specialization) with signaling properties both of cell/cell and cell/matrix junctions. Biol Reprod 2001; 64:396-407.
43. Grima J, Silvestrini B, Cheng CY. Reversible inhibition of spermatogenesis in rats using a new male contraceptive, 1-(2,4-dichlorobenzyl)-indazole-3-carbohydrazide. Biol Reprod 2001; 64:1500-1508.
44. Cheng CY, Silvestrini B, Grima J et al. Two new male contraceptives exert their effects by depleting germ cells prematurely from the testis. Biol Reprod 2001; 65:449-461.
45. Cheng CY, Mruk D, Silvestrini B et al. AF-2364[1-(2,4-dichlorobenzyl)-1H-indazole-3-carbohydrazide] is a potential male contraceptive: A review of recent data. Contraception 2005; 72:251-261.
46. O'Donnell L, McLachlan RI, Wreford NG et al. Testosterone withdrawal promotes stage-specific detachment of round spermatids from the rat seminiferous epithelium. Biol Reprod 1996; 55:895-901.
47. Beardsley A, O'Donnell L. Characterization of normal spermiation and spermiation failure induced by hormone suppression in adult rats. Biol Reprod 2003; 68:1299-1307.

48. Toyama Y, Hosoi I, Ichikawa S et al. β-estradiol 3-benzoate affects spermatogenesis in the adult mouse. Mol Cell Endocrinol 2001; 178:161-168.
49. Wong CH, Xia W, Lee NP et al. Regulation of ectoplasmic specialization dynamics in the seminiferous epithelium by focal adhesion-associated proteins in testosterone-suppressed rat testes. Endocrinology 2005; 146:1192-1204.
50. Zhang J, Wong CH, Xia W et al. Regulation of Sertoli-germ cell adherens junction dynamics via changes in protein-protein interactions of the N-cadherin-β-catenin protein complex which are possibly mediated by c-Src and myotubularin-related protein 2: An in vivo study using an androgen suppression model. Endocrinology 2005; 146:1268-1284.
51. Kobielak A, Pasolli HA, Fuchs E. Mammalian formin-1 participates in adherens junctions and polymerization of linear actin cables. Nat Cell Biol 2004; 6:21-30.
52. Franchi E, Camatini M. Morphological evidence for calcium stores at Sertoli-Sertoli and Sertoli-spermatid interrelations. Cell Biol Int Rep 1985; 9:441-446.
53. Pelletier R, Trifaro JM, Carbajal ME et al. Calcium-dependent actin filament-severing protein scinderin levels and localization in bovine testis, epididymis, and spermatozoa. Biol Reprod 1999; 60:1128-1136.
54. Guttman JA, Janmey P, Vogl AW. Gelsolin—evidence for a role in turnover of junction-related actin filaments in Sertoli cells. J Cell Sci 2002; 115:499-505.
55. Vaid K, Guttman J, Vogl AW. A reevaluation of gelsolin at ectoplasmic specializations in Sertoli cells—The influence of serum in blocking buffers on staining patterns. Mol Biol Cell 2004; 15:427a.
56. Witke W, Sharpe AH, Hartwig JH et al. Hemostatic, inflammatory, and fibroblast responses are blunted in mice lacking gelsolin. Cell 1995; 81:41-51.
57. Russell LD, Goh JC, Rashed RM et al. The consequences of actin disruption at Sertoli ectoplasmic specialization sites facing spermatids after in vivo exposure of rat testis to cytochalasin D. Biol Reprod 1988; 39:105-118.
58. Weber JE, Turner TT, Tung KS et al. Effects of cytochalasin D on the integrity of the Sertoli cell (blood-testis) barrier. Am J Anat 1988; 182:130-147.
59. Russell L, Clermont Y. Anchoring device between Sertoli cells and late spermatids in rat seminiferous tubules. Anat Rec 1976; 185:259-278.
60. Russell LD. Further observations on tubulobulbar complexes formed by late spermatids and Sertoli cells in the rat testis. Anat Rec 1979; 194:213-232.
61. Guttman JA, Takai Y, Vogl AW. Evidence that tubulobulbar complexes in the seminiferous epithelium are involved with internalization of adhesion junctions. Biol Reprod 2004; 71:548-559.
62. Russell LD. Spermatid-Sertoli tubulobulbar complexes as devices for elimination of cytoplasm from the head region late spermatids of the rat. Anat Rec 1979; 194:233-246.
63. Russell LD. Deformities in the head region of late spermatids of hypophysectomized-hormone-treated rats. Anat Rec 1980; 197:21-31.
64. Kierszenbaum AL, Tres LL. The acrosome-acroplaxome-manchette complex and the shaping of the spermatid head. Arch Histol Cytol 2004; 67:271-284.
65. Lock JG, Stow JL. Rab11 in recycling endosomes regulates the sorting and basolateral transport of E-cadherin. Mol Biol Cell 2005; 16:1744-1755.
66. Le TL, Yap AS, Stow JL. Recycling of E-cadherin: A potential mechanism for regulating cadherin dynamics. J Cell Biol 1999; 146:219-232.
67. Akhtar N, Hotchin NA. RAC1 regulates adherens junctions through endocytosis of E-cadherin. Mol Biol Cell 2001; 12:847-862.
68. Ivanov AI, Nusrat A, Parkos CA. Endocytosis of epithelial apical junctional proteins by a clathrin-mediated pathway into a unique storage compartment. Mol Biol Cell 2004; 15:176-188.
69. Izumi G, Sakisaka T, Baba T et al. Endocytosis of E-cadherin regulated by Rac and Cdc42 small G proteins through IQGAP1 and actin filaments. J Cell Biol 2004; 166:237-248.
70. Shen L, Turner JR. Actin depolymerization disrupts tight junctions via caveolae-mediated endocytosis. Mol Biol Cell 2005; 16:3919-3936.
71. Utech M, Ivanov AI, Samarin SN et al. Mechanism of IFN-γ-induced endocytosis of tight junction proteins: Myosin II-dependent vacuolarization of the apical plasma membrane. Mol Biol Cell 2005; 16:5040-5052.
72. Paterson AD, Parton RG, Ferguson C et al. Characterization of E-cadherin endocytosis in isolated MCF-7 and chinese hamster ovary cells: The initial fate of unbound E-cadherin. J Biol Chem 2003; 278:21050-21057.
73. Gaietta G, Deerinck TJ, Adams SR et al. Multicolor and electron microscopic imaging of connexin trafficking. Science 2002; 296:503-507.
74. Berthoud VM, Minogue PJ, Laing JG et al. Pathways for degradation of connexins and gap junctions. Cardiovasc Res 2004; 62:256-267.

75. Matsuda M, Kubo A, Furuse M et al. A peculiar internalization of claudins, tight junction-specific adhesion molecules, during the intercellular movement of epithelial cells. J Cell Sci 2004; 117:1247-1257.
76. Polak-Charcon S, Ben-Shaul Y. Degradation of tight junctions in HT29, a human colon adenocarcinoma cell line. J Cell Sci 1979; 35:393-402.
77. Risinger MA, Larsen WJ. Endocytosis of cell-cell junctions and spontaneous cell disaggregation in a cultured human ovarian adenocarcinoma. (COLO 316). Tissue Cell 1981; 13:413-430.
78. Russell LD. Observations on the inter-relationships of Sertoli cells at the level of the blood- testis barrier: Evidence for formation and resorption of Sertoli-Sertoli tubulobulbar complexes during the spermatogenic cycle of the rat. Am J Anat 1979; 155:259-279.
79. Ng T, Shima D, Squire A et al. PKCα regulates β1 integrin-dependent cell motility through association and control of integrin traffic. EMBO J 1999; 18:3909-3923.
80. Le TL, Joseph SR, Yap AS et al. Protein kinase C regulates endocytosis and recycling of E-cadherin. Am J Physiol Cell Physiol 2002; 283:C489-499.
81. Russell LD, Saxena NK, Turner TT. Cytoskeletal involvement in spermiation and sperm transport. Tissue Cell 1989; 21:361-379.
82. Coulombe PA, Wong P. Cytoplasmic intermediate filaments revealed as dynamic and multipurpose scaffolds. Nat Cell Biol 2004; 6:699-706.
83. Fudge DS, Gardner KH, Forsyth VT et al. The mechanical properties of hydrated intermediate filaments: Insights from hagfish slime threads. Biophys J 2003; 85:2015-2027.
84. Kreplak L, Bar H, Leterrier JF et al. Exploring the mechanical behavior of single intermediate filaments. J Mol Biol 2005; 354:569-577.
85. Fuchs E, Cleveland DW. A structural scaffolding of intermediate filaments in health and disease. Science 1998; 279:514-519.
86. Helfand BT, Chou YH, Shumaker DK et al. Intermediate filament proteins participate in signal transduction. Trends Cell Biol 2005; 15:568-570.
87. Toivola DM, Tao GZ, Habtezion A et al. Cellular integrity plus: Organelle-related and protein-targeting functions of intermediate filaments. Trends Cell Biol 2005; 15:608-617.
88. Lazarides E. Intermediate filaments as mechanical integrators of cellular space. Nature 1980; 283:249-256.
89. Worman HJ, Courvalin JC. Nuclear envelope, nuclear lamina, and inherited disease. Int Rev Cytol 2005; 246:231-279.
90. Franke WW, Grund C, Schmid E. Intermediate-sized filaments present in Sertoli cells are of the vimentin type. Eur J Cell Biol 1979; 19:269-275.
91. Paranko J, Kallajoki M, Pelliniemi LJ et al. Transient coexpression of cytokeratin and vimentin in differentiating rat Sertoli cells. Dev Biol 1986; 117:35-44.
92. Stosiek P, Kasper M, Karsten U. Expression of cytokeratins 8 and 18 in human Sertoli cells of immature and atrophic seminiferous tubules. Differentiation 1990; 43:66-70.
93. Miettinen M, Virtanen I, Talerman A. Intermediate filament proteins in human testis and testicular germ-cell tumors. Am J Pathol 1985; 120:402-410.
94. Frojdman K, Pelliniemi LJ, Lendahl U et al. The intermediate filament protein nestin occurs transiently in differentiating testis of rat and mouse. Differentiation 1997; 61:243-249.
95. Moss SB, Burnham BL, Bellve AR. The differential expression of lamin epitopes during mouse spermatogenesis. Mol Reprod Dev 1993; 34:164-174.
96. Vester B, Smith A, Krohne G et al. Presence of a nuclear lamina in pachytene spermatocytes of the rat. J Cell Sci 1993; 104:557-563.
97. Aumuller G, Steinbruck M, Krause W et al. Distribution of vimentin-type intermediate filaments in Sertoli cells of the human testis, normal and pathologic. Anat Embryol (Berl) 1988; 178:129-136.
98. Getsios S, Huen AC, Green KJ. Working out the strength and flexibility of desmosomes. Nat Rev Mol Cell Biol 2004; 5:271-281.
99. Nievers MG, Schaapveld RQ, Sonnenberg A. Biology and function of hemidesmosomes. Matrix Biol 1999; 18:5-17.
100. Hahn BS, Labouesse M. Tissue integrity: Hemidesmosomes and resistance to stress. Curr Biol 2001; 11:R858-861.
101. Russell L. Desmosome-like junctions between Sertoli and germ cells in the rat testis. Am J Anat 1977; 148:301-312.
102. Johnson KJ, Boekelheide K. Dynamic testicular adhesion junctions are immunologically unique. II. Localization of classic cadherins in rat testis. Biol Reprod 2002; 66:992-1000.
103. Johnson KJ, Boekelheide K. Dynamic testicular adhesion junctions are immunologically unique. I. Localization of p120 catenin in rat testis. Biol Reprod 2002; 66:983-991.

104. Colucci-Guyon E, Portier MM, Dunia I et al. Mice lacking vimentin develop and reproduce without an obvious phenotype. Cell 1994; 79:679-694.
105. Vogl AW, Colucci-Guyon E, Babinet C. Vimentin intermediate filaments are not necessary for the development of a normal differentiated phenotype by mature Sertoli cells. Mol Biol Cell 1996; 7:55a.
106. Allard EK, Johnson KJ, Boekelheide K. Colchicine disrupts the cytoskeleton of rat testis seminiferous epithelium in a stage-dependent manner. Biol Reprod 1993; 48:143-153.
107. Goldstein LS, Yang Z. Microtubule-based transport systems in neurons: The roles of kinesins and dyneins. Annu Rev Neurosci 2000; 23:39-71.
108. Higuchi H, Endow SA. Directionality and processivity of molecular motors. Curr Opin Cell Biol 2002; 14:50-57.
109. Kamal A, Goldstein LS. Principles of cargo attachment to cytoplasmic motor proteins. Curr Opin Cell Biol 2002; 14:63-68.
110. Brinkley BR. Microtubule organizing centers. Annu Rev Cell Biol 1985; 1:145-172.
111. Schroer TA, Sheetz MP. Functions of microtubule-based motors. Annu Rev Physiol 1991; 53:629-652.
112. Hyman A, Karsenti E. The role of nucleation in patterning microtubule networks. J Cell Sci 1998; 111(Pt 15):2077-2083.
113. Russell LD, Malone JP, MacCurdy DS. Effect of the microtubule disrupting agents, colchicine and vinblastine, on seminiferous tubule structure in the rat. Tissue Cell 1981; 13:349-367.
114. Vogl AW, Linck RW, Dym M. Colchicine-induced changes in the cytoskeleton of the golden-mantled ground squirrel (Spermophilus lateralis) Sertoli cells. Am J Anat 1983; 168:99-108.
115. Vogl AW. Changes in the distribution of microtubules in rat Sertoli cells during spermatogenesis. Anat Rec 1988; 222:34-41.
116. Vogl AW, Lin YC, Dym M et al. Sertoli cells of the golden-mantled ground squirrel (Spermophilus lateralis): A model system for the study of shape change. Am J Anat 1983; 168:83-98.
117. Wenz JR, Hess RA. Characterization of stage-specific tyrosinated α-tubulin immunoperoxidase staining patterns in Sertoli cells of rat seminiferous tubules by light microscopic image analysis. Tissue Cell 1998; 30:492-501.
118. Redenbach DM, Vogl AW. Microtubule polarity in Sertoli cells: A model for microtubule-based spermatid transport. Eur J Cell Biol 1991; 54:277-290.
119. Redenbach DM, Boekelheide K. Microtubules are oriented with their minus-ends directed apically before tight junction formation in rat Sertoli cells. Eur J Cell Biol 1994; 65:246-257.
120. Vogl AW, Weis M, Pfeiffer DC. The perinuclear centriole-containing centrosome is not the major microtubule organizing center in Sertoli cells. Eur J Cell Biol 1995; 66:165-179.
121. Guttman J, Lee LE, Vogl AW. Evidence that gmma tubulin is located peripherally in Sertoli cells. FASEB J 2002; 16:A1101.
122. Fleming SL, Shank PR, Boekelheide K. γ-Tubulin overexpression in Sertoli cells in vivo: I. Localization to sites of spermatid head attachment and alterations in Sertoli cell microtubule distribution. Biol Reprod 2003; 69:310-321.
123. Hermo L, Oko R, Hecht NB. Differential post-translational modifications of microtubules in cells of the seminiferous epithelium of the rat: A light and electron microscope immunocytochemical study. Anat Rec 1991; 229:31-50.
124. Lawrence CJ, Dawe RK, Christie KR et al. A standardized kinesin nomenclature. J Cell Biol 2004; 167:19-22.
125. Miki H, Setou M, Kaneshiro K et al. All kinesin superfamily protein, KIF, genes in mouse and human. Proc Natl Acad Sci USA 2001; 98:7004-7011.
126. Ross JL, Wallace K, Shuman H et al. Processive bidirectional motion of dynein-dynactin complexes in vitro. Nat Cell Biol 2006; 8:562-570.
127. Vale RD. The molecular motor toolbox for intracellular transport. Cell 2003; 112:467-480.
128. Goldstein LS, Philp AV. The road less traveled: Emerging principles of kinesin motor utilization. Annu Rev Cell Dev Biol 1999; 15:141-183.
129. Hirokawa N. Kinesin and dynein superfamily proteins and the mechanism of organelle transport. Science 1998; 279:519-526.
130. Neely MD, Boekelheide K. Sertoli cell processes have axoplasmic features: An ordered microtubule distribution and an abundant high molecular weight microtubule-associated protein (cytoplasmic dynein). J Cell Biol 1988; 107:1767-1776.
131. Fawcett DW. Ultrastructure and function of the Sertoli cell. In: Greep RO, ed. Handbook of Physiology. 5(7). Baltimore: Williams and Wilkins, 1975:21-55.
132. Hall ES, Hall SJ, Boekelheide K. 2,5-Hexanedione exposure alters microtubule motor distribution in adult rat testis. Fundam Appl Toxicol 1995; 24:173-182.

133. Hall ES, Eveleth J, Jiang C et al. Distribution of the microtubule-dependent motors cytoplasmic dynein and kinesin in rat testis. Biol Reprod 1992; 46:817-828.
134. Redenbach DM, Hall ES, Boekelheide K. Distribution of Sertoli cell microtubules, microtubule-dependent motors, and the Golgi apparatus before and after tight junction formation in developing rat testis. Microsc Res Tech 1995; 32:504-519.
135. Miller MG, Mulholland DJ, Vogl AW. Rat testis motor proteins associated with spermatid translocation (dynein) and spermatid flagella (kinesin-II). Biol Reprod 1999; 60:1047-1056.
136. Clermont Y, Perey B. The stages of the cycle of the seminiferous epithelium of the rat: Practical definitions in PA-Schiff-hematoxylin and hematoxylin-eosin stained sections. Rev Can Biol 1957; 16:451-462.
137. Clermont Y. Kinetics of spermatogenesis in mammals: Seminiferous epithelium cycle and spermatogonial renewal. Physiol Rev 1972; 52:198-236.
138. Perey B, Clermont Y, Leblond CP. The wave of the seminiferous epithelium in the rat. Am J Anat 1961; 108:47-77.
139. Russell LD. Spermiation—The sperm release process: Ultrastructural observations and unresolved problems. In: Van Blerkom J, Motta PM, eds. Ultrastructure of Reproduction. Boston: Martinus Nijhoff, 1984:46-66.
140. Russell L. Observations on rat Sertoli ectoplasmic ('junctional') specializations in their association with germ cells of the rat testis. Tissue Cell 1977; 9:475-498.
141. Redenbach DM, Boekelheide K, Vogl AW. Binding between mammalian spermatid-ectoplasmic specialization complexes and microtubules. Eur J Cell Biol 1992; 59:433-448.
142. Vogl AW. Spatially dynamic intercellular adhesion junction is coupled to a microtubule-based motility system: Evidence from an in vitro binding assay. Cell Motil Cytoskeleton 1996; 34:1-12.
143. Beach SF, Vogl AW. Spermatid translocation in the rat seminiferous epithelium: Coupling membrane trafficking machinery to a junction plaque. Biol Reprod 1999; 60:1036-1046.
144. Guttman JA, Kimel GH, Vogl AW. Dynein and plus-end microtubule-dependent motors are associated with specialized Sertoli cell junction plaques (ectoplasmic specializations). J Cell Sci 2000; 113(Pt 12):2167-2176.

CHAPTER 12

Blood-Testis Barrier, Junctional and Transport Proteins and Spermatogenesis

Brian P. Setchell*

Functional Evidence for a Blood-Testis Barrier

The term "blood-testis barrier" appears to have been first used by Chiquoine[1] in an article on effects of cadmium on the testis, but evidence for such a barrier already existed, dating back to the early years of the twentieth century (see ref. 2 for early references). In a number of studies, it was shown that some dyes when injected into animals, stained most tissues, with the notable exceptions of the brain and the seminiferous tubules of the testis. The former observation was rapidly taken up and developed to form the basis for the concept of the blood-brain barrier,[3,4] but it was only with the studies of Kormano[5] that the true significance of the earlier observations on the testis was recognized. He showed that dyes which were excluded from the tubules of adult rats readily penetrated those of prepubertal animals. In addition, Kormano noticed that staining of interstitial cells with acriflavine also fell around the time of puberty, suggesting a change in the blood vessels as well. At about the same time as Kormano's studies, Waites and I showed that testis blood flow measured by indicator dilution with rubidium gave much lower values that with iodoantipyrine, while similar values were obtained in most other organs except brain,[6] suggesting that rubidium was also excluded to some extent from parts of the testis, as it was from the brain.

Also around this time, Waites and I devised techniques for collecting fluid from the rete testis (RTF) of sheep[7,8,9] and from the rete testis and seminiferous tubules (STF) of rats,[10] and we found that both RTF and STF differed appreciably in composition from either blood plasma or testicular lymph collected from a vessel in the spermatic cord. That such differences, especially those for small hydrophilic organic compounds such as inositol[11,12] could be maintained provided further evidence that there was not free communication between the various fluid compartments inside the testis, and this was confirmed in studies on the rate of penetration of various radioactive markers from the bloodstream into RTF in rams[13] or RTF and STF in rats.[14-17]

There are three cell types between the fluid inside the blood vessels and that in the lumina of the seminiferous tubules, namely the endothelial cells lining the blood vessels, the peritubular tissue and the Sertoli cells. These last are the only cells to extend all the way from the peritubular tissue to the lumen of the tubule, with the developing germ cells lying either between the base of a Sertoli cell and the peritubular tissue, or in the intercellular space between a pair of Sertoli cells or in crypts in the luminal surface of a Sertoli cell.[18-20] All three cell types could conceivably influence the rate of entry of substances into the tubules,[21] although most attention has been directed to the Sertoli cells (see next section).

*Brian P. Setchell—Department of Anatomical Sciences, University of Adelaide, Adelaide 5005, Australia. Email: brian.setchell@adelaide.edu.au

Molecular Mechanisms in Spermatogenesis, edited by C. Yan Cheng. ©2008 Landes Bioscience and Springer Science+Business Media.

Other techniques used to estimate the effectiveness of the blood-testis barrier include the measurement of the volume of distribution of a marker known to be excluded from STF, such as Cr-EDTA, inulin or sucrose, and relating this either to the volume of the interstitial tissue[22-24] or to the value obtained when the efferent ducts had been ligated 24 h previously, so that the fluid secreted during that time had been retained in the lumina of the seminiferous tubules.[25] Other studies[26,27] used as a marker, hexamethonium iodide, which has been shown not to penetrate the blood-brain barrier,[28] a zinc complex of carnosine labeled with C-14 and Zn-65,[29] or a biotin tracer.[30] Another approach is to relate the amount of a labeled compound to the amount of Tc-99 or I^{125} labeled albumin appearing in the testis and brain of mice following an intravenous injection.[31-39] From these data, an entry rate (K_i) for the marker can be calculated, but this value in the testis could be influenced by changes in vascular permeability as well as in permeability of the tubular barrier.

The latest development has been the use of magnetic resonance imaging of the testis, before and after intravenous injection of gadopentetate dimeglumine.[40,41] Qualitative evidence for a barrier in young animals is provided by the development of a lumen and the secretion of fluid in the tubules.[42-44]

While most evidence for the involvement of the Sertoli cells is morphological (see next section) it should be remembered that when isolated Sertoli cells are cultured at high density on Matrigel in a two-chamber system, they form a confluent layer, which exhibits barrier properties, as shown by an increase in electrical resistance and directional secretion of a number of substances.[45-47] However, the transepithelial resistance (TER) obtained (usually about 100 ohm.cm^2) was usually much less than that seen with MDCK cells or keratinocytes (100-2000 ohm.cm^2).[48] Nevertheless, treatment of Sertoli cell cultures with FSH and testosterone[45] could raise TER to between 580 and 1200 ohm.cm^2, and the cells were usually obtained from prepubertal rats, in which the barrier would not be fully formed (see below).

Structural Evidence for a Barrier

A Sertoli Cells

The existence of specialized junctions between pairs of Sertoli cells was recognised in the 1960's.[49-53] Their significance became apparent when it was shown that electron opaque markers which were injected into the interstitial tissue or reached there from the blood stream, were restricted from entering the tubules to some extent by the peritububular myoid cells, but almost completely by the specialized junctions between pairs of Sertoli cells. The markers used included colloidal carbon, ferritin, horseradish peroxidase, lanthanum salts,[54-58] and more recently biotin.[30]

Peritubular Myoid Cells

Peritubular myoid cells form a single layer in rodents and several layers in primates around the seminiferous tubules.[59] As long ago as 1901, it was suggested[60] that this cell layer formed "a sort of dialysing membrane which regulates the compostion of the fluid contained in the space that it limits" (une sorte de membrane dialysante qui regle la composition du liquide contenu dans l'espace qu'elle limite). The cells change in shape, structure, marker expression and rate of cell division around the time of puberty[61,62] and respond in culture to endothelin[63,64] which as the name implies, is usually produced by endothelial cells, but in the testis is formed mostly by the Sertoli cells.[65] The myoid cells produce PmodS, a protein which has a powerful influence on several Sertoli cell functions,[66,67] although an effect on the blood-testis barrier has not apparently been examined.

The peritubular myoid cells prevented the passage of larger electron-opaque markers like colloidal carbon or thorium, and lanthanum penetrated the myoid cell layer in only about 15% of the tubules in rodent testes.[54,55] However, in primate testes, the peritubular cells have much less effect in restricting the penetration of markers.[56]

Nevertheless, the myoid cells may have an important influence in restricting the entry of retinoic acid (RA) into the tubules. Less than 1% of the RA in the testis is derived from plasma RA, much less than in any other tissue studied.[68] This may be due to the presence in the myoid cells of the RA-degrading enzymes Cyp 26 a1, Cyp 26 b1 and Cyp 26c1,[69] while the first stage of the formation of RA from retinol occurs in the Sertoli cells. It has been known for many years that spermatogenesis is arrested in Vitamin A-deficient animals, and retinoic acid is effective in restoring sperm production only in pharmacological doses (10 mg/week compared with 0.1 to 0.2 mg/week for retinol).[70] The restricted entry of retinoic acid may explain this difference. The myoid cells also contain high levels of cellular retinol binding protein,[71,72] which is probably involved in the transport of retinol into the tubules (see below).

Endothelial Cells

The endothelial cells in the testis are unusual for an endocrine tissue in that they are unfenestrated,[74-76] although in the human testis, some capillaries in the lamina propria do have fenestrations.[77] Endothelial cells in the rat testis also have a much lower density of vesicles than vessels in other tissues, except brain,[78] suggesting that vesicular transport is less important in these tissues than elsewhere in the body.

Structural Constituents of the Sertoli Cell Junctions

In recent times, a large amount of information has appeared about the constituent proteins of the Sertoli cell junctions which constitute that part of the blood-testis barrier (Fig. 1). The main components include occludin, one or more of the claudins, zonula occludens (ZO), and junctional adhesion molecules (JAM's).Occludin, claudin-11 and JAM-1 are transmembrane proteins, the extracellular parts of which join with similar structure on an adjacent Sertoli cell to form a tight junction. In the cytoplasm of the cells, the intracellular tails of the occludin, claudin and JAM molecules are joined to ZO-1 and ZO-2 molecules, which in turn are linked to actin chains.[48]

Occludin is a 60 to 65 kDa protein with four transmembrane domains, one intracellular and two extracellular loops, and is present in the tight junctions between Sertoli cells in rats and mice, but not guinea pig or human.[79] In mice which carry a null mutation of the occludin gene, the testes initially develop normally, but by 40 to 60 weeks of age, the tubules become atrophic, with complete loss of germ cells.[80] Therefore, it is rather surprising that occludin first appears in the fetal testis at about day 13 pc (post-coitus), long before spermatogenesis is initiated, suggesting that occludin has functions other than the establishment of the barrier. In postnatal rats, at about day 5, the reaction for occludin becomes more intense and is then located along the lateral plasma membrane of the Sertoli cells. Then at day 14, the reaction appears as intense focal bands close to the base of the epithelium, near the presumed sites of the tight junctions which are forming at about that time.[81] Injection into rats of a 22-amino acid synthetic peptide corresponding to the second extracellular loop of occludin perturbs the blood-testis barrier and disrupts spermatogenesis.[82]

Claudins are a family of more than 20 proteins, about 22 kDa in size,[83] and claudin-11 is present at tight junctions between Sertoli cells in testes, but again appears first during fetal life. Its concentration in the testis reaches a peak at about 6 days of age, and then appears to decline, probably due to the appearance of claudin-negative germ cells.[84] Claudin-11 null male mice are sterile, and tight junctions appear to be absent in these animals as judged by freeze-fracture.[85] Claudin-5, which is found only in endothelial cells,[86] is present in endothelial cells in the rat testes,[87] but as mice null for this peptide die within a few days of birth,[88] it has not been possible to study the effect of lack of this protein on spermatogenesis.

Integrins are thought to be involved in junctions between testicular cells and extracellular matrix,[48] but there is evidence[89] that integrin $\alpha 6\ \beta 1$ is also present in Sertoli-Sertoli cell junctions, especially at certain stages of spermatogenesis, but also in Sertoli cell-only testes.[90] In testis explants, the development of this suprabasal integrin occurred only in the presence of FSH.[90]

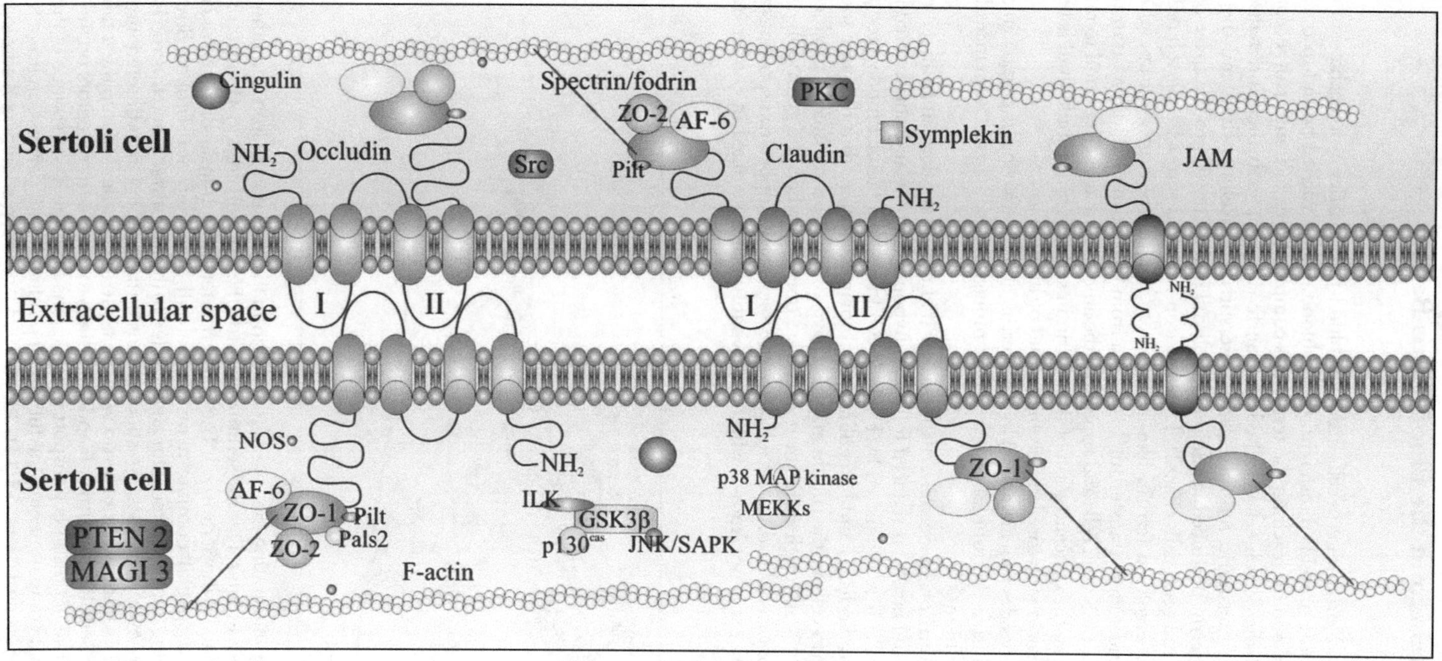

Figure 1. A diagram illustrating the molecular architecture of the three multiprotein complexes found at the Sertoli-Sertoli cell junctions of the blood-testis barrier. The three complexes are: (1) Occludin-ZO1/ZO2; (2) claudin-ZO1/ZO2; and (3) JAM-ZO1. Also shown are the peripheral membrane proteins known to regulate Sertoli cell tight junction dynamics. Reproduced with permission from: Mruk DD, Cheng CY. Endocrin Rev 25:747-806, ©2004 The Endocrine Society.[48]

Transport Proteins and the Blood-Testis Barrier

Transferrin

Iron is transported into the germ cells inside the blood-testis barrier by a mechanism involving a specific transport protein, transferrin. In the blood, iron is carried bound to transferrin secreted by the liver, and on reaching the testis, this complex binds to transferrin receptors on the basal surface of the Sertoli cells.[91] The iron-transferrin complex is then internalised and dissociated, the apo-transferrin returned to the interstitial extracellular fluid and the iron is complexed to transferrin produced inside the Sertoli cell and secreted into the space between the Sertoli cell and the germ cells (Fig. 2). How the iron is moved across the Sertoli cell is still uncertain, but may involve a ferritin-like molecule.[92,93] Sertoli cells in a bicameral culture system synthesize and secrete transferrin,[94] and iron from basally applied human transferrin is transported through rat Sertoli cells and appears in the apical compartment bound to rat transferrin.[95] Nevertheless, the concentration of transferrin in seminiferous tubule fluid is less than one-twentieth of that in interstitial extracellular fluid or blood plasma.[96]

Other elements besides iron are bound by transferrin, and this may be important in causing the accumulation inside the tubules of potentially mutagenic radioactive substances like indium[97,98] and plutonium.[99]

Transferrin production by Sertoli cells is greater if the cells are derived from 17 day old rather than 10 day old rats,[100] is reduced following hypophysectomy and not restored by testosterone treatment.[101] It is stimulated by FSH,[102] cytokines,[103] a factor PmodS produced by the peritubular myoid cells,[104] and heregulins, which may also come from the same source.[105] The presence of germ cells in the tubule may also have an effect on transferrin production by the Sertoli cells,[105,106] although different results were obtained when the germ cells were depleted with methoxyacetic acid.[107] Sertoli cells also secrete an copper-transporting protein, ceruloplasmin,[108] but it is not known whether this substance is involved in copper transport into the tubules.

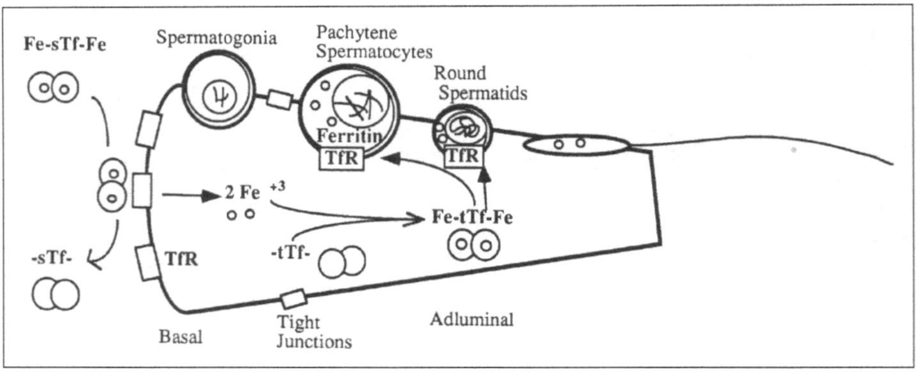

Figure 2. A diagram illustrating the role of transferrin in the transport of iron and other metals into the seminiferous tubules. Diferric serum transferrin (Fe-sTF-Fe) binds to a transferrin receptor on the basal surface of the Sertoli cell. The transferrin-ferric ion-transferrin receptor complex is internalized into special compartments in the cell, acidified and broken down. The apotransferrin and the transferrin receptor are recycled to the cell surface, and the iron is moved through the cell to newly synthesized testicular transferrin (tTf) or is incorporated into ferritin in the Sertoli cell. The testicular transferrin with the ferric ions is released into the intercellular space between the Sertoli and germ cell and then binds to transferrin receptors on the surface of the germ cells. The net result is transport of ferric ions from the basal surface of the Sertoli cell to the adluminal compartment of the tubule. Reproduced with permission from: Sylvester SR, Griswold MD. J Androl 1994; 15:381-385, ©1994 American Society of Andrology.[93]

Another divalent metal transporter DMT1 (Slcl 1a2) is also present in the Sertoli cells of the rat testis, although it is not primarily responsible for translocating iron across the epithelium, but in intracellular handling of iron during spermatogenesis.[109,110]

P-Glycoprotein

P-glycoprotein (Pgp) is the product of the multidrug resistance 1 gene (MDR1 or ABC B1 in humans, and mdr 1a (sometimes called mdr 3) and 1b in mice and rats). It was originally identified in cancer cells which had become resistant to chemotherapeutic drugs.[111-114] Subsequently, it was found that this protein was present in a number of normal tissues, and especially in the endothelial cells of the brain and testis.[115-118] It is also present in other cells in the testis, including Leydig cells, macrophages, peritubular cells, Sertoli cells and late spermatids, although not detectable in spermatogonia, spermatocytes or early spermatids.[119,120] However, the relative concentrations in the various cell types has apparently not yet been determined and another group has detected mdr 1 in germ cells, probably spermatogonia, in rats, as well as in endothelial cells in the testis.[121] In endothelial cells from brain, Pgp is expressed only on the luminal surface, consistent with a role in protecting the brain from circulating lipophilic molecules which would otherwise cross the blood-brain barrier. However, in endothelial cells in the testis, Pgp is expressed on both luminal and abluminal sufaces, which suggests that it acts to exclude substrates of the transporter from the endothelial cells themselves.[122] A mRNA from a related gene mdr 2 is also present in Sertoli cells, but at a lower concentration than in liver.[109]

The testes and brains of mice in which the gene for mdr-1a has been deleted accumulate more ivermectin, digoxin, cyclosporin A, ondasetron, loperamide and vinblastine than controls.[123-126] In other studies,[127,128] similar results were obtained with amitriptyline and some of its metabolites, but not with fluoxetine. In mice in which both mdr 1a and 1b have been knocked out, the entry of the anti-Parkinson drug budipine into the testes and brains was enhanced.[129] In these double knockout mice, the penetration of the steroids, corticosterone, cortisol, aldosterone and progesterone into the testes was also enhanced,[130] although cortisol[131] or prednisolone[132] entry into the testis was unaffected in mdr 1a single knockout mice. Pgp also transports HIV protease inhibitors (HPI) used in the treatment of AIDS[133] and pharmacological inhibition of the transporter enhances the penetration of the HPI nelfinavir into the testes of mice treated with LY-335979, a potent Pgp inhibitor, as well as in mdr-1a knockout mice.[134] The penetration of saquinivir, another HPI into the testes of mice was also enhanced by treatment of the animals with another inhibitor of Pgp, GF120918.[135] However, treatment of mice with a variety of Pgp inhibitors failed to increase the penetration of vinblastine into either testis or brain,[136] and vincristine enters seminiferous tubule fluid reasonably rapidly,[137] although it is a substrate for both Pgp and MRP.[126] The closely related efflux pump, breast cancer resistance protein (BCRP) is also found in the endothelial cells and peritubular myoid cells in the testis,[120] but the structurally related protein encoded by the cystic fibrosis gene is not found in endothelial cells, but is expressed in spermatids in a stage-specific fashion.[121,138]

Multidrug Resistance Protein

Multidrug resistance proteins (MRP) are other members of the ATP-binding cassette superfamily distantly related to Pgp. MRP1 is present in high concentrations in testes[139] and is localized to the Leydig and Sertoli cells in human and mice,[120,140] but cannot be detected in endothelial cells in the rat testis.[141] Mice lacking the gene for this protein are much more sensitive to the damaging effects of etoposide phosphate[141] and methoxychlor[142] than normal mice, suggesting that it acts to exclude these drugs from the seminiferous tubules. MRP1 is also involved in glutathione-mediated transport of sulfated estrogens, and it has been suggested that the high levels of MRP1 in the Leydig cells may be responsible for the efflux of the hydrophilic sulfated conjugates from the cell.[143] The anticancer drug methotrexate, which is transported out of cells by MRP, but poorly by Pgp,[144] is virtually excluded from seminferous tubule fluid.[145]

Other Transport Mechanisms

Endothelial cells in the testis contain high levels of γ-glutamyl transpeptidase,[118,146] an enzyme usually associated with amino acid transport, and it has also been shown that endothelial cells of the larger blood vessels in the rat testis transport leucine with transport kinetics similar to those of brain and much lower than for other tissues.[147] There is also a large amino acid transporter present in rat testis as well as brain and heart, but not other tissues.[148] Endothelial cells in the rat testis also contain an endothelial barrier antigen (EBA), previously thought to be confined to nervous tissue,[149] and an isoform GLUT-1 of the glucose transporter family, usually associated with brain and retina.[118]

The peritubular cells in the mouse testis contain a specialized transporter protein involved in urea movement across plasma membranes, UT-A5, the levels of which are not related to the stage of spermatogenesis in adults but are coordinated with the stage of testis development, increasing around 15 days post partum.[150] In rat Sertoli cells, there are also 4 other urea transporters, UT-A 1, 2, 3 and 4 present at all stages of spermatogenesis, and UT-B is present at stages II and III. UT-A3 was also present in some interstitial cells. Flux of urea across the walls of isolated perfused seminiferous tubules is inhibited by phloretin.[151] It is interesting that there is some evidence for the active accumulation of radioactively labeled urea inside the seminiferous tubules of rats.[152]

Evidence has recently been presented for the presence of a family of saturable nucleoside transporters in isolated Sertoli cells, as primary cultures or as polarized layers on Matrigel, some of which is sodium-dependent and can be inhibited with nitrobenzylthioinosine.[153]

Binding proteins may also be important in the regulating the entry of retinol into the tubules. Homogenates of rat testis bind more retinol and retinoic acid (RA) than any other tissue examined,[154] but in vivo, very little RA enters the tubules from blood.[68] Both myoid and Sertoli cells in the testis contain a cellular retinol-binding protein (CRBP).[155-157] The Sertoli cells also contain a number of retinoic acid receptors.[68,69] Retinol circulates in the plasma bound to a retinol-binding protein (RBP), a 21 kDa protein which normally is present as a 76kDa 1:1 complex with transthyretin. This complex in the testis is confined to the interstitial tissue.[158] When retinol bound to RBP was injected into the testis[158] or under the capsule,[159] it appeared in the tubules only after at least 30 minutes, whereas tritiated retinol injected mixed with albumin, spread rapidly throughout the testis. Early studies could not detect any interaction of RBP with cells in or on the seminiferous tubules.[158] Nevertheless, both peritubular myoid and Sertoli cells appear to be involved in the transport of retinoids to the germ cells. Both cell types in culture are able to accumulate retinol from serum RBP by a saturable and competable process, which involves recognition of the retinol-RBP complex at the cell surface, with subsequent internalization of the retinol but not the RBP. The first step involves the myoid cells, which bind the retinol inside the cell to newly formed CRBP, and the new complex is released into the space between the myoid cells and the Sertoli cells. The latter then take up just the retinol and complex it with new CRBP, before releasing the complex again to reach the germ cells.[71,72,160]

Sertoli cells also contain a prostaglandin D_2 synthetase, which also binds retinoic acid but not retinol.[161] This protein is secreted into rete testis fluid,[162] but its role in the transport of retinoids into the tubules in not yet clear.

Factors Affecting Blood-Testis Barrier Function

Age and Hormones

As already mentioned, studies on the penetration of certain dyes into the seminiferous tubules showed that these dyes were excluded only from the tubules of rats older than about 20 days.[5] Subsequently, it was shown that electron-opaque markers injected into the interstitial tissue of the testes of rats entered the tubules freely up to 16 days of age, but between 16 and 19 days , the occluding junctions between the Sertoli cells appear and the tracers are effectively prevented from reaching the tubular lumen.[163] In immature rat testes, occluding junctions, as demonstrated by freeze-fracture, are absent, although gap junctions are present. Furthermore, perfusion with hypertonic lithium chloride caused the cells outside the Sertoli cells junctions in adult testes to shrivel, with no effect on those inside the junctions, whereas in the testes of 13 day old rats, cellular shrinkage occurred throughout the tubules.[164] Shrinkage of adluminal cells in response to exposure to a hypertonic solution decreased between 14 and 18 days of age.[43] Similarly in guinea pigs, Sertoli cell junctional complexes appeared around 15 days after birth[165] and in mice at about 16 days.[166] In rats around 15 days of age, the barrier appears only in those parts of the tubule where germ cells have reached pachytene.[167]

In seasonal breeders such as mink,[168,169] viscacha,[170] and Djungarian hamsters[171] electron opaque markers are excluded by the Sertoli cell junctions during the breeding season, but during testicular regression, the tracer penetrates throughout the tubules. In the study on mink, the exclusion of the marker from the tubule was associated with the presence of a tubular lumen, rather than any particular type of germ cells. At the other end of life, the barrier in 24 month old rats was grossly deficient, with associated failure in spermatogenesis.[172] The development of the barrier in young rats and mice can be retarded by the neonatal administrations of diethylstilboestrol.[173,174]

The development of a lumen in the tubules is more gradual, beginning at around 10 days after birth, and with the diameter continuing to increase slowly to day 30 and then more rapidly to around day 50.[22,43] Fluid secretion per unit weight of testis also continued to increase until about 45 days of age,[42,44] and the volume of distribution of Cr-EDTA, which is normally excluded from the tubules, continues to fall until after 30 days of age,[22] so the functional barrier appears to develop more gradually than the anatomical one.

The development of transepithelial electrical resistance (TER) in two-compartment Sertoli cell cultures is delayed by FSH for several days, and once established is decreased and then returns to control levels or increases. Testosterone alone caused a rapid increase in TER, and testosterone and FSH together resulted in the highest TER levels. Dihydrotestosterone was more effective than testosterone, whereas estradiol was without effect.[45] Dibutryl cyclic adenosine monophosphate (cAMP) in low concentrations stimulated TER development, whereas higher doses were inhibitory. Cholera toxin mimicked the FSH effects.[175] The effect of cAMP on the Sertoli cell tight junctions is probably mediated by a proteasome-sensitive ubiquitination of occludin.[47] TGF-β3 also regulates blood-testis barrier dynamics, probably by determining the steady-state levels of occludin and ZO-1 via the p38 MAP kinase signaling pathway.[176] Tumour necrosis factor α injected directly into rat testes caused a temporary disruption of the blood-testis barrier, by reducing the levels of occludin, zonula occludens-1 and N-cadherin.[177]

Testosterone, acting through its receptor in the Sertoli cells, regulates the expression of claudin-3, which encodes a transient component of newly formed tight junctions. Sertoli cell-specific ablation of androgen receptor results in increased permeability of the barrier to biotin.[30] The effect of androgen withdrawal on the Sertoli cell junctions was studied either by hypophysectomy or by treatment of rats with ethane dimethane sulfonate to destroy the Leydig cells. These treatments led to degeneration of germ cells and the formation of numerous basally-located vacuoles, formed by multiple focal dilations of the intercellular space associated with the junctional complexes. As this occurred also in Sertoli cell-only testes, produced by fetal irradiation, it cannot be explained by spaces left by degenerating germ cells.[178] The expression of occludin is also reduced by treatment of rats with the anti-androgen, flutamide.[179] In an intratesticular androgen suppression model, using subcutaneous implants of testosterone and estrogen to suppress LH secretion and hence endogenous androgen production, the adherens junctions between the Sertoli cells and spermatids can be disrupted, without affecting blood-testis barrier integrity.[180]

The Sertoli cell barrier to lanthanum develops normally in rats treated in utero with busulfan but at a later age around 30 days of age, at the time of the appearance of the first zygotene and pachytene cells in these animals.[181] However, in prenatally irradiated rats, tight junctions, as detected by freeze fracture, were extensive by 3 months of age, although their ability to block the penetration of markers was not examined.[167] It is probably relevant that the fluid inside the Sertoli cell only tubules of prenatally irradiated or busufan-treated rats was plasma-like in its potassium content, in contrast to the high potassium of normal fluid.[16,183]

Vitamin A Deficiency

In rats made Vitamin A-deficient from weaning (20 days old), Sertoli cell junctions were intact and complete spermatogenesis was maintained up to 80 days of age. However, by 90 days, lanthanum could penetrate through the junctions and by 100 days severe regression of spermatogenesis had occurred.[184] Different results were obtained by Ismail and Morales,[185] who found that the junctions remained impermeable to lanthanum, even when spermatogenesis had failed in rats 104 days old, deficient since 20 days old. In a later study, following long-term deprivation of Vitamin A, the Sertoli cell junctions became permeable to lanthanum when spermatogenesis was arrested and remained so even when spermatogenesis was first reinitiated. Spermatocytes normally found in the adluminal compartment were apoptotic, while spermatocytes normally found in the basal compartment remained normal.[186]

Tissue and Blood Pressures

If the efferent ducts leading from the testis to the epididymis are ligated close to the testis, the fluid normally secreted by the Sertoli cells to transport the immotile spermatozoa is retained inside the seminiferous tubules. These become progressively distended for between 24 and 36 h in rats, so that the testis becomes enlarged and turgid. Then the testis weight falls again and eventually by 21 days, spermatogenesis is completely deranged.[42] During this time the blood-testis barrier, judged by the ratio of the space of distribution of Cr-EDTA to the measured volume of the interstitial tissue remained normal during the phase of fluid accumulation, but increased sharply as testis weight begins to fall again, indicating breakdown of the barrier. Surprisingly, by the time testis weight had returned to control levels, the barrier appeared to be functioning again, and it remained functional even when spermatogenesis was completely disrupted up to 3 weeks later.[24,187] One author[188] found that lanthanum penetrated more readily through the Sertoli cell junctions as early as 24 h after efferent duct ligation. However, other studies with electron opaque markers gave contradictory results.[188-191]

In chronically hypertensive rats, the penetration of sucrose and 2-methyl-4-chlorophenoxyacetic acid into the testis is reduced, while that of the highly permeable antipyrine is unaffected.[192] In rats with testicular degeneration induced by epinephrine, the barrier remains able to exclude lanthanum.[193]

Cadmium and Other Toxic Substances

The testes of most mammals are extremely sensitive to the effects of cadmium salts, in doses which have little effect on other tissues. Early observations[1] concentrated attention on the blood vessels in the testis, and there is no doubt that testis blood flow is reduced in rats as a result of increases in vascular permeability as early as several hours after a single injection of cadmium chloride.[6] Later studies showed that permeability of the blood-testis barrier to rubidium probably preceded the changes in vascular permeability.[194] In guinea pigs on the other hand, increased staining of the interstitial tissue with acriflavine injected subcutaneously occurred before an increase in staining of the seminiferous tubules.[195] However, lower doses of cadmium affect spermatogenesis without noticeable changes in the vascular system, and these effects can be reduced by coadministration of zinc salts.[196]

Exposure of bicameral Sertoli cell cultures to cadmium salts caused a progressive and dose-dependent drop in TER.[197,198] The expression of occludin is decreased and u-plasminogen activator is increased in the presence of cadmium.[198] Treatment of rats with low doses of cadmium chloride caused changes in the tight junction-associated microfilaments in the Sertoli cells by 24 h after injection, although no changes were found after 4 h.[199] The fall in TER in the presence of cadmium was reduced if testosterone and FSH were added.[198] The disruption of the barrier is associated with a transient increase in testicular TGF-β2 and 3 and the phosphorylated p38 mitogen activated protein (MAP) kinase, concomitant with a loss of occludin and ZO-1 from the barrier site.[200] There is also a surge in α_2-macroglobulin at the Sertoli-Sertoli cell junctions at the time of disruption of the barrier.[201]

It is interesting that there are some strains of mice whose testes are much more resistant to the effects of cadmium, and this is associated with reduced transport of cadmium into the testes. The cadmium transporter is saturable and can be competitively inhibited by zinc, but not calcium, and appears not to be associated with any tubular cells, but is probably located in the endothelial cells.[36]

The integrity of the blood-testis barrier is altered by intratesticular treatment of rats with cytochalasin D, a known microfilament inhibitor.[202] Evidence for this was obtained from studies on the penetration of electron-opaque markers, from the effects of perfusion with hypertonic solutions and from the entry of radioactive inulin into seminiferous tubular fluid.

Another substance which has been shown to disrupt the blood-testis barrier is glycerol when injected into the testes of rats. These animals showed increased entry of radioactive inulin and albumin into seminiferous tubular and rete testis fluids,[203] and also disrupted tight junction-associated actin microfilaments, occludin and microtubules in the Sertoli cells.[204]

Other substances which appear to affect the blood-testis barrier include hexanedione,[205] *cis*-platinum,[206] sarin,[26] and DEET[27] but stainless steel corrosion products affects spermatogenesis without apparently interfering with the blood-testis barrier.[207] Other treatments such as bisphenol A[208] or Adjudin (AF 2364)[48] disrupt the junctions between Sertoli cells and spermatids without affecting the blood-testis barrier. Freunds complete adjuvant injected into guinea pigs 7 days previously increased the entry of horseradish peroxidase into the seminiferous tubules.[209]

Temperature and Cryptorchidism

The entry of radioactive albumin into rete testis fluid of rats was unaffected during or following heating of the testes, but the entry of K, Rb, Na, lysine and some steroids was increased during heating.[210] The entry of Cr-EDTA into the tubules was not affected when spermatogenesis had been disrupted in rats by local heating of their testes.[23] In surgically-induced cryptorchidism in rats, the blood-testis barrier appears to remain intact,[211,212] but in spontaneous cases in humans, the penetration of lanthanum between the Sertoli cells depended on the extent of the loss of germ cells.[213] In other conditions of spermatogenic cycle breakdown in humans, lanthanum entry is increased in maturation arrest and in irregular hypospermatogenesis, but in germ cell aplasia the barrier remains efficient.[214]

Mutants and Hybrids

The blood-testis barrier is less efficient in Tfm and Sxr mice, but normal in Mo^{vbr}/Y and Gy/Y mutants.[215] There are defects in both the germ cells and in the blood-testis barrier in *as*-mutant rats, as demonstrated by the distribution of cytochrome-c in the testis, as well as from studies involving spermatogonial transplantation.[216] The blood-testis barrier is deficient in hybrids between blue and silver foxes, and spermatogenesis is arrested at early pachytene.[217]

Significance of the Blood-Testis Barrier

As has already been discussed,[218] there are several obvious consequences of the operation of the blood-testis barrier. The first is immunological. The barrier isolates the developing germ cells from circulating antibodies in the bloodstream. It also means that the body's immunological system does not "see" the haploid germ cells, and therefore a male can be immunized against his own spermatozoa.[219] However, the isolation is not complete and Tung[220] has concluded that "tissue barriers and antigen sequestration are important but not sufficient to protect germ cell antigens and prevent experimental allergic orchitis". Some germ cells outside the barrier can certainly provoke an immunological reaction,[221] even peritubular cells,[222] leading to autoimmune orchitis.[220,223] Furthermore, mice immunized with syngeneic testis antigen have IgG deposits surrounding cells at the periphery of about half the tubule cross-sections, particularly those at stage 7 to 12. Also sera from testis-immune orchidectomized donors are able to transfer IgG passively into the testes of normal syngeneic recipients in an antigen-specific manner,[221] although there is evidence that the rete testis and tubuli recti are the sites of the earliest and most frequent lesions.[224] Therefore, other factors must be involved in making rodent testes, but not those of sheep[225] or monkeys,[226] immunologically privileged sites. Possible factors have been discussed recently by Hedger.[227]

The second effect of the barrier relates to the endocrine system. Peptide hormones such as FSH and LH do not instantaneously pass from the blood even into the extracellular interstitial fluid, so that the Leydig cells begin to respond to a rise in blood LH even before there is any change in the LH levels in the immediate vicinity of these cells.[228] FSH on the other hand acts principally on the Sertoli cells, and therefore must penetrate both the endothelial cell and peritubular cell layers. This is probably less important as the concentration of FSH does not seem to show such pronounced peaks as LH does,[229] and therefore changes in its concentrations in blood are more likely to be reflected in the concentrations at the basal surface of the Sertoli cells.

The situation with steroids is less clear cut. Because of their relatively high lipid solubility, they should pass more readily through the barrier than the hydrophilic peptides, but there is some evidence,[218,230] that the concentration of testosterone in RTF and STF does not change as much as that in blood. This may suggest that there is a transport system for steroids in the tubules, but no further evidence for this idea has been presented. It is clear from the relative concentrations inside and outside the tubules that the androgen-binding protein secreted by the Sertoli cells preferentially inside the barrier certainly does not produce a higher concentration of the total (free plus bound) steroid there. In fact the concentration of free testosterone may be appreciably lower in STF. Conjugated steroids, which are produced in large amounts in the testes of some species such as pig[231] and horse[232] tend to be less lipophilic than the free steroids and therefore remain in higher concentrations in the interstitial extracellular fluid than inside the barrier.

Glucose is transported across the barrier by a transport system the capacity of which appears to be less than the capacity of the Sertoli cells to convert the sugar to lactate. The consequence of this is that there is very little glucose in the fluid inside the tubules[8-12] and the developing germ cells prefer to metabolize lactate even in vitro.[233]

An interesting recent development has been the identification of a number of specific transport proteins for xenobiotics in various cells in the testis. These transporters, Pgp and MDR have important consequences in determining whether a particular toxicant will affect spermatogenesis, but in the case of transferrin, it may result in the accumulation of mutagenic substances in the environment of the germ cells.

One of the most interesting aspects of the function of the blood-testis barrier is the fact that it cannot remain closed all the time, but must open at different points along each tubule at specific times in the spermatogenic cycle to allow developing spermatocytes to pass from the basal to the adluminal compartment.[57] How this is achieved is still a matter of debate. Four theories have been advanced to explain this phenomenon: zipper, intermediate compartment, repetitive removal of membrane segments and junction restructuring. However, junction disassembly and reassembly seems to be the most likely explanation.[48] Opening of the Sertoli-Sertoli cell junctions in a limited part of the tubule must occur without affecting the Sertoli-Sertoli cell junctions elsewhere in that tubule or Sertoli cell-germ cell adherens junctions in the same and other parts of the tubule. It appears that cytokines may be involved[234] and α_2-macroglobulin also appears to play a part.[48,201] One of the most intriguing questions which remains to be answered is how spermatogonia injected into the lumen of a single seminiferous tubule either directly or via the rete testis[235] can pass between pairs of Sertoli cells to take up a position adjacent to the peritubular tissue and repopulate that area of the tubules with developing germ cells. The recipient animals have usually been treated with busulfan or irradiation to eliminate endogenous spermatogenesis, but nothing appears to be known about the efficacy of the barrier in these animals. It is interesting that transmissible leukemic cells, when injected together with testicular cells into the tubules through the rete in normal rats can reach the intertubular tissue where they resume their uncontrolled multiplication and make the recipient animals leukemic.[236]

It has also been repeatedly stated that the specialized environment created by the barrier may be necessary for the germ cells to proceed through meiosis. However, just what these conditions are has yet to be defined, but the fact that spermatogenesis can proceed, albeit to a limited extent, in aggregates of testicular cells encased in alginate[237] may indicate that as long as Sertoli and germ cells are in reasonably close association, that is sufficient.

One fascinating possibility is that retinoic acid (RA), not derived from blood but newly formed from retinol by a two-stage process, may be involved in the switch of the germ cells from mitosis to meiosis in the testis. The first stage of this conversion involves the Sertoli cells and the second the germ cells.[69,238] RA has been shown to cause the germ cells in the fetal ovary to enter meiosis, while in the fetal testis, meiosis is inhibited by destruction of RA by Cyp26 b1[239,240] the same enzyme that in the myoid cells, prevents the entry of RA into the tubules.[68] A premeiotic germ cell-specific cytoplasmic protein encoded by the RA-responsive gene Stra8 is present in only less than half the tubule cross-sections in a mouse testis,[241] although unfortunately these authors did not identify the stage of spermatogenesis at which this protein was expressed. It is interesting that in mice in which the gene for $p27^{kip1}$ is knocked out, spermatocytes were often arrested at preleptotene[242] and this mitotic inhibitor can be induced in cultured Sertoli cells by RA.[243] Furthermore, the expression of mRNA for CRBP is highest in spermatogenic stage IX to XIV, when most of the mitoses in the tubules occur. Preleptotene spermatocytes appear first at stage VII but CRBP mRNA rises significantly only in stage VIII,[157] when the meiotic DNA synthesis is occurring. The expression of mRNA for the retinoic acid receptor RARα is also highest at stage VIII in the rat testis, and this receptor is present in preleptotene spermatocytes as well as in round spermatids.[244] This receptor is required for synchronization of the spermatogenic cycle, and in its absence, preleptotene spermatocytes do not proceed to leptotene in the first, second and third waves.[245,246] However, others have shown that in mice lacking plasma RBP, Vitamin A deficiency does not delay the entry of preleptotene spermatocytes into meiosis, while spermatogenesis is blocked by delayed or arrested differentiation of spermatogonia.[247-250] This suggests that Vitamin A may have several functions in the testis, and furthermore, there may be important difference between mice and rats in the responses of their testes to Vitamin A deficiency.[247]

The observation that when spermatogenesis is restored in previously Vitamin A-deficient rats, spermatocytes progress to pachytene but then degenerate until the barrier is reformed,[186] would add emphasis to the need for the barrier for complete meiosis. Likewise, the finding that the barrier is disrupted by the injection of a 22-amino acid peptide corresponding to the second loop of occludin, accompanied by a cessation of spermatogenesis[82] would strongly emphasise the importance of the barrier for spermatogenesis.

However, as already mentioned, there are a number of conditions in which spermatogenesis is disrupted but the barrier function appears to be intact, suggesting that other factors are also important for normal sperm production. Nevertheless, the blood-testis barrier remains an important factor in the physiology of the testis, in particular in relation to spermatogenesis.

Future Directions

There are a number of lines of research on the blood-testis barrier which could yield important results in the future. First, possible roles of the endothelial and peritubular cells in regulating entry of substances into the testis or of influencing the Sertoli cell barrier need reevaluating. This is because of the many peculiarities of the testicular endothelial cells, many of which they share with brain endothelial cells, the site of the blood-brain barrier[3,4] and the recent demonstration of transport systems for urea in the peritubular cells. Studies on endothelial cells should now be possible following the recent demonstration that these cells can be isolated from rat testes, and that when cocultured with interstitial cells, the endothelial cells enhance the production of testosterone.[251] Techniques for isolation and culture of peritubular cells have been available for some years.[63,64] While cocultures of peritubular and Sertoli cells have been used[252] to study basement membrane gene expression, and the effect of proteins from pachytene spermatocytes[253] and spermatids[254] have been used to study their effects on secretion by Sertoli cells, no-one appears to have used cocultures of peritubular or germ cells and Sertoli cells in bicameral chambers (as illustrated in Fig. 1B,C in ref. 46) to study the effects of other cells on barrier function.

However, probably the most interesting problem in this area is the mechanism by which the Sertoli cell barrier is opened and closed again to allow the passage of the developing germ cells. Various theories have been advanced[48] but more evidence is needed on local factors controlling the distribution of this process in relation to spatially and temporally determined stages of spermatogenesis. Related to this problem is the need for an explanation of the occurrence in fetal testes of the structural proteins associated with the Sertoli-Sertoli cell junctions, occludin and claudin.

One new area of interest in relation to the blood-testis barrier is the involvement of specific transport proteins, such as Pgp and MDR. These may have important toxicological consequences in determining whether a particular compound disrupts spermatogenesis. It is conceivable that toxins could either be normally excluded or concentrated inside the tubules by these transporters, and further information on their distribution and specificity is needed. This may be particularly important for the disruptors of the barrier, cadmium salts and glycerol, and studies on the transport of these substances should be undertaken.

Finally, there is the old question of the role of the barrier in creating the conditions necessary for meiosis which needs further study. Recent progress in stem cell transplantation[235] and in vitro spermatogenesis[237] may provide the tools for further study of this fascinating problem.

References

1. Chiquoine D. Observations on the early events of cadmium necrosis of the testis. Anat Rec 1964; 149:23-36.
2. Setchell BP, Waites GMH. The blood-testis barrier. In: Greep RO, Hamilton DW, eds. Handbook of Physiology Section 7 Vol V. Male Reproductive System. Washington DC: American Physiological Society, 1975:143-172.
3. Davson H, Zlokovic B, Rakic L et al. An Introduction to the Blood-Brain Barrier. London: Macmillan, 1993:1-335.
4. Rubin LL, Staddon JM. The cell biology of the blood-brain barrier. Annu Rev Neurosci 1999; 22:11-28.
5. Kormano M. Dye permeability and alkaline phosphatase activity of testicular capillaries in the post-natal rat. Histochemie 1967; 9:327-338.
6. Waites GMH, Setchell BP. Changes in blood flow and vascular permeability in the testis, epididymis and accessory reproductive organs of the rat after the administration of cadmium chloride. J Endocrinol 1966; 34:329-342.
7. Voglmayr JK, Waites GMH, Setchell BP. Studies on spermatozoa and fluid collected directly from the testis of the conscious ram. Nature 1966; 210:861-863.
8. Voglmayr JK, Scott TW, Setchell BP et al. Metabolism of testicular spermatozoa and characteristics of testicular fluid collected from the conscious ram. J Reprod Fertil 1967; 14:87-99.
9. Setchell BP, Scott TW, Voglmayr JK et al. Characteristics of testicular spermatozoa and the fluid which transports them into the epididymis. Biol Reprod 1969; (Suppl 1):40-66.
10. Tuck RR, Setchell BP, Waites GMH et al. The composition of fluid collected by micropuncture and catheterization from the seminiferous tubules and rete testis of rats. Pflugers Archiv 1970; 318:225-243.
11. Setchell BP, Dawson RMC, White RW. The high concentration of free myo-inositol in rete testis fluid from rams. J Reprod Fertil 1968; 17:329-332.
12. Hinton BT, White RW, Setchell BP. Concentrations of myo-inositol in the luminal fluid of the mammalian testis and epididymis. J Reprod Fertil 1980; 58:395-399.

13. Setchell BP, Voglmayr JK, Waites GMH. A blood-testis barrier restricting passage from blood into rete testis fluid but not into lymph. J Physiol 1969; 200:73-85.
14. Setchell BP, Wallace ALC. The penetration of iodine-labelled FSH and albumin into the seminiferous tubules of sheep and rats. J Endocrinol 1972; 54:67-77.
15. Waites GMH, Jones AR, Main SJ et al. The entry of antifertility and other compounds into the testis. Adv Biosci 1973; 10:101-116.
16. Setchell BP, Hinton BT, Jacks F et al. Restricted penetration of iodinated follicle-stimulating and luteinizing hormone into the seminiferous tubules of the rat testis. Mol Cell Endocrinol 1976; 6:59-69.
17. Howards SS, Jessee SJ, Johnson AL. Micropuncture studies of the blood-seminiferous tubule barrier. Biol Reprod 1976; 14:264-269.
18. Fawcett DM. Ultrastructure and function of Sertoli cells. In: Greep RO, Hamilton DW, eds. Handbook of Physiology Section 7 Vol V. Male Reproductive System. Washington DC: American Physiological Society, 1975:21-55.
19. Russell LD, Clegg ED, Ettlin RA et al. Histological and Histopathological Evaluation of the Testis. Clearwater: Cache River Press, 1990:1-286.
20. Russell LD. Form, dimensions and cytology of mammalian Sertoli cells. In: Russell LD, Griswold MD, eds. The Sertoli cell. Clearwater: Cache River Press, 1993:1-37.
21. Ploen L, Setchell BP. Blood-testis barriers revisited: A homage to Lennart Nicander. Int J Androl 1992; 15:1-4.
22. Setchell BP, Pollanen P, Zupp JL. The development of the blood-testis barrier and changes in vascular permeability at puberty in rats. Int J Androl 1988; 11:225-233.
23. Setchell BP, Tao L, Zupp JL. The penetration of chromium-EDTA from blood plasma into various compartments of rat testes, as an indicator of the blood-testis barrier, following exposure of the testes to heat. J Reprod Fertil 1996; 106:125-133.
24. Tao L, Zupp JL, Setchell BP. Effect of efferent duct ligation on the function of the blood-testis barrier in rats. J Reprod Fertil 2000; 120:13-18.
25. Setchell BP. The entry of substances into the seminiferous tubules. In: Mancini RE, Martini L, eds. Male Fertility and Sterility. New York: Academic Press, 1974:37-57.
26. Jones KH, Dechkonskaia AM, Herrick EA et al. Subchronic effects following a single sarin exposure on blood-brain and blood-testes barrier permeability, acetylcholinesterase, and acetylcholine receptors in the central nervous system of rat: A dose-reponse study. J Toxicol Environ Health A 2000; 61:695-797.
27. Abou-Donia MB, Goldstein LB, Dechovskaia A et al. Effects of daily dermal application of DEET and epermethrin, alone and in combination on sensimotor performance, blood-brain barrier, and blood-testis barrier in rats. J Toxicol Environ Health A 2001; 62:523-541.
28. Malin DH, Lake JR, Schopen CK et al. Nicotine abstinence syndrome precipitated by central but not peripheral hexamethonium. Pharmacol Biochem Behav 1997; 58:695-699.
29. Furuta S, Suzuki M, Toyama S et al. Tissue distribution of polaprezinc in rats determined by the double tracer method. J Pharm Biomed Anal 1999; 19:453-461.
30. Meng J, Holdcraft RW, Shima JE et al. Androgens regulate the permeability of the blood-testis barrier. Proc Nat Acad Sci USA 2005; 102:16696-16700.
31. Banks WA, Kastin AJ. Human interleukin-1α crosses the blood-testis barriers of the mouse. J Androl 1992; 13:254-259.
32. McLay RN, Banks WA, Kastin AJ. Granulocyte macrophage-colony stimulating factor crosses the blood-testis barrier in mice. Biol Reprod 1997; 57:822-826.
33. Banks WA, Kastin AJ, Komaki G et al. Pituitary adenylate cyclase activating polypeptide (PACAP) can cross the vascular component of the blood-testis barrier in the mouse. J Androl 1993; 14:170-173.
34. Banks WA, Kastin AJ, Ehrensing CA. Diurnal uptake of circulating interleukin-1α by brain, spinal cord, testis and muscle. Neuroimmunomodulation 1998; 5:36-41.
35. Banks, WA, McLay RN, Kastin AJ et al. Passage of leptin across the blood-testis barrier. Am J Physiol 1999; 276:E1099-E1104.
36. King LM, Banks WA, George WJ. Differences in cadmium-transport to the testis, epididymis and brain in cadmium-sensitive and -resistant murine strains 129/J and A/J. J Pharm Exp Ther 1999; 289:825-830.
37. King LM, Banks WA, George WJ. Differential zinc transport into testis and brain of cadmium-sensitive and -resistant murine strains. J Androl 2000; 21:656-663.
38. Plotkin SR, Banks WA, Maness LM et al. Differential transport of rat and human interleukin-1α across the blood-brain and blood-testis barrier in rats. Brain Res 2000; 881:57-61.

39. Mizushima H, Nakamura Y, Matsumoto H et al. The effect of cardiac arrest on the blood-testis barrier to albumin, tumor necrosis factor alpha, pituitary adenylate cyclase activating polypeptide, sucrose and verapamil in the mouse. J Androl 2001; 22:255-260.
40. Farghali H, Williams DS, Simplaceanu E et al. An evaluation of the integrity of the blood-testis barrier by magnetic resonance imaging. Magnet Reson Med 1991; 22:81-87.
41. Kim KN, Kim HJ, Lee SD et al. Effect of triolein on the blood-testis barrier in cats. Invest Radiol 2004; 39:445-449.
42. Setchell BP. The secretion of fluid by the testis of rats, rams and goats with some observation on the effects of age, cryptorchidism and hypophysectomy. J Reprod Fertil 1970; 23:79-85.
43. Russell LD, Bartke A, Goh JC. Postnatal development of the Sertoli cell barrier, tubular lumen, and cytoskeleton of Sertoli and myoid cells in the rat, and their relationship to tubular fluid secretion and flow. Am J Anat 1989; 184:179-189.
44. Hinton BT, Setchell BP. Fluid secretion and movement. In: Russell LD, Griswold MD, eds. The Sertoli Cell. Clearwater: Cache River Press, 1993:249-267.
45. Janecki A, Jakubowiak A, Steinberger A. Regulation of transepithelial electrical resistance in two-compartment Sertoli cell cultures: In vitro model of the blood-testis barrier. Endocrinology 1991; 129:1489-1496.
46. Djakiew D, Onoda M. Mutichamber cell culture and directional secretion. In: Russell LD, Griswold MD, eds. The Sertoli Cell. Clearwater: Cache River Press, 1993:181-194.
47. Lui WY, Lee WM. CAMP perturbs inter-Sertoli tight junction permeability barrier in vitro via its effect on proteasome-sensitive ubiquination of occludin. J Cell Physiol 2005; 203:564-572.
48. Mruk DD, Cheng CY. Sertoli-Sertoli and Sertoli-germ cell interactions and their significance in germ cell movement in the seminiferous epithelium during spermatogenesis. Endocrin Rev 2004; 25:747-806.
49. Bawa SR. Fine structure of the Sertoli cell in the human testis. J Ultrastruc Res 1963; 9:459-474.
50. Brokelmann J. Fine structure of germ cells and Sertoli cells during the cycle of the seminiferous epithelium in the rat. Z Zellforsch Mikrosk Anat 1963; 59:820-850.
51. Flickinger C, Fawcett DW. The junctional specializations of Sertoli cells in the seminiferous epithelium. Anat Rec 1967; 158:207-222.
52. Nicander L. An electron microscopical study of cell contacts in the seminiferous tubules of some mammals. Z Zellforsch Mikrosk Anat 1967; 83:375-397.
53. Ross MH. The Sertoli cell and the blood-testicular barrier: An electronmicroscopic study. In: Holstein AF, Horstmann E, eds. Morphological Aspects of Andrology. Grosse, Berlin: 1970:83-86.
54. Fawcett DW, Leak LV, Heidger PM. Electron microscopic observations on the structural components of the blood-testis barrier. J Reprod Fertil 1970; (Suppl 10):105-122.
55. Dym M, Fawcett DW. The blood-testis barrier in the rat and the physiological compartmentation of the seminiferous epithelium. Biol Reprod 1970; 3:308-326.
56. Dym M. The fine structure of the monkey (Macaca) Sertoli cell and its role in maintaining the blood-testis barrier. Anat Rec 1973; 175:639-656.
57. Russell LD. The blood-testis barrier and its formation relative to spermatocyte maturation in the adult rat: A lanthanum tracer study. Anat Rec 1978; 190:99-112.
58. Pelletier RM, Byers SW. The blood-testis barrier and Sertoli cell junctions: Structural considerations. Microsc Res Tech 1992; 20:3-33.
59. Setchell BP, Breed WG. Anatomy, vasculature and innervation of the male reproductive tract. In: Neill JD, ed. Knobil and Neill's Physiology of Reproduction. 3rd ed. Amsterdam: Elsevier, 2006:771-825.
60. Regaud C. Etudes sur la structure des tubes seminiferes et sur la spermatogenesis chez les mammiferes. Arch Anat Microscop 1901; 4:101-154, 231-380.
61. Ross MH. The fine structure and development of the peritubular contractile cell component in the seminiferous tubules of the mouse. Am J Anat 1967; 121:523-558.
62. Palombi F, Farini D, Salanova M et al. Development and cytodifferentiation of peritubular myoid cells in the rat testis. Anat Rec 1992; 233:32-40.
63. Fillipini A, Tripiciano A, Palombi F et al. Rat testicular myoid cells respond to endothelin: Characterization of binding and signal transduction pathway. Endocrinology 1993; 133:1789-1796.
64. Tripiciano A, Fillipini A, Giustiniano Q et al. Direct visualization of rat peritubular myoid cell contraction in response to endothelin. Biol Reprod 1996; 55:25-31.
65. Fantoni G, Morris PL, Firti G et al. A new autocrine/paracrine factor in rat testis. Am J Physiol 1993; 265:E267-E274.
66. Norton JN, Skinner MK. Regulation of Sertoli cell function and differentiation through the actions of a testicular paracrine factor P-Mod-S. Endocrinology 1989; 124:2711-2719.
67. Skinner MK. Cell-cell interaction in the testis. Endocrin Rev 1991; 12:45-77.

68. Kurlandsky SB, Gamble MV, Ramakrishnan R et al. Plasma delivery of retinoic acid to tissues in the rat. J Biol Chem 1995; 270:17850-17857.
69. Vernet N, Dennefeld C, Rochette-Egly C et al. Retinoic acid metabolism and signaling pathways in the adult and developing mouse testis. Endocrinology 2006; 147:96-110.
70. van Pelt AMM, de Rooij DG. Retinoic acid is able to reinitiate spermatogenesis in Vitamin A-deficient rats and high replicate doses support the full development of spermatogenic cells. Endocrinology 1991; 128:697-704.
71. Davis JT, Ong DE. Retinol processing by the peritubular cell from rat testis. Biol Reprod 1995; 52:356-364.
72. Livera G, Rouiller V, Pairault C et al. Regulation and perturbation of testicular functions by vitamin A. Reproduction 2002; 124:173-180.
73. Fawcett DW. Observations on the organization of the interstitial tissue of the testis and on the occluding junctions in the seminiferous epithelium. Adv Biosci 1973; 10:83-99.
74. Duarte HE, de Oliviera C, Orsi AM et al. Ultrastuctural characteristics of the testicular capillaries in the dog (Canis familiaris). Anat Histol Embryol 1995; 24:73-76.
75. Pinart E, Bonet S, Briz MD et al. Morphologic and histochemical study of blood capillaries in boar testes: Effects of abdominal cryptorchidism. Teratology 2001; 63:42-51.
76. Takayama H. Ultrastructure of testicular capillaries as a permeability barrier (in Japanese). Nippon Hinyokika Gakkai Zasshi 1986; 77:1840-1850.
77. Ergun S, Davidoff M, Holstein AF. Capillaries in the lamina propria of human seminiferous tubules are partly fenestrated. Cell Tissue Res 1996; 286:93-102.
78. Stewart PA. Endothelial vesicles in the blood-brain barrier; are they related to permeability? Cell Mol Neurobiol 2000; 20:149-163.
79. Moroi S, Saitou M, Fujimoto K et al. Occludin is concentrated at tight junctions of mouse/rat but not human/guinea pig Sertoli cells in testes. Am J Physiol 1998; 274:C1708-C1717.
80. Saitou M, Furuse M, Sasaki H et al. Complex phenotype of mice lacking occludin, a complex of tight junction strands. Mol Biol Cell 2000; 11:4131-4142.
81. Cyr DG, Hermo L, Egenberger N et al. Cellular immunolocalization of occludin during embryonic and postnatal development of the mouse testis and epididymis. Endocrinology 1999; 140:3815-3825.
82. Chung NPY, Mruk D, Mo MY et al. A 22-amino acid synthetic peptide corresponding to the second extracellular loop of rat occludin perturbs the blood-testis barrier and disrupts spermatogenesis reversibly in vivo. Biol Reprod 2001; 65:1340-1351.
83. Turksen K, Troy TC. Barriers built on claudins. J Cell Sci 2004; 117:2435-2447.
84. Hellani A, Ji J, Mauduit C et al. Developmental and hormonal regulation of the expression of oligodendocyte-specific protein/claudin 11 in mouse testis. Endocrinology 2000; 141:3012-3019.
85. Gow A, Southwood CM, Li JS et al. CNS myelin and Sertoli cell tight junction strands are absent in Osp/Claudin-11 null mice. Cell 1999; 99:649-659.
86. Morita K, Sasaki H, Furuse M et al. Endothelial claudin: Claudin-5/TMVCF constitutes tight junction strands in endothelial cells. J Cell Biol 1999; 147:185-194.
87. Kamimura Y, Chiba H, Utsumi H et al. Barrier function of microvessels and roles of glial cell line-derived neurotrophic factor in the rat testis. Med Electron Microsc 2002; 35:139-145.
88. Nitta T, Hata M, Gotoh S et al. Size-selective loosening of the blood-brain barrier in claudin-5-deficient mice. J Cell Biol 2003; 161:653-660.
89. Salanova M, Stefanini M, De Curtis I et al. Integrin receptor α6 β1 is localized at specific sites of cell-cell contact in rat seminiferous epithelium. Biol Reprod 1995; 52:79-87.
90. Salanova M, Ricci G, Boitani C et al. Junctional contacts between Sertoli cells in normal and aspermatogenic rat seminiferous epithelium contain α6 β1 integrins, and their formation is controlled by follicle stimulating hormone. Biol Reprod 1998; 58:371-378.
91. Kissel K, Hamm S, Schulz M et al. Immunohistochemical localization of the murine transferrin receptor (TfR) on blood-tissue barriers using a novel anti-TfR monoclonal antibody. Histochem Cell Biol 1998; 10:63-72.
92. Sylvester SR, Griswold MD. Molecular biology of iron transport in the testis. In: de Kretser DM, ed. Molecular Biology of the Male Reproductive System. San Diego: Academic Press, 1993:311-326.
93. Sylvester SR, Griswold MD. The testicular iron shuttle: A "nurse" function of the Sertoli cells. J Androl 1994; 15:381-385.
94. Onada M, Suarez-Quian CA, Djakiew D et al. Characterization of Sertoli cells cultures in the bicameral chamber system: Relationship between formation of permeability barriers and polarized secretion of transferrin. Biol Reprod 1990; 43:672-683.

95. Djakiew D, Hadley MA, Byers SW et al. Tranferrin-mediated transcellular transport of ^{59}Fe across confluent epithelial sheets of Sertoli cells grown in bicameral cell culture chambers. J Androl 1986; 7:355-366.
96. Sylvester SR, Griswold MD. Localization of transferrin and transferrin receptors in rat testes. Biol Reprod 1984; 31:196-203.
97. Hoyes KP, Johnson C, Johnston RE et al. Testicular toxicity of the transferrin binding radionuclide ^{114m}In in adult and neonatal rats. Reprod Toxicol 1995; 9:297-305.
98. Hoyes KP, Morris ID, Hendry JH et al. Transferrin-mediated uptake of radionuclides by the testis. J Nucl Med 1996; 37:336-340.
99. Hoyes KP, Bingham D, Hendry JH et al. Transferrin-mediated uptake of plutonium by spermatogenic tubules. Int J Radiat Biol 1996; 70:467-471.
100. Suire S, Fontaine I, Guillou F. Transferrin gene expression and secretion in rat Sertoli cells. Mol Reprod Dev 1997; 48:168-175.
101. Roberts KP, Awonyi CA, Santulli et al. Regulation of Sertoli cell transferrin and sulfated glycoprotein-2 messenger ribonucleic acid levels during restoration of spermatogenesis in the adult hypophysectomized rat. Endocrinology 1991; 129:3417-3423.
102. Suire S, Fontaine I, Guillou F. Follicle stimulating hormone (FSH) stimulates transferrin gene transcription in rat Sertoli cells: Cis and trans-acting elements involved in FSH action via cyclic adenosine 3',5'-monophosphate on the transferrin gene. Mol Endocrinol 1995; 9:756-766.
103. Hoeben E, van Damme J, Put W et al. Cytokines derived from activated human mononuclear cells markedly stimulate transferrin secretion by cultured Sertoli cells. Endocrinology 1996; 137:514-521.
104. Norton JN, Vigne JL, Skinner MK. Regulation of Sertoli cell differentiation by the testicular paracrine factor PmodS: Analysis of common signal transduction pathways. Endocrinology 1994; 134:149-157.
105. Hoeben E, Swinnen JV, Heyns W et al. Heregulins or neu differentiation factors and the interactions between peritubular myoid cells and Sertoli cells. Endocrinology 1999; 140:2216-2223.
106. Roberts KP, Santulli R, Seiden J et al. The effect of testosterone withdrawal and subsequent germ cell depletion on transferrin and sulfated glycoprotein-2 messenger ribonucleic acid levels in the adult rat testis. Biol Reprod 1992; 47:92-96.
107. Maguire SM, Millar MR, Sharpe RM et al. Investigation of the potential role of the germ cell complement in control of the expression of transferrin mRNA in the prepubertal and adult rat testis. J Mol Endocrinol 1997; 19:67-77.
108. Skinner MK, Griswold MD. Sertoli cells synthesize and secrete a ceruloplasmin-like protein. Biol Reprod 1983; 28:1225-1229.
109. Augustine LM, Markelewicz RJ, Boekelheide K et al. Xenobiotic and endobiotic transporter mRNA expression in the blood-testis barrier. Drug Metab Dispos 2005; 33:182-189.
110. Griffin KP, Ward DT, Liu W et al. Differential expression of divalent metal transporter DMT1 (Slc11a2) in the spermatogenic epithelium of the developing and adult rat testis. Am J Physiol 2005; C176-C184.
111. Schinkel AH. The physiological function of drug-transporting P-glycoproteins. Sem Cancer Biol 1997; 8:161-170.
112. Schinkel AH, Jonker JW. Mammalian drug efflux transporter of the ATP binding cassette (ABC) family: An overview. Adv Drug Del Rev 2003; 55:3-29.
113. Fromm MF. Importance of P-glycoprotein at blood-tissue barriers. Trends Pharmacol Sci 2004; 25:423-429.
114. Leslie EM, Deeley RG, Cole SPC. Multidrug resistance proteins: Role of P-glycoprotein, MRP1, MRP2 and BRCP (ABCG2) in tissue defense. Toxicol Appl Pharmacol 2005; 204:216-237.
115. Cordon-Cardo C, O'Brien JP, Casals L et al. Multidrug-resistancce gene (P-glycoprotein) is expressed by endothelial cells at blood-brain barrier sites. Proc Natl Acad Sci USA 1989; 86:695-698.
116. Cordon-Cardo C, O'Brien JP, Boccia J et al. Expression of the multidrug resistance gene product (P-glycoprotein) in human normal and tumor tissues. J Histochem Cytochem 1990; 38:1277-1287.
117. Thiebaut F, Tsuruo T, Hamda H et al. Immunohistochemical localization in normal tissues of different epitopes in the multidrug transport protein P170: Evidence for localization in brain capillaries and crossreactivity of one antibody with a muscle protein. J Histochem Cytochem 1989; 37:159-164.
118. Holash JA, Harik SI, Perry G et al. Barrier properties of testis microvessels. Proc Natl Acad Sci USA 1993; 90:11069-11073.
119. Melaine N, Lienard MO, Dorval I et al. Multidrug resistance genes and p-glycoprotein in the testis of the rat, mouse, guinea pig and human. Biol Reprod 2002; 67:1699-1707.

120. Bart J, Hollema H, Groen HJM et al. The distribution of drug-efflux pumps, Pgp, BCRP, MRP1 and MRP2, in the normal blood-testis barrier and in primary testicular tumours. Eur J Cancer 2004; 40:2064-2070.
121. Trezise AEO, Romano PR, Gill DR et al. The multidrug resistance and cystic fibrosis genes have complementary patterns of epithelial expression. EMBO J 1992; 11:4291-4303.
122. Stewart PA, Beliveau R, Rogers KA. Cellular localization of P-glycoprotein in brain versus gonadal capillaries. J Histochem Cytochem 1996; 44:679-685.
123. Schinkel AH, Smit JJM, van Tellingen O. Disruption of the mouse mdr1a P-glycoprotein gene leads to a deficiency in the blood-brain barrier and to increased sensitivity to drugs. Cell 1994; 77:491-502.
124. Schinkel AH, Wagenaar E, van Deemter L et al. Absence of the mdr1a P-glycoprotein in mice affects tissue distribution and pharmacokinetics of dexamethasone, digoxin and cyclosporin A. J Clin Invest 1995; 96:1698-1705.
125. Schinkel AH, Wagenaar E, Mol CAAM et al. P-Glycoprotein in the blood-brain barrier of mice influences the brain penetration and pharmacological activity of many drugs. J Clin Invest 1996; 97:2517-2524.
126. Van Asperen J, Schinkel AH, Beijenen JH et al. Altered pharmacokinetics of vinblastine in mdr 1a P-glycoprotein deficient mice. J Natl Cancer Inst 1996; 88:994-999.
127. Uhr M, Steckler T, Yassouridis A et al. Penetration of amitriptyline, but not of fluoxetine into brain is enhanced in mice with blood-brain barrier deficiency due to mdr1a P-glycoprotein gene disruption. Neuropsychopharmacology. 2000; 22:380-387.
128. Grauer MT, Uhr M. P-glycoprotein reduces the ability of amitriptyline metabolites to cross the blood-brain barrier in mice after a 10-day administration of amitriptyline. J Psychopharmacol 2004; 18:66-74.
129. Uhr M, Ebinger M, Rosenhagen MC et al. The anti-Parkinson drug budipine is exported actively out of the brain by P-glycoprotein in mice. Neurosci Lett 2005; 383:73-76.
130. Uhr M, Holsboer F, Muller MB. Penetration of endogenous steroid hormones corticosterone, cortisol, aldosterone and progesterone into the brain is enhanced in mice deficient for both mdr1a and mdr1b P-glycoproteins. J Neuroendocrinol 2002; 14:753-759.
131. Karssen AM, Meijer OC, van der Sandt ICJ et al. Multidrug resistance P-glycoprotein hampers the access of cortisol but not of corticosterone to mouse and human brain. Endocrinology 2001; 142:2686-2694.
132. Karssen AM, Meijer OC, van der Sandt ICJ et al. The role of the efflux transporter P-glycoprotein in brain penetration of prednisolone. J Endocrinol 2002; 175:251-260.
133. Huisman MT, Smit JW, Schinkel AH. Significance of P-glycoprotein for the pharmacology and clinical use of HIV protease inhibitors. AIDS 2000; 14:237-242.
134. Choo EF, Leake B, Wandel C et al. Pharmacological inhibition of P-glycoprotein transport enhances the distribution of HIV-1 protease inhibitors into brain and testis. Drug Metab Dispos 2000; 28:655-660.
135. Huisman MT, Smit JW, Wiltshire HR et al. Assessing safety and efficacy of directed P-glycoprotein inhibition to improve the pharmacokinetic properties of saquinavir coadministered with ritonavir. J Pharmacol Exp Ther 2003; 304:596-602.
136. Arboix M, Paz OG, Colombo T et al. Mutidrug resistance-reversing agents increase vinblastine distribution in normal tissues expressing the P-glycoprotein but do not enhance drug penetration into brain and testis. J Pharmacol Exp Ther 1997; 281:1226-1230.
137. Forrest JB, Turner TT, Howard SS. Cyclophosphamide, vincristine and the blood-testis barrier. Invest Urol 1981; 18:443-444.
138. Trezise AEO, Buchwald M. In vivo cell-specific expression of the cystic fibrosis transmembrane conductance regulator. Nature 1991; 353:434-437.
139. Stride BD, Valdimarsson G, Gerlach JH et al. Structure and expression of the messenger RNA encoding the murine multidrug resistance protein, an ATP cassette transporter. Mol Pharmacol 1996; 49:962-971.
140. Flens MJ, Zaman GJR, van der Valk P et al. Tissue distribution of the multidrug resistance protein. Am J Path 1996; 148:1237-1247.
141. Wijnholds J, Scheffer GL, van der Valk M et al. Mutidrug resistance protein 1 protects the oropharanygeal mucosal layer and the testicular tubules against drug-induced damage. J Exp Med 1998; 188:797-808.
142. Tribull TE, Bruner RH, Bain LJ. The multidrug resistance-associated protein 1 transports methoxychlor and protects the seminiferous epithelium from injury. Toxicol Lett 2003; 142:61-70.
143. Qian YM, Song WC, Cui H et al. Glutathione stimulated sulfated estrogen transport by multidrug resistance protein 1. J Biol Chem 2001; 276:6404-6411.

144. Borst P, Oude Elferink R. Mammalian ABC transporter in health and disease. Ann Rev Biochem 2002; 71:537-592.
145. Riccardi, R, Vigersky RA, Barnes S et al. Methotrexate in the interstitial space and seminiferous tubules of rat testis. Cancer Res 1982; 42:1617-1619.
146. Niemi M, Setchell BP. Gamma glutamyl transpeptidase in the vasculature of the rat testis. Biol Reprod 1986; 35:385-391.
147. Bustamante JC, Setchell BP. The uptake of amino acids, in particular leucine, by isolated perfused testes of rats. J Androl 2000; 21:452-463.
148. Duelli R, Enerson BE, Gerhardt DZ et al. Expression of large amino acid transporter LAT1 in rat brain endothelium. J Cereb Blood Flow Metab 2000; 20:1557-1562.
149. Ghabriel MN, Lu JJ, Hermanis G et al. Expression of a blood-brain barrier specific antigen in the male reproductive tract. Reproduction 2002; 123:389-397.
150. Fenton RA, Howorth A, Cooper GJ et al. Molecular characterization of a novel UT-A urea transporter isoform (UT-A5) in testis. Am J Physiol 2000; 279:C1425-C1431.
151. Fenton RA, Cooper GJ, Morris ID et al. Coordiated expression of UT-A and UT-B urea transporters in rat testis. Am J Physiol 2002; 282:C1492-C1501.
152. Turner TT, Hartmann PK, Howards SS. Urea in the seminiferous tubule: Evidence for active transport. Biol Reprod 1979; 20:511-515.
153. Kato R, Maeda T, Akaike T et al. Nucleoside transport at the blood-testis barrier studied with primary-cultured Sertoli cells. J Pharmacol Exp Ther 2005; 312:601-608.
154. Ong DE, Chytil F. Retinoic acid-binding protein in rat tissue. J Biol Vhem 1975; 250:6113-6117.
155. Kato M, Sung WK, Kato K et al. Immunohistochemical studies on the localization of cellular retinol-binding protein in rat testis and epididymis. Biol Reprod 1985; 32:173-189.
156. Davis JT, Ong DE. Synthesis and secretion of retinal-binding protein by cultured rat Sertoli cells. Biol Reprod 1992; 47:528-533.
157. Rajan N, Sung WK, Goodman DS. Localization of cellular retinol-binding protein mRNA in rat testis and epididymis and its stage-dependent expression during the cycle of the seminiferous epithelium. Biol Reprod 1990; 43:835-842.
158. McGuire BW, Orgebin-Crist MC, Chytil F. Autoradiographic localization of serum retinal-binding protein in rat testis. Endocrinology 1981; 108:658-667.
159. Rajguru SU, Kang YH, Ahluwalia BS. Localization of retinol (Vitamin A) in rat testes. J Nutr 1982; 112:1881-1891.
160. Shingleton JL, Skinner MK, Ong DE. Characteristics of retinol accumulation from serum retinal-binding protein by cultured Sertoli cells. Biochemistry 1989; 28:9641-9647.
161. Samy ET, Li JCH, Grima J et al. Sertoli cell prostaglandin D_2 synthetase is a multifunctional molecule: Its expression and regulation. Endocrinology 2000; 141:710-721.
162. Gerena RL, Irikura D, Urade Y et al. Identification of a fertility-associated protein in bull seminal plasma as lipocalin-type prostaglandin D synthase. Biol Reprod 1998; 58:826-833.
163. Vitale R, Fawcett DW, Dym M. The normal development of the blood-testis barrier and the effects of clomiphene and estrogen treatment. Anat Rec 1973; 176:333-344.
164. Gilula NB, Fawcett DW, Aoki A. The Sertoli cell occluding junctions and gap junctions in mature and developing mammalian testis. Dev Biol 1976; 50:142-168.
165. Pelletier RM, Friend DS. The Sertoli cell junctional complex: structure and permeability to filipin in the neonatal and adult guinea pig. Am J Anat 1983; 168:213-228.
166. Nagano T, Suzuki F. The postnatal development of the junctional complexes of the mouse Sertoli cells as revealed by freeze-fracture. Anat Rec 1976; 185:403-418.
167. Bergmann M, Dierichs R. Postnatal formation of the blood-testis barrier in the rat with special reference to the initiation of meiosis. Anat Embryol 1983; 168:269-275.
168. Pelletier RM. Cyclic formation and decay of the blood-testis barrier in the mink (Mustela vison), a seasonal breeder. Am J Anat 1986; 175:91-117.
169. Pelletier RM. Blood barriers of the epididymis and vas deferens act asynchronously with the blood barrier of the testis in the mink (Mustela vison). Microsc Res Tech 1994; 27:333-349.
170. Morales A, Cavicchia JC. Seasonal changes of the blood-testis barrier in viscacha (Lagostomus maximus maximus): A freeze-fracture and lanthanum tracer study. Anat Rec 1993; 236:459-464.
171. Bergmann M. Photoperiod and testicular function in Phodopus sungorus. Adv Anat Embryol Cell Biol 1987; 105:1-76.
172. Levy S, Serre V, Hermo L et al. The effects of aging on the seminiferous epithelium and the blood-testis barrier of the Brown Norway rat. J Androl 1999; 20:356-365.
173. Toyama, Y, Ohkawa M, Oku R et al. Neonatally administered diethylstilbestrol retards the development of the blood-testis barrier in the rat. J Androl 2001; 22:413-423.

174. Hosoi I, Toyama Y, Maekawa M et al. Development of the blood-testis barrier in the mouse is delayed by neonatally administered diethylstilbestrol but not by β-estradiol 3-benzoate. Andrologia 2002; 34:255-262.
175. Janecki A, Jakubowiak A, Steinberger A. Effects of cyclic AMP and phorbol ester on transepithelial electrical resistance of Sertoli cell monolayers in two-compartment culture. Mol Cell Endocrinol 1991; 82:61-69.
176. Xia W, Cheng CY. TGF-β3 regulates anchoring junction dynamics in the seminiferous epithelium of the rat testis via the Ras/ERK signaling pathway: An in vivo study. Dev Biol 2005; 280:321-343.
177. Li MWM, Xia W, Mruk DD et al. Tumor necrosis factor α reversibly disrupts the blood-testis barrier and impairs Sertoli-germ cell adhesion in the seminiferous epithelium of adult rat testes. J Endocrinol 2006; 190:313-329.
178. Kerr JB, Savage GN, Millar M et al. Response of the seminiferous epithelium of the rat testis to withdrawal of androgen; evidence for direct effect upon intercellular spaces associated with Sertoli cell junctional complexes. Cell Tissue Res 1993; 274:153-161.
179. Gye MC, Ohsako S. Effects of flutamide in the rat testis on the expression of occludin, an integral member of the tight junctions. Toxicol Lett 2003; 143:217-222.
180. Xia W, Wong CH, Lee NP et al. Disruption of Sertoli-germ cell adhesion function in the seminiferous epithelium of the rat testis can be limited to adherens junctions without affecting the blood-testis barrier integrity: An in vivo study using an androgen suppression model. J Cell Physiol 2005; 205:141-157.
181. Cavicchia JC, Sacerdote FL. Correlation between blood-testis barrier development and onset of the first spermatogenic wave in normal and busulfan-treated rats; a lanthanum and freeze-fracture study. Anat Rec 1991; 230:361-368.
182. Ribiero AF, David-Ferreira JF. The inter-Sertoli cell tight junctions in germ cell-free seminiferous tubules from prenatally irradiated rats: A freeze-fracture study. Cell Biol Int 1996; 20:513-522.
183. Levine N, Marsh DJ. Micropuncture study of the fluid composition of "Sertoli cell-only" seminiferous tubules in rats. J Reprod Fertil 1975; 43:547-549.
184. Huang HFS, Yang CS, Meyenhofer M et al. Disruption of sustentacular (Sertoli) cell tight junctions and regression of spermatogenesis in vitamin-A-deficient rats. Acta Anat 1988; 133:10-15.
185. Ismail N, Morales CR. Effects of vitamin A deficiency on the inter-Sertoli cell tight junctions and on the germ cell population. Microsc Res Tech 1992; 20:43-49.
186. Morales A, Cavicchia JC. Spermatogenesis and blood-testis barrier in rats after long-term vitamin A deprivation. Tissue Cell 2002; 34:349-355.
187. Setchell BP. The movement of fluids and substances in the testis. Aust J Biol Sci 1986; 39:193-207.
188. Neaves WB. Permeability of Sertoli cell tight junctions to lanthanum after ligation of ductus deferens and ductuli efferentes. J Cell Biol 1973; 59:559-572.
189. Ross MH. Permeability of Sertoli-Sertoli junctions and Sertoli-spermatid junctions after efferent duct ligation and lanthanum treatment. Am J Anat 1977; 148:49-56.
190. Osman DI, Ploen L. The terminal segment of the seminiferous tubules and the blood-testis barrier before and after efferent duct ligation in the rat. Int J Androl 1978; 1:235-249.
191. Anton E. Preservation of the rat blood-testis barrier after ligation of the ductuli efferentes, as demonstrated by intra-arterial perfusion with peroxidase. J Reprod Fertil 1982; 66:227-230.
192. Porsti I, Ylitalo P. Penetration of some compounds through blood-brain and blood-testis barriers in chronically hypertensive rats. Acta Physiol Scand 1984; 120:387-391.
193. Gravis CJ, Chen I, Yates RD. Stability of the intra-epithelial component of the blood-testis barrier in epinephrine-induced testicular degeneration in Syrian hamsters. Am J Anat 1977; 148:19-32.
194. Setchell BP, Waites GMH. Changes in the permeability of testicular capillaries and of the "blood-testis barrier" after injection of cadmium chloride in the rat. J Endocrinol 1970; 41:81-86.
195. Johnson MH. The effect of cadmium chloride on the blood-testis barrier of the guinea-pig. J Reprod Fertil 1969; 551-553.
196. Lee IP, Dixon RL. Effects of cadmium on spermatogenesis studied by velocity sedimentation cell separation and serial mating. J Pharmacol Exp Ther 1973; 187:641-652.
197. Janecki A, Jakubowiak A, Steinberger A. Effect of cadmium chloride on transepithelial electrical resistance of Sertoli cell monolayers in two-compartment cultures—A new model for toxicological investigations of the "blood-testis" barrier in vitro. Toxicol Appl Pharmacol 1992; 112:51-57.
198. Chung NPY, Cheng CY. Is cadmium chloride-induced inter-Sertoli tight junction permeability barrier disruption a suitable in vitro model to study the events of junction disassembly during spermatogenesis in the rat testis. Endocrinology 2001; 142:1878-1888.
199. Hew KW, Heath GL, Jiwa AH et al. Cadmium in vivo causes disruption of tight junction-associated microfilaments in rat Sertoli cells. Biol Reprod 1993; 49:840-849.

200. Wong CH, Mruk DD, Lui WY et al. Regulation of blood-testis barrier dynamics: An in vivo study. J Cell Sci 2004; 117:783-798.
201. Wong CH, Mruk DD, Siu MKY et al. Blood-testis barrrier dynamics are regulated by α-macroglobulin via the c-jun N-terminal protein kinase pathway. Endocrinology 2005; 146:1893-1908.
202. Weber JE, Turner TT, Tung KSK et al. Effects of cytochalasin D on the integrity of the Sertoli cell (blood-testis) barrier. Am J Anat 1988; 182:130-147.
203. Eng F, Wiebe JP, Alima LH. Long-term alteration in the permeability of the blood-testis barrier following a single intratesticular injection of dilute aqueous glycerol. J Androl 1994; 15:311-317.
204. Wiebe JP, Kowalik A, Gallardi RL et al. Glycerol disrupts tight junction-associated actin microfilaments, occludin, and microtubules in Sertoli cells. J Androl 2000; 21:625-635.
205. Hall ES, Eveleth J, Boekelheide K. 2,5-Hexadione exposure alters the rat Sertoli cell cytoskeleton. II. Intermediate filaments and actin. Toxicol Appl Pharmacol 1991; 111:443-453.
206. Pogach LM, Lee Y, Gould S et al. Characterization of cis-platinum-induced Sertoli cell dysfunction in rodents. Toxicol Appl Pharmacol 1989; 98:350-361.
207. Pereira ML. Studies on the permeability of the blood-testis barrier in stainless steel-administered mice. Cell Biol Int 1995; 19:619-624.
208. Toyama Y, Suzuki-Toyota F, Maekawa M et al. Adverse effects of bisphenol A to spermiogenesis in mice and rats. Arch Histol Cytol 2004; 67:373-381.
209. Willson JT, Jones NA, Katxh S et al. Penetration of the testicular-tubular barrier by horseradish peroxidase induced by adjuvant. Anat Rec 1973; 176:85-100.
210. Main SJ, Waites GMH. The blood-testis barrier and temperature damage to the testis of the rat. J Reprod Fertil 1977; 51:439-450.
211. Stewart RJ, Boyd S, Brown S et al. The blood-testis barrier in experimental unilateral cryptorchidism. J Path 1990; 160:51-55.
212. Hagenas L, Ploen L, Ritzen EM et al. Blood-testis barrier: Maintained function of inter-Sertoli cell junction in experimental cryptorchidism in the rat, as judged by a simple lanthanum-immersion technique. Andrologia 1976; 9:3-7.
213. Cavicchia JC, Sacerdote FL, Ortiz L. The human blood-testis barrier in impaired spermatogenesis. Ultrastuct Path 1996; 20:211-218.
214. Meyer JM, Mezrahid P, Vignon F et al. Sertoli cell barrier dysfunction and spermatogenic breakdown in the human testis: A lanthanum tracer investigation. Int J Androl 1996; 19:190-198.
215. Fritz IB, Lyon MF, Setchell BP. Evidence for a defective seminiferous tubule barrier in testes of Tfm and Sxr mice. J Reprod Fertil 1983; 67:359-363.
216. Noguchi J, Toyama Y, Yuasa S et al. Hereditary defects in both germ cells and the blood-testis barrier system in as-mutant rats: Evidence from spermatogonial transplantation and tracer permeability analysis. Biol Reprod 2002; 67:880-888.
217. Berg KA. The blood-testis barrier in sterile blue fox-silvr fox hybrids compared with that in normal foxes of both species. Int J Androl 1984; 7:167-175.
218. Setchell BP. The functional significance of the blood-testis barrier. J Androl 1980; 1:2-10.
219. Teuscher C, Wild GC, Tung KSK. Immunochemical analysis of guinea pig sperm autoantigens. Biol Reprod 1982; 26:218-229.
220. Tung KSK, Teuscher C. Mechanisms of autoimmune disease in the testis and ovary. Hum Reprod Update 1995; 1:35-50.
221. Yule TD, Montoya GD, Russell LD et al. Autoantigenic cells exist outside the blood testis barrier. J Immunol 1988; 141:1161-1167.
222. Lustig L, Satz ML, Sztein MB et al. Antigens of the basement membranes of the seminferous tubules induce autoimmunity in Wistar rats. J Reprod Immunol 1982; 4:79-90.
223. Rival C, Guazzone VA, Theas MS et al. Pathomechanism of autoimmune orchitis. Andrologica 2005; 37:226-227.
224. Yule TD, Tung KSK. Experimental autoimmune orchitis induced by testis and sperm antigen-specific T cell clones: An important pathogenic cytokine in tumor necrosis factor. Endocrinology 1993; 133:1098-1107.
225. Maddocks S, Setchell BP. The rejection of thyroid allografts in the ovine testis. Immunol Cell Biol 1988; 66:1-8.
226. Setchell BP, Granholm T, Ritzen EM. Failure of thyroid allografts to function in the testes of cynomolgous monkeys. J Reprod Immunol 1995; 28:75-80.
227. Hedger M. Immunophysiology of the male reproductive tract. In: Neill JD, ed. Knobil and Neill's Physiology of Reproduction. 3rd ed. Amsterdam: Elsevier, 2006:1195-1286.
228. Setchell BP, Pakarinen P, Huhtaniemi I. How much LH do the Leydig cells see? J Endocrinol 2002; 175:375-382.

229. Lincoln GA. Seasonal aspects of testicular function. In: Burger H, de Krester D, eds. The Testis, 2nd edition. New York: Raven Press, 1989:329-385.
230. Setchell BP, Laurie MS, Main SJ et al. The mechanism of transport of testosterone through the walls of the seminiferous tubules of the rat testis. Int J Androl 1978; (Suppl 2):506-512.
231. Setchell BP, Laurie MS, Flint APF et al. Transport of free and conjugated steroids from the boar testis in lymph, venous blood and rete testis fluid. J Endocrinol 1983; 96:127-136.
232. Setchell BP, Cox JE. Secretion of free and conjugated steroids by the horse testis into lymph and venous blood. J Reprod Fertil 1982; (Suppl. 32):123-127.
233. Jutte NH, Jabseb R, Grootegoed JA et al. Regulation of survival of rat pachytene spermatocytes by lactate supply from Sertoli cells. J Reprod Fertil 1982; 65:431-438.
234. Xia W, Mruk DD, Lee WM et al. Cytokines and junction restructuring during spermatogenesis—A lesson to learn from the testis. Cytokine Growth Factor Rev 2005; 16:469-493.
235. Brinster RL, Zimmermann JW. Spermatogenesis following male germ-cell transplantation. Proc Natl Acad Sci USA 1994; 91:11298-11302.
236. Jahnukainen K, Hou M, Petersen C et al. Intratesticular transplantation of testicular cells from leukemic rats causes transmission of leukemia. Cancer Res 2001; 61:706-710.
237. Parks JE, Lee DR, Huang S et al. Prospects for spermatogenesis in vitro. Theriogenology 2003; 59:73-86.
238. Zhai Y, Sperkova Z, Napoli JL. Cellular expression retinal dehydrogenase types 1 and 2: Effects of Vitamin A status on testis mRNA. J Cell Physiol 2001; 186-232.
239. Bowles J, Knight D, Smith C et al. Retinoid signaling determines germ cell fate in mice. Science 2006; 312:596-600.
240. Koubova J, Menke DB, Zhou Q et al. Retinoic acid regulates sex-specific timing of meiotic initiation in mice. Proc Nat Acad Sci USA 2006; 103:2474-2479.
241. Oulad-Abdelghani M, Bouillet P, Decimo D et al. Characteriation of a premeiotic germ cell-specific cytoplasmic protein encoded by Stra8, a novel retinoic acid-responsive gene. J Cell Biol 1996; 135:469-477.
242. Beumer TL, Kiyokawa H, Roepers-Gajadien HL et al. Regulatory role of $p27^{kip1}$ in the mouse and human testis. Endocrinology 1999; 140:1834-1840.
243. Buzzard JJ, Wreford NG, Morrison JR. Thyroid hormone, retinoic acid and testosterone suppress proliferation and induce markers of differentiation in cultured rat Sertoli cells. Endocrinology 2006; 144:3722-3731.
244. Akmal KM, Dufour JM, Kim KH. Retinoic acid receptor α gene expression in the rat testis: Potential role during the prophase of meiosis and in the transition from round to elongating spermatids. Biol Reprod 1997; 56:549-556.
245. Chung SSW, Wolgemuth DJ. Role of retinoid signaling in the regulation of spermatogenesis. Cytogenet Genome Res 2004; 105:189-202.
246. Chung SSW, Sung W, Wang X et al. Retinoic acid receptor α is required for synchronization of spermatogenic cycles and its absence results in progressive breakdown of the spermatogenic process. Dev Dynam 2004; 230:754-766.
247. Ghyselinck NB, Vernet N, Dennefeld et al. Retinoids and spermatogenesis: Lessons from mutant mice lacking the plasma retinal binding protein. Dev Dynam 2006; 235:1608-1622.
248. de Rooij DG, van Pelt AMM, Van de Kant HJG et al. Role of retinoids in spermatogonial proliferation and differentiation and the meiotic prophase. In: Bartke A, ed. Function of Somatic Cells in the Testis. New York: Springer Verlag, 1994:345-361.
249. van Pelt AMM, van Dissel-Emiliani FMF, Gaemers IC et al. Characteristics of A spermatogonia and preleptotene spermatocytes in the Vitamin A-deficient rat testis. Biol Reprod 1995; 53:570-578.
250. Gaemers IC, Sonneveld E, van Pelt AMM et al. The effect of 9-cis-retinoic acid on proliferation and differentiation of A spermatogonia and retinoid receptor gene expression in the Vitamin A-deficient mouse testis. Endocrinology 1998; 139:4269-4276.
251. Setchell BP, Palombi F. Isolation of endothelial cells from the rat testis, and their effect on testosterone secretion by interstitial cells. Miniposter 13th European Workshop on Molecular and Celular Endocrinology of the Testis. 2004; C6.
252. Richardson LL, Kleinman HK, Dym M. Basement membrane gene expression by Sertoli and peritubular myoid cells in vitro in the rat. Biol Reprod 1995; 52:320-330.
253. Onoda M, Djakiew D. Pachytene spermatocyte protein(s) stimulate Sertoli cells grown in bicameral chambers: Dose-dependent secretion of ceruloplasmin, sulfated glucoprotein-1, sulfated glycoprotein-2 and transferring. In Vitro Cell Dev Biol 1991; 27A:215-222.
254. Onoda M, Djakiew D. A 29,000M® protein derived from round spermatids regulates Sertoli cell secretion. Mol Cell Endocrinol 1993; 93:53-61.

Chapter 13

Cross-Talk between Tight and Anchoring Junctions—Lesson from the Testis

Helen H.N. Yan,* Dolores D. Mruk, Will M. Lee and C. Yan Cheng

Abstract

Spermatogenesis takes place in the seminiferous tubules in adult testes such as rats, in which developing germ cells must traverse the seminiferous epithelium while spermatogonia (2n, diploid) undergo mitotic and meiotic divisions, and differentiate into elongated spermatids (1n, haploid). It is conceivable that this event involves extensive junction restructuring particularly at the blood-testis barrier (BTB, a structure that segregates the seminiferous epithelium into the basal and the adluminal compartments) that occurs at stages VII-VIII of the seminiferous epithelial cycle. As such, cross-talk between tight (TJ) and anchoring junctions [e.g., basal ectoplasmic specialization (basal ES), adherens junction (AJ), desmosome-like junction (DJ)] at the BTB must occur to coordinate the transient opening of the BTB to facilitate preleptotene spermatocyte migration. Interestingly, while there are extensively restructuring at the BTB during the epithelial cycle, the immunological barrier function of the BTB must be maintained without disruption even transiently. Recent studies using the androgen suppression and Adjudin models have shown that anchoring junction restructuring that leads to germ cell loss from the seminiferous epithelium also promotes the production of AJ (e.g., basal ES) proteins (such as N-cadherins, catenins) at the BTB site. We postulate the testis is using a similar mechanism during spermatogenesis at stage VIII of the epithelial cycle that these induced basal ES proteins, likely form a "patch" surrounding the BTB, transiently maintain the BTB integrity while TJ is "opened", such as induced by TGF-b3 or TNFa, to facilitate preleptotene spermatocyte migration. However, in other stages of the epithelial cycle other than VII and VIII when the BTB remains "closed" (for ~10 days), anchoring junctions (e.g., AJ, DJ, and apical ES) restructuring continues to facilitate germ cell movement. Interestingly, the mechanism(s) that governs this communication between TJ and anchoring junction (e.g., basal ES and AJ) in the testis has remained obscure until recently. Herein, we provide a critical review based on the recently available data regarding the cross-talk between TJ and anchoring junction to allow simultaneous maintenance of the BTB and germ cell movement across the seminiferous epithelium.

Introduction

In adult rats, spermatogenesis takes place in the seminiferous tubules in testes, in which spermatozoa (1n, haploid) differentiate from spermatogonia (type A, 2n, diploid) in the seminiferous epithelium in ~58 days via six mitotic and two meiotic divisions consecutively.[1,2] During this time, germ cells also undergo different phases of cellular differentiation with changes

*Corresponding Author: Helen H.N. Yan—Center for Biomedical Research, The Population Council, 1230 York Avenue, New York, NY 10021, USA. Email: hyan@pathology.hku.hk

Molecular Mechanisms in Spermatogenesis, edited by C. Yan Cheng. ©2008 Landes Bioscience and Springer Science+Business Media.

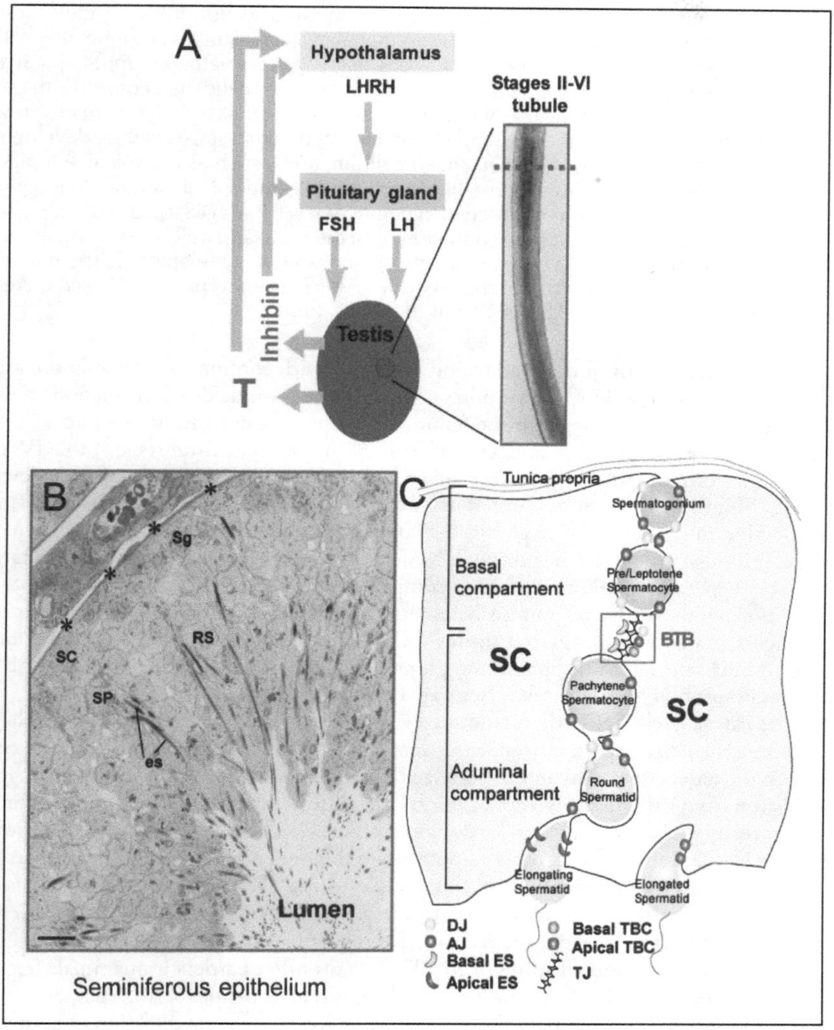

Figure 1. The physiological relationship along the hypothalamic-pituitary-testicular axis that regulates testicular function, and the intimate structural relationship between Sertoli and germ cells in the seminiferous epithelium during spermatogenesis. A) This is a schematic drawing that shows the hormonal regulation of spermatogenesis in the testis via the hypothalamic-pituitary-testicular axis. LHRH released from the hypothalamus stimulates the production of LH and FSH by the pituitary gland, which in turn regulates Leydig and Sertoli cell functions, residing in the interstitium and the seminiferous epithelium, respectively. Testosterone (T) and inhibin (and others, e.g., follistatin) released by Leydig and Sertoli cells, respectively, provide the necessary feed-back loops to maintain the endogenous levels of LH and FSH to regulate spermatogenesis. Any changes in the homeostasis of these hormones can perturb spermatogenesis. For instance, a reduction of intra-testicular T level can suppress spermatid (step 8 and beyond) adhesion, leading to spermatid depletion from the epithelium without disrupting the blood-testis barrier (BTB) integrity.[60-62] The right panel represents a stage II-VI seminiferous tubule dissected from the testis by using a transilluminating stereomicroscope as described.[1] Legend continued on following page.

Figure 1, continued from previous page. B) A semi-thin cross-section from an adult rat testis showing a seminiferous tubule at stage V of the epithelial cycle, illustrating the intimate relationship between Sertoli (SC) and different germ cells (e.g., sg, spermatogonium; SP, pachytene spermatocyte; RS, round spermatid; es, elongating/elongate spermatid) that constitute the seminiferous epithelium, resting on the basement membrane (see asterisks). C) A schematic drawing of the seminiferous epithelium that illustrates germ cells at different stages of their development are associated with Sertoli cells via specialized cell junctions, such as AJ, apical ectoplasmic specialization (apical ES) and desmosome-like junctions (DJ), and apical tubulobulbar complex (apical TBC). The BTB, which is composed of tight junction (TJ), basal ES, basal TBC, DJ, and AJ, anatomically divides the seminiferous epithelium into the basal and adluminal compartments. However, the BTB must "open" to accommodate the movement of preleptotene spermatocytes across the barrier at stage VIII of the epithelial cycle.[7] This figure was prepared based on recent findings and reviews in the field.[6,17,45,110] Bar in (B), 10 μm.

in morphology particularly at the head region associated with chromatin condensation, as well as tail elongation (see Fig. 1). Earlier studies using PAS (periodic acid-Schiff reaction) staining has divided these cellular changes in the seminiferous epithelium in adult rats into 14 stages, which, in turn, are comprised of one seminiferous epithelial cycle, from stages I to XIV. Each stage displays a unique pattern of association of germ cells at different stages of their development with Sertoli cells in the seminiferous epithelium.[1-6] If an investigator is visualizing a specific section of the tubule at stage I in the epithelium under a transillumination stereomicroscope, this stage progresses to II through XIV and returns to stage I in ~12.9 days in rats. As such, a type A spermatogonium requires to complete the epithelial cycle 4.5 times in ~58 days utilizing much of these time for mitosis before it divides and matures into 256 spermatozoa.[1,4] This process is precisely regulated under FSH, LH, and testosterone via coordination between the hypothalamus, pituitary gland, and the testis, which is known as the hypothalamic-pituitary-testicular axis (see Fig. 1).

Besides these well defined hormonal events that occur along the hypothalamic-pituitary-testicular axis, spermatogenesis cannot proceed unless preleptotene spermatocytes residing in the basal compartment can traverse the blood-testis barrier (BTB) at late stage VII through early stage VIII (these two cycles combined last for ~3.5 days in rats), entering into the adluminal compartment for further development[7] (Fig. 1). The BTB is a functional term initially coined by Chiquoine[8] and others[9] to illustrate the presence of a physiological barrier in the testis. The tightness of the BTB is comparable to the blood-brain barrier. It prevented staining of the seminiferous tubules when dyes (e.g., acriflavine used by Kormano[9]) were injected into animals (for a review, see ref. 10). Subsequent studies by Setchell and colleagues have illustrated many unique features of the BTB versus other barriers in mammals (e.g., the blood-brain barrier or the blood-retina barrier).[10] For instance, besides Sertoli cells, peritubular myoid cells in rodents contribute to the BTB function by limiting the diffusion of lanthanum and colloidal carbon,[11,12] however, in other blood-tissue barriers, the barrier function is contributed almost exclusively by the epithelial or endothelial cells alone.

Several hypotheses regarding the movement of germ cells across the BTB have been suggested. For instance, the "zipper theory" proposes that during germ cell migration across the BTB, new occluding fibrils form below the preleoptotene/leptotene spermatocytes, to be followed by the break down of occluding fibrils above these spermatocytes.[3,13] The "intermediate cellular compartment theory" of Russell[7,14] suggests the presence of a unique compartment inhabited by the preleptotene/leptotene spermatocytes in transit where these spermatocytes are trapped in between two occluding zonules as confirmed by electron microscopy. The "repetitive removal of membrane segments theory" of Pelletier[15] suggests that the upward movement of the migrating germ cells create stresses on the Sertoli cell junctional complexes, which, in turn, induces the formation of intercellular pockets. Each developing germ cell (except elongating spermatid) is trapped in one of these intercellular pockets, sealed at both ends by tight junction (TJ), and anchoring junctions [e.g., adherens junction (AJ) and desmosome-like junctions (DJ). Note: while DJ is an intermediate filament-based anchoring junction that localizes to the BTB, virtually no functional study is found in the literature regarding this junction type. Also, the molecular composition is virtually unknown, and as such, DJ is not included in our remaining discussion herein] and moves progressively across the seminiferous epithelium until it is internalized in autophagic vesicles. However, neither the "zipper", the "intermediate cellular compartment", nor the "repetitive removal of membrane segment" theories can perfectly describe the processes of preleptotene spermatocyte migration across the BTB during stage VIII of the epithelial cycle, taking into account the interactions between integral membrane proteins at the BTB, their peripheral adaptors, kinases, phosphatases, cytokines, proteases and protease inhibitors.[3,5,6,14-17] This is not entirely unexpected since these postulates by and large were based on morphological studies without any biochemical and/or molecular data available at the time. A recent hypothesis known as the "junction restructuring theory" has provided a more solid basis in delineating the complicated biochemical and molecular cascade of events behind this phenomenon (for a review, see refs. 6,17). The essence of this hypothesis suggests that germ cell movement is composed of waves of junction disassembly and reassembly that occur under the influence of cytokines (e.g., TGF-β3 and TNF-α) that are released by Sertoli and/or germ cells into the microenvironment to facilitate cell movement. For instance, these cytokines regulate the steady-state levels of proteins at the BTB (e.g., occludin, ZO-1, cadherins and catenins) and the homeostasis of proteases and protease inhibitors in the epithelium.[17] The net result of these interactions determines the "opening" or the "closing" state of the BTB to facilitate germ cell movement. This biochemical theory, if confirmed and adequately characterized, should provide new clues for developing novel male contraceptives, such as by "shutting-down" the BTB to prohibit the migration of preleptotene spermatocytes from the basal to the adluminal compartment. Recent studies have also illustrated that this hypothesis fits quite well with the "zipper theory" (see below for further discussion).

The Concept of Endocytosis in BTB Dynamics

In other epithelia, endocytosis has been shown to play a pivotal role in junction restructuring to facilitate cell migration.[18-20] This mechanism also provides the efficient means for restructuring junctional complexes at the TJ-barrier by perturbing its permeability without requiring de novo protein synthesis.[18] For instance, it is suggested that intercellular movement is achieved by coendocytosis of apposing TJ-integral membrane proteins into the adjacent cells in a study using mouse Eph4 cells in vitro.[19] Besides, there is growing evidence that the "leaky" intestinal epithelia in chronic disorders is mediated by abnormal internalization of TJ-integral membrane proteins via endocytosis.[21,22] Interferon-γ (IFNγ), a proinflammatory cytokine, was shown to increase the intestinal permeability through its effects on TJ proteins such as occludin, junctional adhesion molecule-A (JAM-A) and claudin-1 in T84 cells.[22,23] For instance, TJ proteins were internalized into large vacuoles via the RhoA/ROCK signaling pathway.[22]

In the testis, endocytosis is also employed by Sertoli cells for house-keeping activities, such as phagocytosis of germ cells undergoing apoptosis or anoikis. This process is also used to eliminate residual bodies from elongating spermatids prior to spermiation when fully mature spermatids (spermatozoa) are emptied into the tubular lumen.[17] At present, it is not clear if testes employ similar mechanism as other epithelia to regulate the rapid turnovers of TJ- and AJ-integral membrane proteins at the BTB to facilitate germ cell migration. Obviously, this can certainly be possible. Cytokines, such as TGF-β and TNF-α, have been shown to increase BTB permeability via different signaling pathways.[24,25] However, the mechanism(s) that reduces the TJ protein levels following cytokine treatment is not known. Does this simply the result of a decline in de novo protein synthesis or involve internalization of TJ-integral membrane proteins? Recent findings have suggested that endocytosis does occur in the testis at the apical ES to facilitate spermiation. For instance, the formation of tubulobulbar complexes (TBC, another testis-specific AJ type) at the Sertoli cell-elongated spermatid interface at late stage VIII of the epithelial cycle prior to spermiation by replacing the apical ES has been speculated to assist the release of mature spermatids via internalization of TBC-junction molecules.[16] This postulate has been confirmed in a recent study[26] which showed that the TBC indeed appeared at the concave surface of the head of spermatids that was previously occupied by apical ES. Furthermore, the adhesion domains of nectin-2 and 3 were found to be internalized as membrane vesicles near the TBC at spermiation.[26] The fate of these internalized adhesion molecules at TBC remains to be determined; they can either be degraded or recycled back to the cell surface. In other epithelia, most of the endocytosed molecules (e.g., E-cadherin and occludin) enter the recycling pathway so that they can be rapidly recycled back to the cell surface to maintain junction integrity, especially in unstable cell-cell contacts. For instance, a significant increase in E-cadherin recycling was detected in MDCK cells during [Ca^{2+}]-depletion-induced loss of cell adhesion.[27,28]

It is conceivable that internalization of TJ and/or AJ integral membrane proteins takes place at the BTB between adjacent Sertoli cells. However, this would be a more complicated event since TJ, AJ (e.g., basal ES and basal TBC), and desmosome-like junctions are coexisting at the BTB (see Figs. 1, 2). In other epithelia, it is believed that endocytic recycling of TJ proteins (e.g., occludin) is mediated by Rab GTPases,[28] and Rab8B was shown to structurally associate

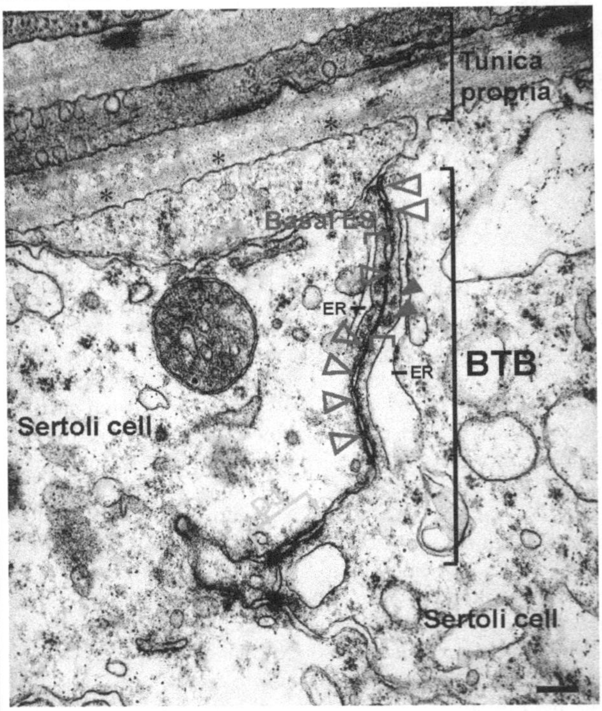

Figure 2. Electron micrograph of normal rat testes illustrating the typical BTB ultrastructural features. The features shown herein for BTB from an adult rat are applicable to mice and most other mammals. The basement membrane (asterisk), which is part of the tunica propria, appears as a homogeneous substance. This is a modified form of extracellular matrix (ECM)[42] and is clearly visible underneath the collagen (type 1) fibrils. The BTB is composed of coexisting tight junction (TJ, blue arrowheads), basal ES (bracketed in red), desmosome-like junction (DJ, bracketed in green, see electron dense substances on both sides of the apposing Sertoli cell plasma membranes typified of desmosome), and adherens junction (AJ, bracketed in yellow). Basal ES refers to the ultrastructure between two adjacent Sertoli cells typified by the presence of actin bundles (red arrowheads) sandwiched between the endoplasmic reticulum (ER) and the plasma membrane that are found on both sides of the two adjacent Sertoli cells (SC). Bar, 0.2 μm.

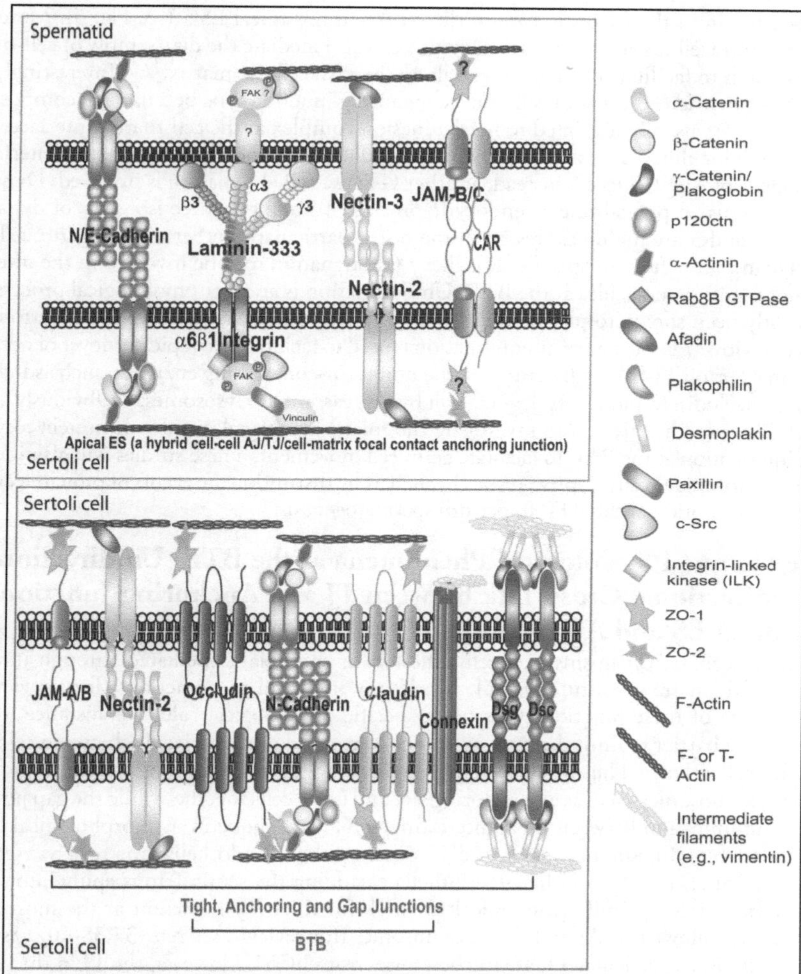

Figure 3. A schematic drawing depicting the currently known protein complexes at the apical ectoplasmic specialization (ES) and the BTB. Apical ES (top panel) is limited to the interface between Sertoli cells and spermatids (step 8 and beyond) in the apical compartment of the seminiferous epithelium in adult rat testes. As discussed in the text, the apical ES is a testis-specific hybrid cell-cell actin-based adherens junction (AJ), tight junction (TJ), and cell-matrix focal contact anchoring junction type since it contains protein complexes that are found in AJ (e.g., cadherins/catenins, nectins/afadins), TJ (e.g., JAM/CAR/ZO-1), and focal adhesion complex (FAC) (e.g., α6β1 integrin/laminin-333) of other epithelia. Some of the peripheral adaptors (e.g., α- and β-catenins, ZO-1), kinases (c-Src) and signaling molecules (e.g., p120ctn) that are known to associate with these complexes in adult rat testes are also shown. The BTB (bottom panel) is found between two adjacent Sertoli cells near the basement membrane that segregates the seminiferous epithelium into the adluminal and the basal compartments (see Figs. 1C, 2). In adult rat testes, the BTB is constituted by coexisting tight and anchoring junctions (see Figs. 1C, Fig. 2). The BTB is composed of protein complexes that are found in TJ (e.g., JAMs/ZO-1, claudins/ZO-1, occludin/ZO-1), AJ/basal ES/basal TBC (e.g., N-cadherin/catenin), desmosome-like junction [e.g., connexins, desmogleins (Dsg), desmocollins (Dsc)] of other epithelia. This drawing was prepared based on several recent papers and reviews.[17,74,89,111-113] Because of space limitation, only the integral membrane proteins and some of the better studied adaptors, kinases and signaling molecules are shown.

with E-cadherin in the rat testis at both the BTB and the apical ES[29] (see Fig. 3). Moreover, other than intracellular movement, endocytosis can also mediate the disassembly of cell-matrix focal adhesion to facilitate cell movement along the extracellular matrix.[30,31] Interestingly, the basal ES is a hybrid cell-cell and cell-matrix anchoring junction type because it is composed of proteins that are usually restricted to focal adhesion complex at the cell-matrix interface, such as FAK and vinculin.[32] The disassembly of focal adhesion at the fibroblast-matrix interface is independent of Rho GTPases, instead, another GTPase called dynamin is involved. Dynamin is known to play a pivotal role in endocytic process. Among the three isoforms of dynamin, dynamin-2 and 3 are highly expressed in the testis, particularly in Sertoli and germ cells[33,34] while dynamin-1 is neuron-specific. It is likely that dynamin may be involved in the internalization of junction molecules at the BTB. Ubiquitination is another physiological process that has recently been shown to play a crucial role in junction protein turnover using Sertoli cells cultured in vitro.[35] For instance, ubiquitination is used to facilitate the rapid turnover of occludin at the inter-Sertoli TJ-barrier by targeting the ubiquitin-conjugating enzymes, such as Itch and UBC4, to occludin to induce its degradation by proteasomes or lysosomes.[35] Obviously, much research is needed in this area to investigate the role(s) of integral membrane protein recycling and ubiquitination at the BTB to facilitate germ cell movement. These studies will also identify new targets for male contraceptive research, such as by disrupting the events of protein recycling and/or internalization at the BTB to perturb spermatogenesis.

Some Unique Physiological Phenomena at the BTB: Unidirectional and Bidirectional Cross-Talk between TJ and Anchoring Junction (e.g., Basal ES and AJ)

In multi-cellular organisms, cell-cell adhesion in epithelia is mediated through junction complexes which are constituted by TJ, AJ, desmosomes and gap junctions (for a review, see ref. 36). Each of these junction types has a specific physiological role. For instance, the TJ functions as a barrier to limit the passage of ions, water and other molecules between cells, and maintains cell polarity. The AJ links neighboring cells together by forming a continuous adhesion belt, desmosomes serve as an anchoring site and unite cells together while the gap junction is for communication between cells. Interestingly, BTB is unique in its morphological layout versus other blood-tissue barriers found in other epithelia/endothelia (for reviews, see refs. 2,3,5,6). In brief, in other epithelia/endothelia excluding the seminiferous epithelium, junctions are organized typically from apical to basal, in which TJ is present at the most apical region, to be followed by AJ and then desmosomes (for reviews, see refs. 37,38-40). As such, these junctions, in particular TJ, are furthest away from ECM. However, the TJ in the testis is located at the basal compartment of the seminiferous epithelium, closest to the basement membrane, a modified form of ECM[41,42] and coexisting with AJ, basal ES, basal TBC (both basal ES and basal TBC are testis-specific AJ types restricted to the Sertoli-Sertoli cells interface at the BTB), gap junctions, and desmosome-like junctions (see Figs. 1, 2).[3,16,17,43-45]

Apart from the unique morphological features of BTB, the testis apparently is using a specialized junction restructuring mechanism in assisting preleptotene spermatocytes to migrate across the BTB, such that the post-meiotic germ cell antigens can be sequestered from the immune system while permitting continuous restructuring of the TJ-barrier and/or anchoring junction (e.g., basal ES and AJ) at the BTB. This apparently is in contrast to other blood-tissue barriers (e.g., blood-brain and blood-retina barriers), even though they are suggested to be dynamic in nature.[18] Unlike the BTB, these blood-tissue barriers do not undergo such drastic restructuring to facilitate the migration of preleptotene spermatocytes which are 10-15 μm in diameter. Besides, except for stage VIII of the epithelial cycle, the BTB remains closed to limit the entry of preleptotene spermatocytes into the adluminal compartment. This implicates that there are unique molecules and mechanisms in place to coordinate these events.

In the past decade, different in vivo models have been used to study BTB dynamics and regulation.[17] There are a number of interesting observations stemming from this body of work.

For instance, studies using $CdCl_2$,[46-48] an environmental toxicant, and glycerol[49-51] have shown that these toxicants can irreversibly perturb TJ which, in turn, lead to anchoring junction damage, dislodging germ cells of all classes from the epithelium. These studies thus illustrate the presence of cross-talk between tight and anchoring junctions that a disruption in TJ can spread to anchoring junction such as apical ES, which is located at the opposite end of the TJ in the seminiferous epithelium (see Fig. 1C). These findings are consistent with the cellular physiology in other epithelia, such as the skin, in which a disruption of TJ leads to underlying AJ damage and vice versa,[52-54] illustrating bi-directional cross-talk between TJ and anchoring junction. However, in studies using antispermatogenic drugs such as Adjudin[55] and lonidamine,[56] it was shown that anchoring junction (e.g., apical ES) disruption could be limited to the interface between Sertoli cells and elongating spermatids/elongate spermatids/round spermatids/spermatocytes (but not spermatogonia) without compromising anchoring (e.g., basal ES) and tight junctions between Sertoli cells at the BTB,[17,57,58] illustrating unidirectional cross-talk between TJ and anchoring junction in the testis. These findings were also supported in a recent study using the model of McLachlan and O'Donnell by suppressing the endogenous testosterone level in the testis using testosterone/estradiol (TE) implants.[59,60] For instance, suppression of intratesticular androgen level by using TE implants in adult rats can lead to disruption of apical ES at the Sertoli-germ cell interface (step 8 spermatids and beyond) without perturbing the BTB nor anchoring junctions between Sertoli cells and round spermatids/spermatocytes/spermatogonia.[60,61] Indeed, using the androgen suppression model, we have confirmed that a disruption of apical ES can be limited to the Sertoli cell-spermatid interface without compromising the BTB integrity nor the anchoring junction between Sertoli cells and round spermatids/spermatocytes in the seminiferous epithelium.[62] In short, these findings are drastically different from other blood-tissue barriers (e.g., in the skin) since AJ disruption in these barriers always leads to TJ damage,[53,54] and the assembly and integrity of TJ depend on AJ.[63,64] For instance, when the reassembly of junctional complexes in intestinal cells is initiated by an incubation of high-calcium medium, AJ is reassembled within ~30 min prior to TJ assembly.[65] As such, these results illustrated that this unidirectional cross-talk mechanism is operating at the BTB in which a disruption of Sertoli-germ cell adhesion can be restricted to anchoring junction (e.g., apical ES) without interfering with TJ nor anchoring junction (e.g., basal ES) at the BTB.

Changes in Protein-Protein Interactions between Integral Membrane Proteins and Their Adaptors, and Cross-Talk between Junctions at the BTB in the Regulation of BTB Dynamics

To address the observations regarding the cross-talk between TJ and AJ (e.g., basal ES) at the BTB that regulate its timely opening to facilitate preleptotene spermatocyte migration at stage VIII of the cycle, recent studies have shifted the focus on the role of protein-protein interactions in BTB dynamics.

Studies based on two different in vivo models, namely the Adjudin[32,55,57] and the androgen suppression model have yielded some interesting observations that leads to a hypothesis to be tested in future studies. First, in the testosterone suppression model of O'Donnell[60,61] in which subdermal testosterone/estradiol implants were placed in adult rats to suppress the intratesticular T level, it was shown that a loss of testosterone in the seminiferous epithelium selectively perturbed apical ES junction (from step 8 spermatids and beyond), leading to spermatid depletion from the seminiferous epithelium. While the BTB integrity and functionality were not compromised,[62] there were significant changes at the BTB as well, reminiscence of the seminiferous epithelium during spermatogenesis, such as stage VIII of the epithelial cycle. For instance, at the time of apical ES restructuring that led to spermatid depletion from the epithelium, there were enhanced production of several basal ES proteins (e.g., cadherins, integrins, JAM-A).[57,66,74] Second, these observations were consistent with other findings using the Adjudin model in which the Adjudin-induced anchoring junction restructuring in the seminiferous epithelium also led to progressive depletion of germ cells from the seminiferous epithelium, beginning with elongating/elongate spermatids, to be followed by round spermatids and spermatocytes.[6,75] However, the BTB apparently remained "intact".[17] Likewise, an induction of an array of proteins at the BTB was also detected, such as cadherins, cateneins, integrins,[32,74-76] illustrating restructuring indeed occurred at the BTB, but unlike the apical ES at the Sertoli cell-spermatid interface that led to spermatid loss from the epithelium, such BTB restructuring did not lead to functional damage which compromise the immunological barrier, reminiscent of the seminiferous epithelium at stage VIII of the epithelial cycle. We thus postulate that these transiently induced basal ES proteins that form a "patch" are being used to temporarily "reinforce" the TJ-barrier function at the BTB during androgen suppression- or Adjudin-induced junction restructuring in the seminiferous epithelium so that the BTB integrity can be maintained as observed in these models. However, this transient induction in basal ES proteins can also "supersede" the TJ-barrier function temporarily when TJ must open to accommodate preleptotene spermatocyte migration at stage VIII of the epithelial cycle. This speculation was also supported by a study using fluorescent microscopy. For instance, in studies using the androgen suppression model, it was shown that during the androgen depletion-induced spermatid (step 8 and beyond) loss, the increased basal ES proteins (e.g., N-cadherin, β-catenin) at the BTB had surrounded the entire basal compartment, forming a transient "patch", and extended into the seminiferous epithelium well beyond the BTB site.[57,62,66] As such, these basal ES proteins could "patch" the TJ-barrier, reinforcing the BTB integrity, which is also the mechanism being used to maintain the transiently disrupted TJ-barrier at the Sertoli-Sertoli interface at stage VIII of the cycle, facilitating preleptotene spermatocyte migration while maintaining the immunological barrier at the BTB. It is obvious that this possibility must be carefully evaluated and investigated in future studies.While functional data are not yet available to support this "patch" hypothesis, recent findings in the field seem to favor this postulate. For instance, several TJ proteins, such as JAM-C and coxsackievirus and adenovirus receptor (CAR) are putative integral membrane proteins at the TJ of multiple epithelia,[67-70] yet recent studies have shown that they are also putative Sertoli and/or germ cell products that are restricted to the apical ES.[71,72] A recent report has also identified the presence of JAM-A in germ cells,[73] which is also detected at the BTB colocalizing with ZO-1 by fluorescent microscopy,[62] suggesting that it is likely a component of the basal ES at the BTB. These findings are significant because they illustrate that ectoplasmic specialization (e.g., apical and basal ES), a testis-specific AJ type, is indeed a hybrid of AJ and TJ as it consists components of TJ-integral membrane proteins. Thus, these TJ component proteins at the basal ES can confer the necessary tight junction functionality, however, when the TJ fibrils are disrupted, the transiently induced basal ES proteins serve as a transient "patch". Nonetheless, this concept must be vigorously investigated in future studies.

One may argue that since there was a surge in anchoring junction proteins in the seminiferous epithelium, and these proteins were being used to "reinforce" the TJ-barrier function at the BTB, why would such an increase in anchoring junction protein levels (e.g., cadherins and catenins) in the seminiferous epithelium fail to retain germ cells outside the BTB. Based on limited available data, it seems that this loss of cell adhesion is the result of a loss of protein-protein association between cadherins and catenins at the Sertoli-germ cell interface.[66] This is likely mediated by a surge in tyrosine phosphorlyation of β-catenin, resulting in a reduction in its adhesive activity.[66] Other studies have shown that tyrosine phosphorylation of AJ proteins (e.g., cadherins) facilitates junction disassembly in various epithelia,[77,78] as well as in pathological conditions, such as tumor metastasis[79] whereas Ser/Thr phosphorylation, on the contrary, promotes adhesion. In addition, other molecules are operating side-by-side to regulate BTB. For instance, the integrity of endothelial TJ-barrier was found to be partly regulated by reactive oxygen species, such as hydrogen peroxide. These reactive oxygen species up-regulate tyrosine phosphorylation of FAK and paxillin (note: these are cell-matrix focal adhesion proteins but have now been found at the apical and basal ES, such as the BTB), as well as β-catenin and VE-cadherin in the vascular endothelium.[80] Likewise, recent studies have shown that NO, a reactive oxygen species produced by NOS, regulates Sertoli cell TJ-barrier and Sertoli-germ cell anchoring junction function via the cGMP/PKG signaling pathway[81,82] which is also associated with a significant decline in cadherin-NOS and catenin-NOS interaction.[74,76] It is likely that these changes can lead to an increase in phosphorylation of the cadherin/catenin complex via the action of PKG.[76,82] These observations thus support the notion that as preleptotene spermatocytes traverse the BTB, there must be a coordination in the disintegration of TJ and anchoring junction. We speculate that when TJ is "opened" to accommodate cell migration, the transiently induced basal ES proteins form a "patch" to supersede the temporarily loss TJ-barrier function (see text above). Thereafter, cell adhesion complexes in the "patch" also transiently "open" to facilitate cell movement by altering their phosphorylation status so that preleptotene spermatocytes can continue their migration. However, one may also argue if the basal ES and perhaps AJ transiently loss their adhesion function at the BTB to facilitate preleptotene spermatocyte migration, how can BTB maintains its cell adhesion and TJ-barrier function at the time. Interestingly, in studies using the Adjudin and the androgen suppression model, it was shown that there was a transient induction in TJ-proteins (e.g., occludin, ZO-1, JAMs) at the BTB when spermatids were depleting from the epithelium.[57,62,66,73] We speculate that these induced TJ-proteins are being used to supersede the temporal loss of AJ function at the BTB to confer adhesion between migration preleptotene spermatocytes and Sertoli cells. For instance, it is known that the first extracellular domain of occludin can confer cell adhesion function.[83] In short, it is likely that TJ and basal AJ at the BTB are working in concert to facilitate preleptotene spermatocyte migration while maintaining the TJ-barrier function and cell adhesion in this microenvironment.

In the testis, apical ES is considered to be a hybrid cell-cell actin-based AJ and cell-matrix focal contact anchoring junction type restricted to the interface between Sertoli cells and developing spermatids in adult rat testes.[32,84,85] This conclusion is reached since several focal contact proteins usually restricted to the cell-martix interface to facilitate cell movement (e.g., macrophages and fibroblasts) in other epithelia are also found at the apical ES. For instance, FAK is localized at the basal ES near the basement membrane while its phosphorylated and activated form, p-FAK-Tyr^{397}, is detected almost exclusively at the apical ES and is structurally associated with a nonreceptor protein tyrosine kinase, c-Src.[32] Furthermore, their protein levels are significantly induced when germ cells are depleting from the seminiferous epithelium, as illustrated in the Adjudin and testosterone-suppression models.[32,86] Other protein kinases, including Csk, CK2 and Fer kinases have also been found to associate with N-cadherin and catenin at the basal and apical ES.[74,75,87] Integrin-linked kinase (ILK) was also reported to be associated with β1 integrin at the apical ES.[85] Collectively, these findings coupled with recent reports that TJ proteins are also integral components of the apical and basal ES (see discussion above) thus illustrate that ES is indeed a unique hybrid anchoring junction type of AJ, focal contact, and TJ, that can confer AJ functionality (i.e., cell adhesion) while facilitate cell movement (e.g., focal contact function) and transiently confer TJ functionality (e.g., during BTB restructuring in which the induced basal ES proteins form a "patch" at the BTB). Thus, it is not entirely unlikely that basal ES can supersede the function of TJ and vice versa as discussed herein.

Cross-Talk between TJ and Anchoring Junctions at the BTB That Regulates BTB Dynamics

The coexistence of TJ and AJ at the BTB has been illustrated by studies using electron and freeze-fracture microscopy since the 1970s.[12,16,41,88] Recent studies using fluorescent microscopy have also colocalized TJ and AJ to the same site at the BTB. Even though occludin and cadherin at the BTB have no direct protein-protein interaction as demonstrated by coimmunoprecipitation, they are linked via their peripheral adaptors, such as ZO-1 and catenins.[89] This finding is not entirely unexpected since at the early stage of TJ assembly, ZO-1 was shown to associate with catenins in MDCK cells.[90] Besides, ZO-1 also serves as a cross-linker between the cadherin/catenin protein complex and the actin-based cytoskeleton in nonepithelial cells.[91,92] In a more current study, ZO-1 was found to use the same domain for its interaction with occludin and α-catenin.[93] As such, ZO-1 is not only a TJ adaptor; in fact, it shuffles between TJ and AJ and links these two junction types to cytoskeleton.

Using an in vivo model to study junction dynamics involving Adjudin, rats were treated with a single dose of this compound at 50 mg/kg b.w. by gavage to induce germ cell depletion from the seminiferous epithelium.[17] The drug is targeted at the apical ES with minimal effect to TJs and basal ES.[57] Interestingly, at the time of germ cell loss, the association between the protein complexes at TJ (e.g., occludin/ZO-1) and AJ (e.g., cadherin/catenin) via their corresponding adaptors was temporarily abolished, namely ZO-1 and α- and γ-catenins. In essence, ZO-1 was no longer associated with catenins, and as such, occludin and N-cadherin as well as their adaptors, ZO-1 and γ-catenin were diffusing away from the BTB site.[89] Yet, their association was reestablished by day 7 after treatment when germ cells (e.g., elongating/elongate spermatids and some round spermatids) were depleted from the epithelium. Based on such timely dissociation between TJ and AJ protein complexes in the seminiferous epithelium, an "*engagement and disengagement*" theory was proposed to describe the unique mechanism employed by the testis to facilitate germ cell movement pertinent to spermatogenesis[89] (Fig. 4). It is likely that under physiological conditions, such as at stages other than VII and VIII of the epithelial cycle, TJ and AJ (e.g., basal ES) are structurally "engaged" via their peripheral adaptors at the BTB to reinforce barrier integrity (Fig. 4). At the time of spermiation and when preleptotene spermatocytes must traverse the BTB,[6,88] which occur concurrently at stage VIII of the epithelial cycle, a transient "disengagement" between adaptors (e.g., ZO-1 and catenins) of the corresponding TJ and AJ protein complexes takes place to facilitate germ cell movement across the barrier, avoiding the unnecessary damage to TJ during AJ (e.g., basal ES) restructuring. This novel mechanism thus preserves barrier integrity while facilitating germ cell movement (Fig. 4). After spermiation and the movement of preleptotene spermatocytes across the BTB, the adaptors, namely ZO-1 and α-/γ-catenins become "engaged" again to strengthen the barrier. This theory not only provides a solid biochemical basis regarding the mechanism of germ cell movement across the BTB, it also provides the rationale for the coexisting TJ and AJ at the BTB. However, the identity of the protein(s) that "pulls" ZO-1 away from catenins to maintain the "disengaged" state and facilitate germ cell movement remains to be determined. Recent studies have shown that dynamins (e.g., dynamin II), large GTPases that serve as "pinchase-like mechanoenzymes" to facilitate the formation of endocytic vesicles by severing nascent endocytic pits from the plasma membrane,[94,95] are likely to maintain such a "disengaged" state at the BTB.[73] This work must be vigorously validated and expanded in future studies.

In this context, it is of interest to note that this theory does not account for the temporal disruption of TJ at the BTB, which must occur to accommodate preleptotene spermatocyte migration. Recent studies have unequivocally demonstrated that TNFα and TGF-β3 produced and secreted by Sertoli and/or germ cells into the BTB microenvironment can induce reversible disruption of the barrier[58,96] as receptors for these cytokines are mostly resided in Sertoli cells.[6,17] This is illustrated in a functional BTB assay by monitoring the diffusion of a small molecular dye (e.g., fluorescein 5'-isothiocyanate, Mr 389) from the systemic circulation into the adluminal compartment behind the BTB following TNFα treatment.[96] Thus, it is highly plausible that these cytokines at the BTB perturb TJs, transiently open the barrier to facilitate preleptotene spermatocyte migration at stage VIII of the epithelial cycle. Indeed, the expression levels of both TNFα and TGF-β3 are highest at stage VIII of the cycle.[25,58]

Other studies using Sertoli cell cultures have shown that TGF-β3 regulates TJ-barrier function via the p38 and ERK MAP kinase signaling pathways.[97,98] Furthermore, studies using the in vivo $CdCl_2$ model have unequivocally demonstrated that BTB dynamics are regulated by TGF-β3[24,47] via its effects, at least in part, on the steady-state protein levels of protease inhibitors (e.g., α_2-macroglobulin), and proteases (e.g., cathepsin L),[47,99] which, in turn, assist BTB restructuring. Other studies have shown that MMPs and TIMPs are both present at the ES and BTB, and whose actions are coordinated by TNFα.[25] Collectively, these data suggest that at the time preleptotene spermatocytes traverse the BTB, it is initially mediated by a transient loss in

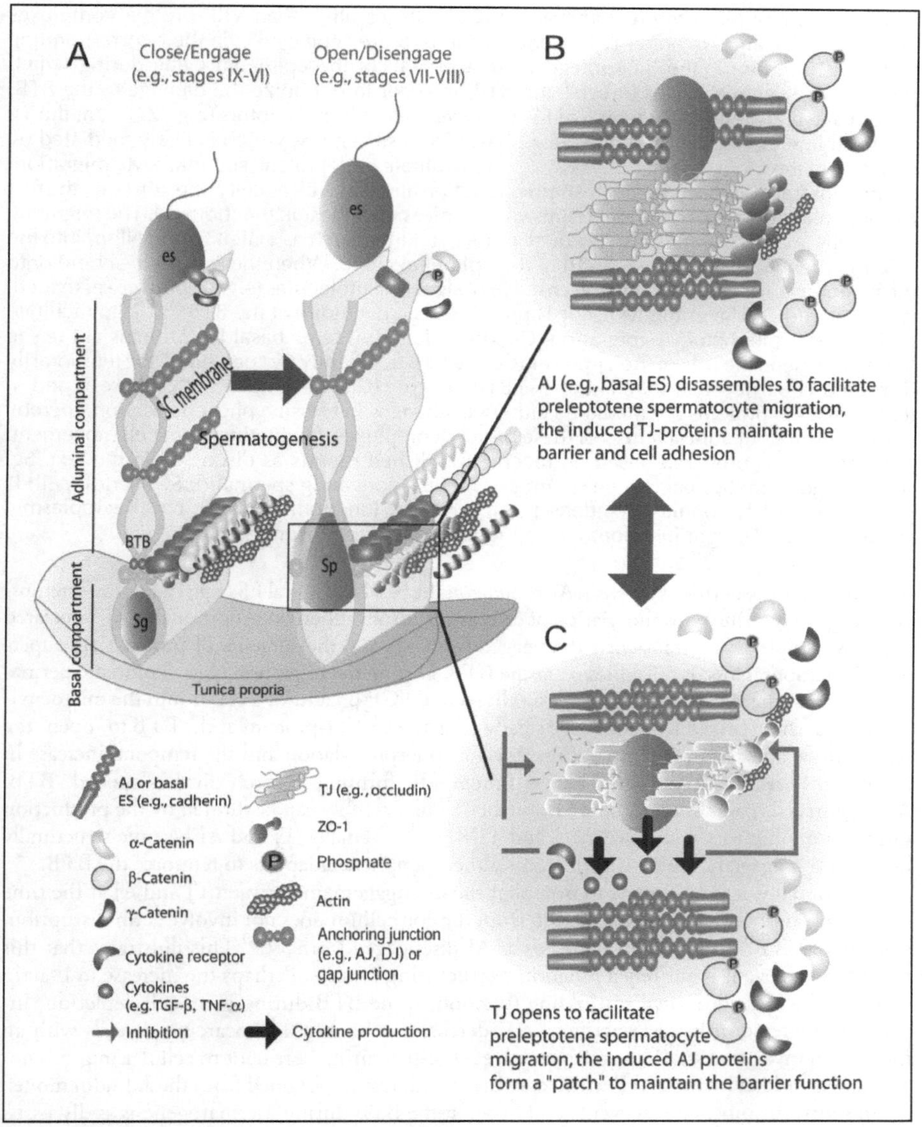

Figure 4. A-C) A schematic drawing that illustrates the engagement and disengagement mechanism between TJ and AJ at the BTB to facilitate preleptotene spermatocyte migration. A) The restructuring of TJs and AJs (e.g., basal ES) at the BTB are regulated by the "engagement (close)" and "disengagement (open)" mechanism to facilitate preleptotene spermatocyte migration across the BTB with minimal damaging effects on the barrier integrity. The left top panel shows the spatial arrangement of the seminiferous epithelium in which the BTB separates the epithelium into the basal and adluminal compartments. TJs (e.g., occludin/ZO-1) and basal ES (e.g., N-cadherin/γ-catenin) that coexist at the BTB are structurally associated with each other via the peripheral adaptors (e.g., ZO-1 and catenins). At stage VIII of the epithelial cycle, spermiation occurs when elongated spermatids emptying into the tubule lumen, and when preleptotene spermatocytes traverse the BTB, a transient opening of BTB must occur. Figure legend continued on following page.

Figure 4, continued from previous page. B,C) In stages other than VIII, protein complexes occludin/ZO-1 and N-cadherin/β-catenin at the BTB are "engaged" via their corresponding adaptors to reinforce the BTB integrity. At stage VIII of the epithelial cycle during which preleptotene spermatocytes traverse the BTB, in order to minimize the damage to the BTB, adaptors (e.g., catenins) at the apical ES are 'disengaged' from adaptors (e.g., ZO-1) at the TJ. We postulate that at the time of AJ (e.g., basal ES) disassembly, which is likely mediated by TGF-β3 via the ERK signaling pathway,[57,58] to facilitate preleptotene spermatocyte migration, TJ-proteins transiently maintain the barrier function alone as well as cell adhesion (e.g., the first extracellular domain of occludin is known to confer cell adhesion function) (B). The migrating germ cells and Sertoli cells also produce more cytokines, such as TGF-β3 and TNF-α, into the BTB microenvironment at stage VIII of the epithelial cycle. When these cytokines bind onto the receptors on the Sertoli cell, the cascade of signaling molecules (e.g., p-p38) are activated, which, in turn, reduces the levels of TJ proteins (e.g., occludin) at the BTB[24,47,58] to facilitate preleptotene spermatocyte migration (C). The induced AJ (e.g., basal ES) proteins at the site likely supersede the role of the TJ-proteins at the BTB transiently by "patching" the temporarily disrupted TJ-barrier so as to maintain the BTB integrity (C). The "unpairing" of these TJ and AJ (e.g., basal ES) proteins are mediated either via changes in tyrosine phosphorylation, thereby causing the loss of adhesiveness of these protein complexes, facilitating germ cell movement. This model was prepared based on recently published reports as discussed in the text. Sg, spermatogonium; Sp, pachytene spermatocyte; es, elongating spermatid; SC, Sertoli cell; P, phosphate; ZO-1, zonula occludens-1; AJ, adherens junction; basal ES, basal ectoplasmic specialization; TJ, tight junction; GJ, gap junction; DJ, desmosomes.

protein-protein associations between AJ-proteins at the basal and apical ES (e.g., cadherins/catenins) via a surge in tyrosine phosphorylation of catenins (and/or cadherins). Additionally, AJ-associated proteins complexes are transiently disengaged from TJs and the surge in TJ proteins can supersede the temporal loss of cell adhesion at the BTB. During the migration of preleptotene spermatocytes across the BTB, Sertoli and germ cells secrete TGF-β3 and/or TNF-α into the microenvironment at the BTB, which reduce the steady-state levels of TJ-proteins at the BTB to "open" the barrier to facilitate germ cell migration. Ser/Thr phosphorylation and the temporal increase in AJ-proteins can substitute the TJ-barrier function by forming a "patch" in the "opened" BTB. After germ cells pass through the BTB, further TJ disassembly can be limited by the production of protease inhibitors such as α_2-MG and TIMPs.[99,100] Finally, TJ and AJ become structurally linked and "engaged", which is mediated via their peripheral adaptors to reinforce the BTB.

Additionally, it is of interest to note that the disengagement between TJ and AJ at the time of Adjudin-induced germ cell depletion from the epithelium does not involve actin disruption, since the level of F to G-actin increases as AJ disengaged from TJ.[89] This illustrates that this germ cell loss event is entirely a junction restructuring process. Perhaps the increase in F-actin content provides additional scaffolding function to the BTB during germ cell depletion. Indeed, an increase in F- to G-actin ratio is detected in human adenocarcinoma cells with an increase in invasiveness,[101] illustrating active AJ restructuring pertinent to cellular migration is associated with an increase in F-actin, consistent with results obtained from the Adjudin model.

In short, the biochemical events that occur at the BTB during spermatogenesis as discussed above are in agreement with the "junction restructuring theory".[17] Also, these recent biochemical findings do not negate the "zipper theory"[3,13] or the "intermediate cellular compartment theory".[7,14] Indeed, these three theories are not mutually exclusive. In essence, the "junction restructuring theory" is a biochemical version of the combined "zipper" and "intermediate cellular compartment" theories, taking into account the molecular players in the junction restructuring events that occur during spermatogenesis. For instance, in the "zipper theory", the "old" TJ fibrils above the migrating preleptotene spermatocytes must be broken down after the formation of the nascent TJ fibrils below these migrating cells as illustrated in the "intermediate cellular compartment theory" in which preleptotene spermatocytes were shown to be trapped between TJ fibrils in the seminiferous epithelium.[14] The "disengagement" between TJs and AJs at the BTB as discussed above (see also ref. 89) thus offers the biochemical mechanism to facilitate preleptotene spermatocyte migration across the BTB.

Table 1. *Junction types and their molecular components at the BTB of adult rodent testes*

Junction Type	Component Proteins	Mr (kDa)	Interacting Partners
TJ	***- Integral membrane proteins***		
	Occludin, occludin IB	60-65	***ZO-1, ZO-2***, ZO-3, ***cingulin, NOS***
	Claudin-1, 2, 3, 4, 5, 6, 7, 8, 9, 10, 11, 12-24	20-25	***ZO-1, ZO-2***, ZO-3
	JAM-A, B	40	***ZO-1, cingulin***, AF-6/afadin, PAR3, PAR6, aPKC, PICK-1, CASK, MUPP-1
	CAR	46	ZO-1, MUPP-1, MAGI-1
	CLMP (CAR-liked membrane protein)	44-48	Occludin, ZO-1
	BT-IgSF (Brain- and testis-specific immunoglobulin superfamily)	43.77-52	n.k.
	Tricellulin	66-72	n.k.
	- Peripheral membrane proteins		
	ZO-1, 2, 3	210-225	***Occludin, claudin, JAM, α and γ-cateinins***, connexin 43, ***actin***, afadin, 4.1R
	Clingulin	140	***JAM-A, ZO-1, ZO-2***, ZO-3, myosin,
Basal ES and/or AJ	***- Integral membrane proteins***		
	N- or E-Cadherin	127-135	***α, β and γ-Catenins, p120^ctn^, c-Src, NOS-2,3, ponsin, α-actinin, actin, Rab8b***
	Celsr cadherins 1,2	320	***Protocadherin a, Rab7***
	Nectin-1, 2, 4	70-85	***Afadin, ponsin, α2-macroglobulin***, ZO-1, PAR3, PAR6, aPKC, PICK-1
	- Peripheral membrane proteins		
	α-Catenin	100-104	***N-Cadherin, β and γ-catenins, ZO-1, p120ctn, α-actinin, actin***, afadin
	β-Catenin	92	***N-Cadherin, α and γ-catenins, p120ctn α-actinin, actin, NOS-2,3, PRKG***
	γ-Catenin	82	***N-Cadherin, α and β-catenins, ZO-1, p120ctn, α-actinin, actin, Rab8b***
	p120^{ctn}	65-120	***N-Cadherin, β and γ-catenins, α-actinin, actin,***
	Afadin/AF-6	205	***Nectin, ponsin, α2-macroglobulin, actin***, P-cadherin
Basal TBC	MN7	90	
	Actin	42	
	Cofilin	20	

continued on next page

Table 1. Continued

Junction Type	Component Proteins	Mr (kDa)	Interacting Partners
Desmosome-like junction	Connexins 26, 30.2, 30.3, 31, 31.1, 32, 33, 36, 37, 40, 43, 45, 46, 50, 57	27-70	***Occludin***, ZO-1, ZO-2, N-cadherin, α and β-catenins, p120ctn
	Desmocollin-1, -2 ,-3	107-115	Plakophilin, desmoplakin vimentin
	Desmoglein-1α, -1β, -1γ, -2, -3, -4	110	Plakoglobin, desmoplakin, vimentin
Others	4.1B*	110	n.k.
	4.1G*	130-140	Cadherin
	LYRIC**	80	Occludin, ZO-1
	P-glycoprotein (P-gp)	n.k.	n.k.
	Multidrug resistance-associated protein (MRP1)	n.k.	n.k.

This table was prepared based on current findings in the field as discussed in the text. References given here are not exhaustive due to the limited page space. As such, only selected references are given herein and additional references can be found in the text and earlier reviews.[6,17,30,39,40,46,108-110,113-124] In the column for "Component proteins", proteins that have been positively identified in the testis are underlined. In the column for "Interacting partners", underlined proteins that are **bold** and ***italic*** are those that were shown to interact with the corresponding integral membrane proteins at the BTB; proteins that are underlined only are found in testes but were shown to interact with the corresponding target proteins in other epithelia; proteins that are included in the table but not underlined are those that were found in similar blood-tissue barriers other than the testis. n.k. = not known. *These proteins are found at the Sertoli cell-spermatogonia interface near the basal compartment, and may not be a component of the BTB; **, Protein that has not been identified in the BTB but it is known to interact with TJ-associated proteins.

Cross-Talk between TJ, Anchoring Junction, and GJ in the Seminiferous Epithelium Is Crucial to Spermatogenesis

In other epithelia, cross-talk between different junctions has been the subject of active investigation in recent years. For instance, cross-talk between cadherins and integrins is likely mediated by Rap1 GTPase. It was shown that the disassembly of AJ through endocytosis activated Rap1, which, in turn, enhanced the integrin cell-matrix adhesion by redistributing intergrins to new adhesion sites. This thus avoids uncontrolled cell dissemination.[102] Direct association between AJ proteins (e.g., nectin-1 and 3) and PAR-3 (a signaling molecule usually restricted to TJ and crucial to cell polarization working in concert with aPKC and PAR-6[103]) was also reported in neural epithelial cells in which the affinity of nectins toward afadin (an adaptor of nectin) and PAR-3 was found to be similar.[104,105] Protein interacting with C-kinase-1 (PICK-1), a scaffolding protein, interacts with both AJ (e.g., nectin) and TJ proteins (e.g., JAM-A, B & C but not claudins) in CHO cells.[106] It is believed that PICK-1 is an adaptor which coordinates cross-talk between TJ and AJ in epithelial cells. However, the significance (and its presence in the testis) of PICK-1 in cross-talk between TJ and anchoring junction (e.g., basal ES) at the BTB and between apical ES and BTB remains to be determined. Gap junctions (GJ) (e.g., connexin-43) are recently shown to associate with TJ (e.g., ZO-1 & 2)[107,108] and AJ proteins (e.g., N-cadherin, α-catenin, β-catenin and p120^{ctn}).[109] These findings thus demonstrate the potential inter-dependent relationship between junction types in various epithelia including the BTB, which is likely mediated via peripheral adaptors. In some cases, their roles can be temporarily superseded by each other, as illustrated in the engagement and disengagement theory in the BTB.[89] In others, the formation of a junction type requires the coassembly of another type. For instance, when either connexin-43 (GJ) or N-cadherin (AJ) was disrupted by RNA silencing, gap junctional communication as well as the mobility of NIH3T3 cells was reduced,[109] illustrating a functional AJ and GJ linkage.

Concluding Remarks—Lesson from the Testis

In the past decade, much work has been done in dissecting the role of TJ and anchoring junction dynamics in spermatogenesis, however, the crucial information is still lacking in the field as highlighted in this review. For instance, how is the cross-talk between TJ and anchoring junctions initiated and regulated? Is the cross-talk limited between TJ and AJ (e.g., basal ES and apical ES) or is it extended to the desmosome-like junctions? What are the signaling molecules and pathways that are involved in this cross-talk? Answers to some of these questions will also unravel potential targets for male contraception and may offer an explanation for unexplained infertility. Nonetheless, recent findings regarding the regulation of different junction types at the BTB as reviewed herein have illustrated that the testis has a unique mechanism in place in which anchoring junction (e.g., basal ES) and TJ can be functionally segregated so that preleptotene spermatocytes can traverse the BTB without compromising the TJ-barrier function. Additionally, cytokines (e.g., TGF-β3 and TNFα) produced locally by Sertoli and/or germ cells and secreted into the microenvironment of BTB are also being used to transiently "open" the TJ-barrier to facilitate germ cell movement. It will be of interest and physiologically important to determine if this mechanism is used to facilitate food absorption across the epithelial TJ-barrier in small intestine or to facilitate transepithelial migration of neutrophils across the endothelial TJ-barrier in microvessels at the inflammation site.

Acknowledgements

This work was supported in part by grants from the National Institutes of Health (NIH, NICHD U01 HD045908 and U54 HD29990 Project 3), and the CONRAD Program (CICCR CIG 96-05-A/B, CIG 01-72, and CIG 01-74). W.M.L. was supported by a grant from the Hong Kong Research Grant Council (HKU 7599/06M). H.H.N.Y. was supported by a University of Hong Kong Postgraduate Research Fellowship Award.

References

1. Parvinen M. Regulation of the seminiferous epithelium. Endocr Rev 1982; 3:404-417.
2. Russell L, Ettlin R, Sinha Hikim A et al. Histological and Histopathological Evaluation of the Testis. Clearwater: Cache River Press, 1990.
3. Russell L, Peterson R. Sertoli cell junctions: Morphological and functional correlates. Int Rev Cytol 1985; 94:177-211.
4. Hess RA, Schaeffer DJ, Eroschenko VP et al. Frequency of the stages in the cycle of the seminiferous epithelium in the rat. Biol Reprod 1990; 43:517-524.
5. Vogl AW, Pfeiffer DC, Redenbach DM et al. Sertoli cell cytoskeleton. In: Russell LD, Griswold MD eds. The Sertoli Cell. Clearwater: Cache River Press, 1993:39-86.
6. Cheng CY, Mruk DD. Cell junction dynamics in the testis: Sertoli-germ cell interactions and male contraceptive development. Physiol Rev 2002; 82:825-874.
7. Russell L. Movement of spermatocytes from the basal to the adluminal compartment of the rat testis. Am J Anat 1977; 148:313-328.
8. Chiquoine AD. Observations on the early events of cadmium necrosis of the testis. Anat Rec 1964; 149:23-35.
9. Kormano M. Dye permeability and alkaline phosphatase activity of testicular capillaries in the post-natal rat. Histochemie 1967; 9:327-338.
10. Setchell BP, Waites GMH. The blood-testis barrier. Washington DC: American Physiological Society, 1975.
11. Dym M, Fawcett DW. The blood-testis barrier in the rat and the physiological compartmentation of the seminiferous epithelium. Biol Reprod 1970; 3:308-326.
12. Fawcett DW, Leak LV, Heidger PMJ. Electron microscopic observations on the structural components of the blood-testis barrier. J Reprod Fertil Suppl 1970; 10:105-122.
13. Dym M, Cavicchia J. Further observations on the blood-testis barrier in monkeys. Biol Reprod 1977; 17:390-403.
14. Russell L. Morphological and functional evidence for Sertoli-germ cell relationships. In: Russell LD, Griswold MD, eds. The Sertoli Cell. Clearwater: Cache River Press, 1993:365-390.
15. Pelletier RM. The tight junctions in the testis, epididymis, and vas deferens. Tight Junctions. New York: CRC Press, 2001:599-628.
16. Pelletier RM, Byers SW. The blood-testis barrier and Sertoli cell junctions: Structural considerations. Microsc Res Tech 1992; 20:3-33.
17. Mruk DD, Cheng CY. Sertoli-Sertoli and Sertoli-germ cell interactions and their significance in germ cell movement in the seminiferous epithelium during spermatogenesis. Endocr Rev 2004; 25:747-806.
18. Ivanov AI, Nusrat A, Parkos CA. Endocytosis of the apical junctional complex: Mechanisms and possible roles in regulations of epithelial barriers. Bioessays 2005; 27:356-365.
19. Matsuda M, Kubo A, Furuse M et al. A peculiar internalization of claudins, tight junction-specific adhesion molecules, during the intercellular movement of epithelial cells. J Cell Sci 2004; 117:1247-1257.
20. Ivanov AI, Nusrat A, Parkos CA. Endocytosis of epithelial apical junctional proteins by a clathrin-mediated pathway into a unique storage compartment. Mol Biol Cell 2004; 15:176-188.
21. Hopkins AM, Walsh SV, Verkade P et al. Constitutive activation of Rho proteins by CNF-1 influences tight junction structure and epithelial barrier function. J Cell Sci 2003; 116:725-742.
22. Utech M et al. Mechanism of IFN-γ-induced endocytosis of tight junction proteins: Myosin II-dependent vacuolarization of the apical plasma membrane. Mol Biol Cell 2005; 16:5040-5052.
23. Watson CJ, Hoare CJ, Garrod DR et al. Interferon-γ selectively increases epithelial permeability to large molecules by activating different populations of paracellular pores. J Cell Sci 2005; 118:5221-5230.
24. Lui WY, Wong CH, Mruk DD et al. TGF-β3 regulates the blood-testis barrier dynamics via the p38 mitogen activated protein (MAP) kinase pathway: An in vivo study. Endocrinology 2003; 144:1139-1142.
25. Siu MKY, Lee WM, Cheng CY. The interplay of collagen IV, tumor necrosis factor-α, gelatinase B (matrix metalloprotease-9), and tissue inhibitor of metalloproteases-1 in the basal lamina regulates Sertoli cell-tight junction dynamics in the rat testis. Endocrinology 2003; 144:371-387.
26. Guttman JA, Takai Y, Vogl AW. Evidence that tubulobulbar complexes in the seminiferous epithelium are involved with internalization of adhesion junctions. Biol Reprod 2004; 71:548-559.
27. Le TL, Yap AS, Stow JL. Recycling of E-cadherin: A potential mechanism for regulating cadherin dynamics. J Cell Biol 1999; 146:219-232.
28. Morimoto S et al. Rab 13 mediates the continuous endocytic recycling of occludin to the cell surface. J Biol Chem 2005; 280:2220-2228.

29. Lau ASN, Mruk DD. Rab8B GTPase and junction dynamics in the testis. Endocrinology 2003; 144:1549-1563.
30. Burridge K. Foot in mouth: Do focal adhesions disassemble by endocytosis? Nat Cell Biol 2005; 7:545-547.
31. Ezratty EJ, Partridge MA, Gundersen GG. Microtubule-induced focal adhesion disassembly is mediated by dynamin and focal adhesion kinase. Nat Cell Biol 2005; 7:581-590.
32. Siu MKY, Mruk DD, Lee WM et al. Adhering junction dynamics in the testis are regulated by an interplay of β1-integrin and focal adhesion complex-associated proteins. Endocrinology 2003; 144:2141-2163.
33. Cook TA, Urrutia R, McNiven MA. Identification of dynamin 2, an isoform ubiquitously expressed in rat tissues. Proc Natl Acad Sci USA 1994; 91:644-648.
34. Kamitani A et al. Distribution of dynamins in testis and their possible relation to spermatogenesis. Biochem Biophys Res Commun 2002; 294:261-267.
35. Lui WY, Lee WM. cAMP perturbs inter-Sertoli tight junction permeability barrier in vitro via its effect on proteasome-sensitive ubiquitination of occludin. J Cell Physiol 2005; 203:564-572.
36. Alberts B et al. The Molecular Biology of the Cell. New York: Garland Publishing Inc., 1994.
37. Denker BM, Nigam SK. Molecular structure and assembly of the tight junction. Am J Physiol 1998; 274:F1-F9.
38. Tsukita S, Furuse M, Itoh M. Structural and signalling molecules come together at tight junctions. Curr Opin Cell Biol 1999; 11:628-633.
39. Tsukita S, Furuse M, Itoh M. Multifunctional strands in tight junctions. Nat Rev Mol Cell Biol 2001; 2:285-293.
40. Wolburg H, Lippoldt A. Tight junctions of the blood-brain barrier: Development, composition and regulation. Vasc Pharmacol 2002; 38:323-337.
41. Dym M. The mammalian rete testis—A morphological examination. Anat Rec 1976; 186:493-523.
42. Dym M. Basement membrane regulation of Sertoli cells. Endocr Rev 1994; 15:102-115.
43. Bart J et al. An oncological view on the blood-testis barrier. Lancet Oncol 2002; 3:357-363.
44. Toyama Y, Maekawa M, Yuasa S. Ectoplasmic specializations in the Sertoli cell: New vistas based on genetic defects and testicular toxicology. Anat Sci Int 2003; 78:1-16.
45. Vogl AW, Pfeiffer DC, Mulholland DJ et al. Unique and multifunctional adhesion junctions in the testis: Ectoplasmic specializations. Arch Histol Cytol 2000; 63:1-15.
46. Prozialeck WC. Evidence that E-cadherin may be a target for cadmium toxicity in epithelial cells. Toxicol Appl Pharmacol 2000; 164:231-249.
47. Wong CH, Mruk DD, Lui WY et al. Regulation of blood-testis barrier dynamics: An in vivo study. J Cell Sci 2004; 117:783-798.
48. Hew KW, Heath GL, Jiwa AH et al. Cadmium in vivo causes disruption of tight junction-associaetd microfilaments in rat Sertoli cells. Biol Reprod 1993; 49:840-849.
49. Wiebe JP, Barr KJ. The control of male fertility by 1,2,3-trihydroxypropane (THP; glycerol): Rapid arrest of spermatogenesis without altering libido, accessory organs, gonadal steroidogenesis, and serum testosterone, LH and FSH. Contraception 1984; 29:291-302.
50. Wiebe JP, Barr KJ. Sustained azoospermia in squirrel, monkey, Saimiri sciureus, resulting from a single intratesticular glycerol injection. Contraception 1989; 39:447-457.
51. Wiebe JP, Kowalik A, Gallardi RL et al. Glycerol disrupts tight junction-associated actin microfilaments, occludin, and microtubules in Sertoli cells. J Androl 2000; 21:625-635.
52. Troxell ML, Chen Y, Cobb N et al. Cadherin function in junctional complex rearrangement and post-translational control of cadherin expression. Am J Physiol Cell Physiol 1999; 276:C404-C418.
53. Guo X et al. Regulation of adherens junctions and epithelial paracellular permeability: A novel function for polyamines. Am J Physiol Cell Physiol 2003; 285:C1174-C1187.
54. Man Y, Hart VJ, Ring CJA et al. Loss of epithelial integrity resulting from E-cadherin dysfunction predisposes airway epithelial cells to adenoviral infection. Am J Respir Cell Mol Biol 2000; 23:610-617.
55. Cheng CY et al. AF-2364, [1-(2,4-dichlorobenzyl)-1H-indazole-3-carbohydrazide] is a potential male contraceptive: A review of recent data. Contraception 2005; 72:251-261.
56. Traina ME et al. Lonidamine transiently affects spermatogenesis in pubertal CD1 mice. Contraception 2005; 72:262-267.
57. Xia W, Cheng CY. TGF-β3 regulates anchoring junction dynamics in the seminiferous epithelium of the rat testis via the Ras/ERK signaling pathway: An in vivo study. Dev Biol 2005; 280:321-343.
58. Xia W, Mruk DD, Lee WM et al. Differential interactions between transforming growth factor-β3/TβR1, TAB1, and CD2AP disrupt blood-testis barrier and Sertoli-germ cell adhesion. J Biol Chem 2006; 281:16799-16813.

59. McLachlan RI, Wreford NG, Meachem SJ et al. Effects of testosterone on spermatogenic cell populations in the adult rat. Biol Reprod 1994; 51:945-955.
60. O' Donnell L, McLachlan RI, Wreford NG et al. Testosterone withdrawal promotes stage-specific detachment of round spermatids from the rat seminiferous epithelium. Biol Reprod 1996; 55:895-901.
61. Beardsley A, O'Donnell L. Characterization of normal spermiation and spermiation failure induced by hormone suppression in adult rats. Biol Reprod 2003; 68:1299-1307.
62. Xia W, Wong CH, Lee NPY et al. Disruption of Sertoli-germ cell adhesion function in the seminiferous epithelium of the rat testis can be limited to adherens junctions without affecting the blood-testis barrier integrity: An in vivo study using an androgen suppression model. J Cell Physiol 2005; 205:141-157.
63. Gumbiner B, Stevenson B, Grimaldi A. The role of the cell adhesion molecule uvomorulin in the formation and maintenance of the epithelial junctional complex. J Cell Biol 1988; 107:1575-1587.
64. Yap AS, Brieher WM, Gumbiner BM. Molecular and functional analysis of cadherin-based adherens junctions. Annu Rev Cell Dev Biol 1997; 13:119-146.
65. Ivanov AI, Hunt D, Utech M et al. Differential roles for actin polymerization and a myosin II motor in assembly of the epithelial apical junctional complex. Mol Biol Cell 2005; 16:2636-2650.
66. Zhang J et al. Regulation of Sertoli-germ cell adherens junction dynamics via changes in protein-protein interactions of the N-cadherin-β-catenin complex which are possibly mediated by c-Src and myotubularin-related protein 2: An in vivo study using an androgen suppression model. Endocrinology 2005; 146:1268-1284.
67. Martin-Padura I et al. Junctional adhesion molecule, a novel member of the immunoglobulin superfamily that distributes at intercellular junctions and modulates monocyte transmigration. J Cell Biol 1998; 142:117-127.
68. Palmeri D, van Zante A, Huang CC et al. Vascular endothelial junction-associated molecule, a novel member of the immunoglobulin superfamily, is localized to intercellular boundaries of endothelial cells. J Biol Chem 2000; 275:19139-19145.
69. Raschperger E et al. The coxsackie- and adenovirus receptor (CAR) is an in vivo marker for epithelial tight junctions, with a potential role in regulating permeability and tissue homeostasis. Exp Cell Res 2006; 312:1566-1580 .
70. Bergelson JN et al. Isolation of a common receptor for Coxsackie B viruses and adenoviruses 2 and 5. Science 1997; 275:1320-1323.
71. Gliki G, Ebnet K, Aurrand-Lions M et al. Spermatid differentiation requires the assembly of a cell polarity complex downstream of junctional adhesion molecule-C. Nature 2004; 431:320-324.
72. Mirza M et al. Coxsackievirus and adenovirus receptor (CAR) is expressed in male germ cells and forms a complex with the differentiation factor JAM-C in mouse testis. Exp Cell Res 2006; 312:817-830.
73. Lie P et al. Dynamin II interacts with the cadherin- and occludin-based protein complexes at the blood-testis barrier in adult rat testes. J Endocrinol 2006; 191:571-586.
74. Lee NPY, Cheng CY. Protein kinases and adherens junction dynamics in the seminiferous epithelium of the rat testis. J Cell Physiol 2005; 202:344-360.
75. Chen YM, Lee NPY, Mruk DD et al. Fer kinase/Fer T and adherens junction dynamics in the testis: An in vitro and in vivo study. Biol Reprod 2003; 69:656-672.
76. Lee NPY, Mruk DD, Wong CH et al. Regulation of Sertoli-germ cell adherens junction dynamics in the testis via the nitric oxide synthase (NOS/cGMP/protein kinase G (PRKG)/β-catenin (CATNB) signaling pathway: An in vitro and in vivo study. Biol Reprod 2005; 73:458-471.
77. Gumbiner BM. Regulation of cadherin adhesive activity. J Cell Biol 2000; 148:399-404.
78. Lilien J, Balsamo J. The regulation of cadherin-mediated adhesion by tyrosine phosphorylation/dephosphorylation of β-catenin. Curr Opin Cell Biol 2005; 17:459-465.
79. Matsuyoshi N et al. Cadherin-mediated cell-cell adhesion is perturbed by v-src tyrosine phosphorylation in metastatic fibroblasts. J Cell Biol 1992; 118:703-714.
80. Usatyuk PV, Natarajan V. Regulation of reactive oxygen species-induced endothelial cell-cell and cell-matrix contacts by focal adhesion kinase and adherens junction proteins. Am J Physiol Lung Cell Mol Physiol 2005; 289:L999-L1010.
81. Lee NPY, Cheng CY. Regulation of Sertoli cell tight junction dynamics in the rat testis via the nitric oxide synthase/soluble guanylate cyclase/3',5'-cyclic guanosine monophosphate/protein kinase G signaling pathway: An in vitro study. Endocrinology 2003; 144:3114-3129.
82. Sarkar O, Xia W, Mruk DD. Adjudin-mediated junction restructuring in the seminiferous epithelium leads to displacement of soluble guanylate cyclase from adherens junctions. J Cell Physiol 2006; 208:175-187.

83. Van Itallie CM, Anderson JM. Occludin confers adhesiveness when expressed in fibroblasts. J Cell Sci 1997; 110:1113-1121.
84. Siu MKY, Cheng CY. Interactions of proteases, protease inhibitors, and the β1 integrin/laminin γ3 protein complex in the regulation of ectoplasmic specialization dynamics in the rat testis. Biol Reprod 2004; 70:945-964.
85. Mulholland DJ, Dedhar S, Vogl AW. Rat seminiferous epithelium contains a unique junction (ectoplasmic specialization) with signaling properties both of cell/cell and cell/matrix junctions. Biol Reprod 2001; 64:396-407.
86. Wong CH et al. Regulation of ectoplasmic specialization dynamics in the seminiferous epithelium by focal adhesion-associated proteins in testosterone-suppressed rat testes. Endocrinology 2005; 146:1192-1204.
87. Wine RN, Chapin RE. Adhesion and signaling proteins spatiotemporally associated with spermiation in the rat. J Androl 1999; 20:198-213.
88. Russell L. Observations on rat Sertoli ectoplasmic ('junctional') specializations in their association with germ cells of the rat testis. Tissue Cell 1977; 9:475-498.
89. Yan HHN, Cheng CY. Blood-testis barrier dynamics are regulated by an engagement/disengagement mechanism between tight and adherens junctions via peripheral adaptors. Proc Natl Acad Sci USA 2005; 102:11722-11727.
90. Rajasekaran AK, Hojo M, Huima T et al. Catenins and zonula occludens-1 form a complex during early stages in the assembly of tight junctions. J Cell Biol 1996; 132:451-463.
91. Kniesel U, Wolburg H. Tight junctions of the blood-brain barrier. Cell Mol Neurobiol 2000; 20:57-76.
92. Itoh M, Nagafuchi A, Moroi S et al. Involvement of ZO-1 in cadherin-based cell adhesion through its direct binding to α-catenin and actin filaments. J Cell Biol 1997; 138:181-192.
93. Muller SL et al. The tight junction protein occludin and the adherens junction protein α-catenin share a common interaction mechanism with ZO-1. J Biol Chem 2005; 280:3747-3756.
94. Thompson H, McNiven M. Dynamin: Switch or pinchase? Curr Biol 2001; 11:R850.
95. Cao H et al. Cortactin is a component of clathrin-coated pits and participates in receptor-mediated endocytosis. Mol Cell Biol 2003; 23:2162-2170.
96. Li MWM et al. Tumor necrosis factor α reversibly disrupts the blood-testis barrier and impairs Sertoli-germ cell adhesion in the seminiferous epithelium of adult rat testes. J Endocrinol 2006; 190:313-329.
97. Lui WY, Lee WM, Cheng CY. Transforming growth factor β3 regulates the dynamics of Sertoli cell tight junctions via the p38 mitogen-activated protein kinase pathway. Biol Reprod 2003; 68:1597-1612.
98. Lui WY, Lee WM, Cheng CY. Transforming growth factor-β3 perturbs the inter-Sertoli tight junction permeability barrier in vitro possibly mediated via its effects on occludin, zonula occludens-1, and claudin-11. Endocrinology 2001; 142:1865-1877.
99. Wong CH, Mruk DD, Siu MKY et al. Blood-testis barrier dynamics are regulated by α_2-macroglobulin via the c-Jun N-terminal protein kinase pathway. Endocrinology 2005; 146:1893-1908.
100. Mruk DD et al. Role of tissue inhibitor of metalloproteases-1 in junction dynamics in the testis. J Androl 2003; 24:510-523.
101. Nowak D, Krawczenko A, Dus D et al. Actin in human colon adenocarcinoma cells with different metastatic potential. Acta Biochem Pol 2002; 49:823-828.
102. Balzac F et al. E-cadherin endocytosis regulates the activity of Rap1: A traffic light GTPase at the crossroads between cadherin and integrin function. J Cell Sci 2005; 118:4765-4783.
103. Ohno S. Intercellular junctions and cellular polarity: The PAR-aPKC complex, a conserved core cassette playing fundamental roles in cell polarity. Curr Opin Cell Biol 2001; 13:641-648.
104. Takekuni K et al. Direct binding of cell polarity protein PAR-3 to cell-cell adhesion molecule nectin at neuroepithelial cells of developing mouse. J Biol Chem 2003; 278:5497-5500.
105. Ozaki-Kuroda K et al. Nectin couples cell-cell adhesion and the actin scaffold at heterotypic testicular junctions. Curr Biol 2002; 12:1145-1150.
106. Reymond N, Garrido-Urbani S, Borg J et al. PICK-1: A scaffold protein that interacts with nectins and JAMs at cell junctions. FEBS Lett 2005; 579:2243-2249.
107. Singh D, Solan JL, Taffet SM et al. Connexin 43 interacts with Zona Occludens-1 and -2 proteins in a cell cycle stage-specific manner. J Biol Chem 2005; 280:30416-30421.
108. Hunter AW, Barker RJ, Zhu C et al. ZO-1 alters connexin 43 gap junction size and organization by influencing channel accretion. Mol Biol Cell 2005; 16:5686-5698.

109. Wei C, Francis R, Xu X et al. Connexin43 associated with an N-cadherin-containing multiprotein complex is required for gap junction formation in NIH3T3 cells. J Biol Chem 2005; 280:19925-19936.
110. Vogl AW, Vaid KS, Guttman JA. The Sertoli cell cytoskeleton. In: Cheng CY, ed. Molecular Mechanisms in Spermatogenesis. Austin: Landes Bioscience, 2007.
111. Yan HHN, Cheng CY. Laminin α3 forms a complex with β3 and γ3 chains that serves as the ligand for α6β1-integrin at the apical ectoplasmic specialization in adult rat testes. J Biol Chem 2006; 281:17286-17303.
112. Cyr DG et al. Cellular immunolocalization of occludin during embryonic and postnatal development of the mouse testis and epididymis. Endocrinology 1999; 140:3815-3825.
113. Green KJ, Bohringer M, Gocken T et al. Intermediate filament associated proteins. Adv Protein Chem 2005; 70:143-202.
114. Beall SA, Boekelheide K, Johnson KJ. Hybrid GPCR/cadherin (Celsr) proteins in rat testis are expressed with cell type specificity and exhibit differential Sertoli cell-germ cell adhesion activity. J Androl 2005; 26:529-538.
115. Inagaki M et al. Roles of cell-adhesion molecules nectin 1 and nectin 3 in ciliary body development. Development 2005; 132:1525-1537.
116. Pointis G, Segretain D. Role of connexin-based gap junction channels in testis. Trends Endocrinol Metab 2005; 16:300-306.
117. Terada N et al. Immunohistochemical study of a membrane skeletal molecule, protein 4.1G, in mouse seminiferous tubules. Histochem Cell Biol 2005; 124:303-311.
118. Yin T, Green KJ. Regulation of desmosome assembly and adhesion. Semin. Cell Dev Biol 2004; 15:665-677.
119. Britt DE et al. Identification of a novel protein, LYRIC, localized to tight junctions of polarized epithelial cells. Exp Cell Res 2004; 300; 134-148.
120. Bart J et al. The distribution of drug-efflux pumps, P-gp, BCRP, MRP1 and MRP2, in the normal blood-testis barrier and in primary testicular tumours. Eur J Cancer 2004; 40:2064-2070.
121. Terada N et al. Immunohistochemical study of protein 4.1B in the normal and W/W^{v} mouse seminiferous epithelium. J Histochem Cytochem 2004; 52:769-777.
122. Whittock NV, Bower C. Genetic evidence for a novel human desmosomal cadherin, desmoglein 4. J Invest Dermatol 2002; 120:523-530.
123. Ikenouchi J et al. Tricellulin constitutes a novel barrier at tricellular contacts of epithelial cells. J Cell Biol 2005; 171:939-945.

Chapter 14

The Role of the Leydig Cell in Spermatogenic Function

Renshan Ge, Guorong Chen and Matthew P. Hardy*

Introduction

Two anatomically distinct compartments, respectively, the interstitium where Leydig cells reside and the seminiferous tubules contribute the major functions of the testis, testosterone secretion and sperm production. This structural partitioning is achieved by peritubular myoid cells, which surround the seminiferous tubules. Despite the anatomic separation of the two compartments, they are functionally coupled by endocrine and paracrine inter-communication. For example, the testosterone secreted by Leydig cells under the stimulus of luteinizing hormone (LH), diffuses into seminiferous tubules and drives spermatogenesis together with another gonadotropic hormone, follicle-stimulating hormone (FSH). This dependency of the seminiferous epithelium on testosterone illustrates the significance of the Leydig cell in spermatogenesis.

Leydig cells are polygonal in shape and are the major cell type within the interstitium where they are often found adjacent to blood vessels and the seminiferous tubules.[1] In addition to Leydig cells, other cell types such as fibroblasts, macrophages and small numbers of mast cells are also present in the interstitial space.[2] The Leydig cell is the principal source for the testosterone in systemic circulation in males. In rodents, there are two generations of Leydig cells, fetal and adult, and in humans, there is a middle generation of neonatal Leydig cells.[3] The first generation is designated as fetal not because of a functional immaturity but rather due to its embryonic origin (see ref. 4, for review). Fetal Leydig cells originate from stem cells in embryo that have yet to be identified, and go on to become fully competent in androgen synthesis prior to birth, leading to fetal masculinization (see ref. 5 for review). Fetal Leydig cells remain in the testis after birth but do not proliferate or contribute significantly to androgen levels thereafter, and are gradually lost from the testis by attrition.[6] The next generation (in the rodent) referred to as the adult Leydig cells forms during pubertal development. Adult Leydig cells are not derived from preexisting fetal Leydig cells but from undifferentiated stem cells that are present in the interstitium. Conceptually, development of adult Leydig cells can be divided into four stages: stem, progenitor, immature and adult Leydig cell, according to their morphological and biochemical characteristics.[7-9] Stem Leydig cells are spindle-shaped and do not express Leydig cell markers such as LH receptor and steroidogenic enzyme proteins.[8,9] However, given their status as stem cells, they are capable of self-renewal and commitment to differentiation into progenitor Leydig cells. Progenitor Leydig cells, which are also spindle-shaped have a low capacity for steroidogenesis and mainly produce androsterone.[7,10-12] Progenitor develop into

*Corresponding Author: Matthew P. Hardy—Population Council and The Rockefeller University, 1230 York Avenue, New York, NY 10021, USA.
Email: m-hardy@popcbr.rockefeller.edu

Molecular Mechanisms in Spermatogenesis, edited by C. Yan Cheng. ©2008 Landes Bioscience and Springer Science+Business Media.

immature Leydig cells which are round and have a well-developed smooth endoplasmic reticulum and abundant cytoplasmic lipid droplets.[13] Immature Leydig cells secrete 5α reduced androgens and primarily 5α-androstane-3α, 17β-diol (3αDIOL) and 5α-androstane-3β, 17β-diol (3βDIOL).[10,14] Immature Leydig cells ultimately develop into adult Leydig cells at the completion of puberty, whereupon testosterone is the predominant androgen end product.[10] The pubertal rise in testosterone levels and initiation of spermatogenesis are coincident and interdependent, as will be discussed in this review.

Abbreviations

Genes: CYP11A1, cytochrome P450 cholesterol side-chain cleavage enzyme; CYP17A, cytochrome P450 17α-hydroxylase/$C_{17\text{-}20}$-lyase; HSD3B2, 3β-hydroxysteroid dehydrogenase 2; HSD17B3, 17β-hydroxysteroid dehydrogenase 3; Gnrh, gonadotrophin releasing hormone; Lhcgr, luteinizing hormone receptor; ESR1, estrogen receptor α; CYP19A1, cytochrome P450 aromatase; ESR2, estrogen receptor β.

Proteins: LH, luteinizing hormone; FSH, follicle stimulating hormone; $P450_{c17}$, cytochrome P450 17α-hydroxylase/$C_{17\text{-}20}$-lyase; $P450_{scc}$, cytochrome P450 cholesterol side-chain cleavage enzyme; StAR, Steroidogenic acute regulatory protein; PBR, peripheral-type benzodiazepine receptor; 3β-HSD, 3β-hydroxysteroid dehydrogenase; 17βHSD3, 17β-hydroxysteroid dehydrogenase 3; $P450_{arom}$, cytochrome P450 aromatase; GnRH, gonadotrophin releasing hormone; 3α-HSD, 3α-hydroxysteroid dehydrogenase; hCG, human chorionic gonadotropin; INSL3, Insulin-like protein 3.

Chemicals: T, testosterone; 3αDIOL, 5α-androstane-3α, 17b-diol; 3βDIOL, 5a-androstane-3β, 17β-diol; E_2, estradiol.

Androgen and Spermatogenesis

Testosterone Biosynthesis

Leydig cells have a cyto-architecture that is typical for a steroid secreting cell, in that they possess an abundant smooth endoplasmic reticulum and numerous mitochondria, which have tubular cristae. They are able to synthesize cholesterol from acetate or to take up this substrate for steroidogenesis from lipoproteins present in circulation.[15] The cytochrome P450 17α-hydroxylase/$C_{17\text{-}20}$-lyase ($P450_{c17}$) enzyme, which catalyzes later steps in testosterone biosynthesis may be active in cholesterol synthesis, because it has recently been shown to exhibit squalene epoxidase activity.[15] The movement of cholesterol to the inner mitochondrial membrane, the location of the cholesterol side-chain cleavage enzyme ($P450_{scc}$), is the rate-limiting step of androgen synthesis. Transport of cholesterol is acutely regulated by LH and occurs in two steps: mobilization of cholesterol from cellular stores such as lipid droplets or the plasma membrane to the outer mitochondrial membrane and then the transfer of cholesterol from the outer to the inner mitochondria membranes.[16] Steroidogenic acute regulatory (StAR) protein has been viewed as indispensable in the second phase of this process.[17] StAR is expressed in steroidogenic tissues in response to agents that stimulate steroid production, and mutations in the StAR gene result in steroidogenic failure such as occur in the disease of congenital lipoid adrenal hyperplasia. The mechanism by which StAR mediates cholesterol transfer in the mitochondria has not been fully characterized.[18] Another mitochondrial protein, peripheral-type benzodiazepine receptor (PBR), has been shown to be involved in intra-mitochondrial transport of cholesterol.[19] Further research will be necessary to establish a definitive mechanism of cholesterol transport, but it may be that the function of StAR is convey cholesterol to PBR, which in turn forms a pore from the external face in the outer mitochondrial membrane for its internal conveyance.

P450scc is located on the matrix (or internal) side of the inner mitochondrial membrane. The side-chain cleavage reaction uses three molecules of oxygen and three molecules of

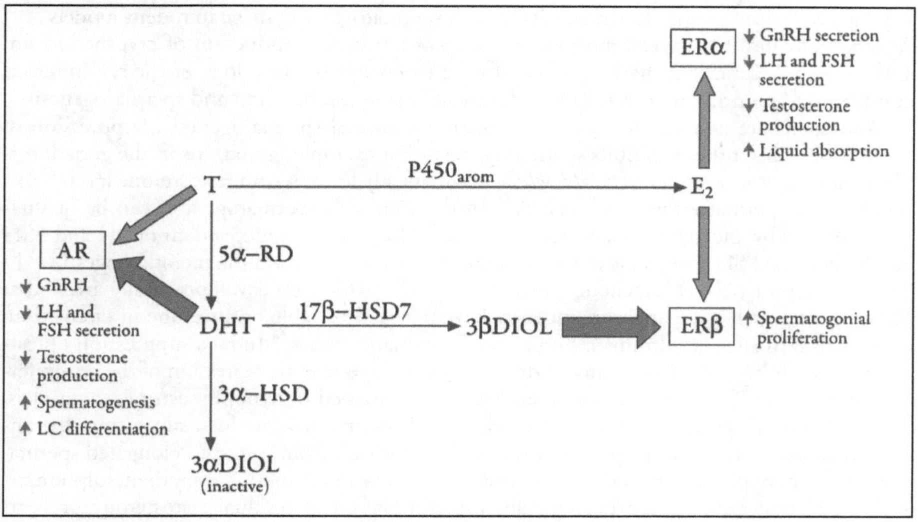

Figure 1. Physiological actions of testosterone (T) and its metabolites on the male reproductive axis. T and its 5α-reduced metabolite, DHT, bind to the androgen receptor (AR) thereby exerting androgen action. The $P450_{arom}$ metabolite of T, E_2, binds either ERα or ERβ causing estrogenic activity. The metabolite of DHT formed by 17β-HSD7, 3βDIOL, binds to ERβ with downstream effects in spermatogonia. The metabolite of DHT formed by 3α-HSD, 3αDIOL, is inactive. The thin dark arrows depict the catalytic direction of each steroidogenic enzyme. The blue thicker arrows show the interaction between steroid hormone and receptors (the widths of these arrows represent the biopotency of the ligand receptor complex). The green small arrows represent the stimulatory action, and the red small arrows show the inhibitory action. A color version of this figure is available online at www.eurekah.com.

NADPH and a mitochondrial electron transfer system resulting in the formation of pregnenolone.[20] The enzymes required for subsequent steps of steroidogenesis are located in the smooth endoplasmic reticulum (SER) membranes in the cytoplasm. The bulk of the pregnenolone formed in the mitochondrion diffuses into the SER and serves as a substrate for progesterone synthesis by the 3β-hydroxysteroid dehydrogenase (3β-HSD) enzyme. However, recent evidence shows that once pregnenolone is formed, it may be converted within the mitochondria to progesterone by a mitochondrial form of the enzyme 3β-HSD.[21] Although multiple isoforms of 3β-HSD have been identified, the testicular 3β-HSD is coded by type I and II 3β-HSD gene (*HSD3b2*).[22] Once formed progesterone is converted by P450c17 into androstenedione by two steps: 17α-hydroxylation and C17-C20 cleavage.[23,24] In the human, the gene for P450c17, *CYP17A*, is located on chromosome 10.[25] The final step of androgen synthesis, conversion of androstenedione into testosterone is catalyzed by 17β-hydroxysteroid dehydrogenase (17β-HSD). There are multiple isoforms of 17β-HSD, and the testicular isoform is type III 17β-HSD (17β-HSD3), coded by 17β-HSD3 gene (*hsd17b3*).[26] Testosterone either associates with androgen binding protein and moves into the seminiferous tubule lumen to regulate spermatogenesis or is further metabolized into different steroids, some of which are more biologically active such as dihydrotestosterone in reactions catalyzed by types 1 and 2 5α-reductase (Fig. 1).

Androgen and Spermatogenesis

Spermatogenic dysfunction is often associated with impaired Leydig cell dysfunction. Between 12 and 15% of men with diminished spermatogenesis have lower testosterone levels.[27]

Leydig cell dysfunction is clearly associated with spermatogenic damage in rodent models.[28,29] Agents that cause Leydig cell dysfunction, such as irradiation, induction of cryptorchidism, and vitamin A deficiency, have also been found to disrupt the histology of the seminiferous epithelium,[29] pointing to a clear linkage between Leydig cell function and spermatogenesis.

Androgens are essential for the maintenance of normal spermatogenesis. Suppression of testosterone biosynthesis inhibits spermatogenesis. For example, mutations in the gonadotrophin releasing hormone gene (*Gnrhhpg/hpg*) dramatically lower serum testosterone levels[30] to a point where spermatogenesis is blocked.[31] In these animals spermatogenesis can be qualitatively rescued by androgen replacement therapy.[30] This rescue is independent of LH and FSH action, because FSH alone fails to promote spermatogenesis beyond the meiotic stages.[32,33] In the LH receptor (*Lhcgr*) knockout mouse Leydig cells, which are developmentally arrested at the progenitor cell stage and consequently have barely detectable testosterone in circulation, exogenous testosterone administration restores spermatogenesis.[34] In rats, suppression of testosterone levels by hypophysectomy leads to an acute, stage-specific regression of the seminiferous epithelium.[35-37] If testosterone levels are not maintained in hypophysectomized animals, mid-stage round spermatids and mature, elongated spermatozoa are lost, suggesting that androgen action is involved in spermiation and the transition from round to elongated spermatids. When hypophysectomized rats are treated further with ethane 1,2-dimethanesulphonate, a chemical that destroys the Leydig cells, the elimination of residual testosterone prevents spermatogenesis from proceeding beyond meiosis.[36,38]

Intratesticular levels of testosterone are very high compared to blood and the question arises as to how much testosterone is required for maintenance of spermatogenesis. Spermatogenesis is maintained, at a reduced level, when testicular concentrations are only 5% of control.[39] Suppression of FSH release induced by high dose administration of testosterone or estradiol (E_2), or by anti-LH or -GnRH immunization, lowers intratesticular testosterone levels to 20% to 40% of normal while allowing spermatogenesis to proceed in a quantitatively normal manner.[40,41] Recently, it has been shown that intratesticular testosterone levels as low as 2% of normal are compatible with the continuation of spermatogenesis in LH receptor knockout mice.[42]

Stimulation by androgen is a prerequisite for the differentiation of germ cells. However, evidence also points to a negative regulation of spermatogonial stem cells by androgen. Testosterone inhibits spermatogonial proliferation and differentiation, and this can be reversed by the androgen receptor antagonist flutamide.[43,44] A similar phenomenon has been observed in juvenile spermatogonial depletion (*jsd*) mice, in which germ cells regress to a spermatogonia-only phenotype following the first wave of spermatogenesis. Treatments that oppose androgen action, such as GnRH antagonist or flutamide administration, stimulate proliferation and differentiation of spermatogonia.[45] The inhibition of spermatogonial differentiation by testosterone in jsd mutant mice is achieved only at the normal scrotal temperature.[46]

Androgen Receptor-Mediated Regulation of Spermatogenesis

Testosterone binds to the androgen receptor thereby initiating nuclear translocation of the ligand-bound receptor complex and the regulatory functions of the androgen receptor in modulating gene transcription.[47] Spermatogenesis is dependent on a constant level of androgen receptor mediated activity, seen by the fact that a null mutation in the X chromosome-linked gene that encodes the androgen receptor causes complete Androgen Insensitivity Syndrome (AIS) in both humans and mice, with consequent small, abdominally positioned testes and spermatogenic blockade early in meiosis.[48,49] In the testis, the androgen receptor is expressed in somatic cells including Leydig, myoid, and Sertoli cells[50,51] and, in human males, in spermatogonia.[51-53] Immunocytochemical localization studies of rat testes had placed androgen receptor expression in spermatogonia, but direct androgen action on these cells is apparently not a requirement for fertility: androgen receptor null germ cells have the capacity to form sperm when transplanted into the testes of wild type males.[54,55]

A role for androgen receptor-mediated activity is seen in Leydig cells where it is to promote maturation of the steroidogenic pathway. In rodents it has been observed that Leydig cells do complete differentiation both in the naturally occurring androgen receptor loss-of-function, testicular feminization mutant and in conditional knockout mice in which androgen receptor expression is selectively deleted in Leydig cells.[56,57] Due to the reduction of androgen action on the Leydig cell, testosterone production is sharply reduced in these animals, which causes an arrest of spermatogenesis.

Sertoli cells are the only somatic cell type in the testis that is in direct contact with differentiating germ cells. Testosterone withdrawal causes retention of mature spermatids and premature release of round spermatids,[35,37,58,59] and this led to the general postulate that Sertoli cells are the primary mediators of androgen receptor-mediated regulation of spermatogenesis. The androgen receptor is expressed in a stage-specific manner in Sertoli cells as a function of the seminiferous cycle,[50,60] which can be maintained (in the absence of gonadotropic stimulation) by administration of exogenous androgen. Androgen receptor expression in Sertoli cells is highest at stages VII-VIII.[35,37] Upstream of the androgen receptor gene is an androgen response element.[61]

Results of the selective knockout of androgen receptor expression in Sertoli cells[62-64] suggest the existence of multiple androgen receptor-dependent steps in spermatogenesis. While there is no apparent defect in meiosis, the germ cells are defective in making the transition from round to elongating spermatids. A requirement for androgen receptor activity in Sertoli cells exists at three points: (A) progression through meiosis I; (B) transition from the round to elongating spermatid; and (C) in the terminal phases of spermatogenesis (spermiogenesis). Androgen action is evidently not needed for passage of the germ cell through meiosis.[62-64]

Other Leydig Cell-Derived Biologically Active Steroids and Spermatogenesis

Estrogen

Testosterone can be considered a prohormone that is converted in target tissues into the more potent androgen, dihydrotestosterone. In addition, however, testosterone can be metabolized into other active steroids including estrogens. It has long been known that estrogens affect spermatogenesis (see ref. 65 for review). More recently, it has been established that both estrogen receptor α (*ESR1*)[66] and aromatase[67] knockout mice are infertile. Moreover, the presence of both estrogen receptor (ER) α and β isotypes in the male reproductive tract[65] indicates the importance of estrogen action in male reproduction. E_2 is believed to be the endogenous ligand of both ER isotypes, and has the same affinity in each case. Other ligands exhibit selectivity in ER binding. For example, one of the endogenous metabolites of androgen, 3βDIOL, binds ERβ with higher affinity compared to E_2,[68] and must therefore be considered as an estrogen.

Testosterone is metabolized to E_2 via the microsomal P450 aromatase (P450arom), which is encoded by the *CYP19A1* gene. The P450arom reaction uses three molecules of oxygen and three molecules of NADPH for every molecule of testosterone catalyzed.[69] *CYP19A1* has an age-dependent pattern of expression in the testis. In prepubertal and immature testis, Sertoli cells are the major sources of estradiol, whereas localization in Leydig cells becomes predominant as animals mature.[70,71] LH stimulates the formation of E_2 form in Leydig cells.[72] *CYP19A1* mRNA and activity is also found in germ cells from the pachytene spermatocyte stage to round spermatids.[73-77] P450arom also is higher in mature spermatids than in earlier stage germ cells.[73,78]

Thirty years ago, it was noted that 3βDIOL is an estrogenic metabolite of dihydrotestosterone.[79] The synthesis of 3βDIOL from dihydrotestosterone is catalyzed by 17β-hydroxysteroid dehydrogenase 7 (17β-HSD7) (Fig. 1), with the enzyme functioning in this instance as a 3β-HSD.[80] During the puberty, when Leydig cells are still immature, they express higher levels of 5α reductase and 3α-hydroxysteroid dehydrogenase (3α-HSD) and 17β-HSD7, and expression of these enzymes declines significantly with the transition to adulthood.[10] From postnatal days 10 to 20, 3αDIOL is the major metabolite released from the testes, and later on 3βDIOL secretion becomes predominant.[81] In the human testis, metabolism of testosterone to 5α-reduced products is also notable prior to puberty and, in contrast to rats, 3βDIOL is the major end product.

Estrogens and Spermatogenesis

In instances where spermatogenesis is inhibited and testosterone levels are lowered, estrogen levels are typically elevated.[82] A subset of male infertility patients has been described that have an endocrinopathic increase in serum E_2 concentrations.[27] The change in estradiol activity can often be detected as an abnormally low testosterone to estradiol (T: E_2) ratio, which is considered indicative of increased aromatase activity. It appears that either LH or human chorionic gonadotropin (hCG) can stimulate increased P450arom activity levels in Leydig cells, implicating overexposure to gonadotropin as a factor in abnormally high T: E2 ratios. Local synthesis of E_2 in the Leydig cell blocks steroidogenesis at the P450c17. Men that have spermatogenic failure in association with an increased T: E2 ratio can be treated with P450arom inhibitors thereby improving their fertility status. There is, however, limited direct evidence that estrogen directly disrupts spermatogenesis (reviewed in ref. 65). Indeed, at the low concentration at which it is normally present in the male, estrogen may be physiologically beneficial for spermatogenesis. Consistent with this hypothesis the knockout of P450arom in mice (ArKO), causes an arrest at the round spermatid stage.[67] Similarly, mice lacking *ESR1*[66,83-86] and *CYP19A1*[67,87] expression all have fertility problems. *ESR2* is widely expressed in the male reproductive tract but has yet to be assigned a functional role in spermatogenesis.[88-92] Male mice with an *ESR2* knockout are fertile, but this does not exclude the possibility that ERβ-mediated signaling is involved in spermatogenesis. In this regard it has been noted that E2 stimulates proliferation of spermatogonia.[93] The positive and negative aspects of estradiol's effects on the testis must be taken into consideration when considering the impact of environmental estrogens on male reproductive health. Exposures of laboratory animals and wildlife to high levels of estrogenic chemicals including industrial chemicals such as pesticides (e.g., DDT, methoxychor), industrial chemicals (e.g., DES, tamoxifen) and phytoestrogens (e.g., genisterin) resulted in a number of abnormalities, including reduced gonad size, feminization of genetic males, and low sperm count and quality.[94-96] For example, estrogen administration during the neonatal period or adulthood can impair the production and maturation of sperm.[97,98]

Estrogen Receptor-Mediated Regulation of Spermatogenesis

Throughout postnatal development, ERα is mainly expressed in Leydig cells and is not present in the seminiferous tubules.[99-101] In rodents, ERα is abundantly expressed in the rete testis,[101] efferent ductules[99,101] and epididymis.[99-101] It remains unclear whether ERα is expressed in sperm. There are no reports of ERα localization in rodent and human germ cells with the exception of a single study reporting its presence in rat spermatocytes and spermatids.[102] ERβ is present at relatively low levels in spermatogonia[92,103] and immature Sertoli cells[92,103] relative to ERα. By day 21, ERβ is abundantly expressed in pachytene spermatocytes[92] but not in other germ cells.[103] In the mouse, ERβ is also specifically immunolocalized to the spermatocytes by day 12, but decreases to the undetectable level by day 26.[104] ERβ expression is also seen in the epididymis from day 21 onward.[104,105] Localization runs from the efferent ducts to the epididymis in the mouse[106,107] and rat.[85,100] In adult males of certain species, mouse, primate and human,[102,107-109] Leydig cells are observed to express ERβ, although other reports put this in dispute.[91,110] Expression of ERβ in rat, monkey and human spermatogonia[103,108,109,111] appears to be established. It is unclear whether ERβ remains present at later stages of sperm differentiation and further exploration of differences between species will need additional investigation.[92,103,108,110,112,113]

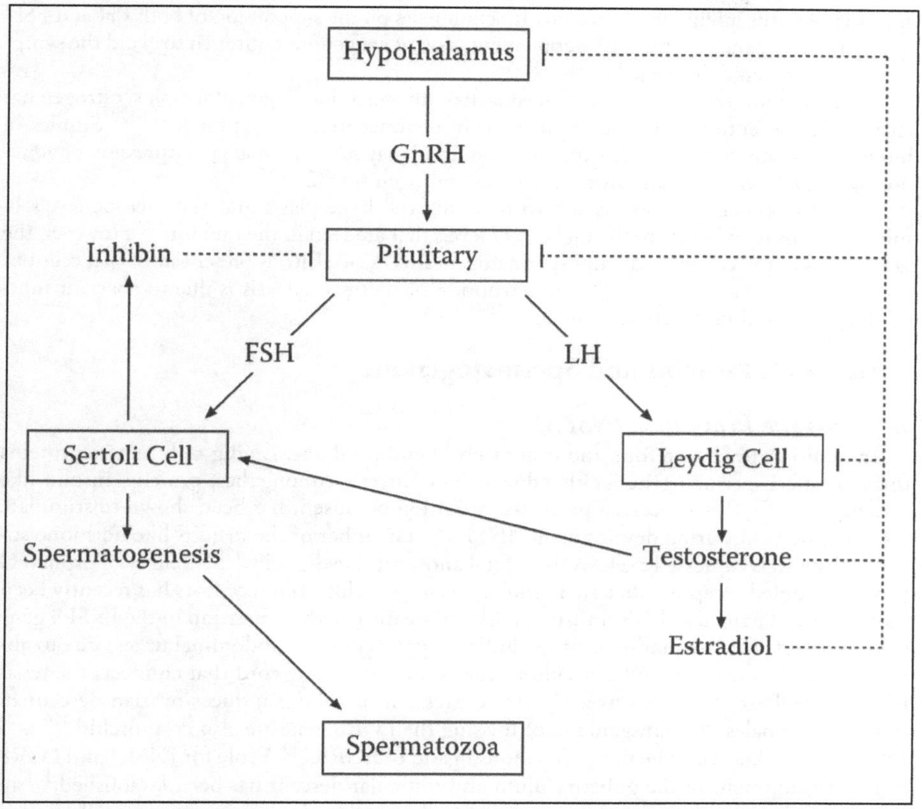

Figure 2. Stimulatory (—) and inhibitory (---) pathways exploited in male hormonal contraception. Testosterone and its metabolite estradiol exert negative feedback inhibition on the hypothalamic-pituitary axis. Based on the negative feedback, androgens alone or in combination with other sex steroids have been developed to suppress spermatogenesis.

E_2 is thought to be the natural ligand of both ERα and β. Receptor binding analyses have shown that 3βDIOL can activate both ERα and ERβ with a Kd of 1.9×10^{-8} M, and that it has a negligible affinity for the androgen receptor.[114] Other studies have shown that 3βDIOL may have a much higher potency when bound to ERβ, as measured by transcriptional activation, relative to ERα.[115]

The Leydig Cell as Target for Hormonal Contraception

The hypothalamus secretes gonadotropin-releasing hormone (GnRH), which is transported to pituitary where it stimulates gonadotropins secretion (LH and FSH). LH and FSH are required to initiate and maintain spermatogenesis. Testosterone secreted by Leydig cells has a negative feedback effect on the hypothalamus and the pituitary inhibiting LH and FSH secretion (Fig. 2). In humans, the negative feedback of testosterone on the hypothalamic-pituitary axis serves to inhibit secretion of both LH and FSH, which is the basis for the current hormonal approach to male contraception (Fig. 2).[116] In mice, selective immuno-vaccination against LH receptor leads to the suppression of fertility in about 60% of treated mice.[117] Administration of an antiserum against LH (passive immunization) disrupts spermatogenesis in rats.[118] However, it is increasingly clear that inactivation of Leydig cell testosterone production will not be sufficient to suppress spermatogenesis. The current approach towards inhibition of testicular function relies on the suppression of both LH and FSH secretion and in parallel, often with supplementation of exogenous androgen to avoid the symptoms of androgen deficiency.[119]

Of the steroids that exert negative feedback on the secretion of gonadotropins, estrogen has received less attention from the stand point of contraceptive development.[120-122] Studies in humans have shown that administration of estradiol may further enhance suppression of gonadotropin levels when coadministered with an androgen (Fig. 2).[116]

The ERα knockout is associated with Leydig cell hyperplasia and testosterone levels in mice, and this may be due to the higher LH levels that are seen in the mutant.[123] However, the same knockout is known to disrupt spermatogenesis.[84] Since ERα is present in Leydig cells but not in seminiferous tubules,[99-101] the disruption of spermatogenesis is due to aberrant morphology observed in the efferent ductules.[124]

Leydig Cell Proteins and Spermatogenesis

Insulin-Like Protein 3 (INSL3)

In addition to testosterone and other steroid end products, Leydig cells secrete proteins that may affect spermatogenesis either directly or indirectly. Among these proteins, insulin-like protein 3 (INSL3) has received particular attention because it has been shown to stimulate testicular descent during development. INSL3 is a member of the insulin-like hormone superfamily and is expressed exclusively in fetal and adult Leydig cells.[125] A family of orphan G protein-coupled receptors that are homologous to gonadotropin receptors has recently been identified and named as LGR 4 through 8.[126] Male mice with a mutation in the INSL3 gene exhibit defects in testicular descent, including cryptorchidism (abdominal testes) due to abnormal development the gubernaculum (the connective tissue cord that connects the testis to the scrotal sac).[127,128] Conversely, overexpression of INSL3 induces ovarian descent in transgenic females.[129] Transgenic mice missing the LGR8 gene are also cryptorchid,[126] and INSL3 is now known to be the endogenous ligand of LGR8.[130] A role for INSL3 and LGR8 in the development of the gubernaculum and testicular descent has been established,[131] in that disruption of either gene causes cryptorchidism and leads to spermatogenic failure (due to the lowering of intratesticular testosterone levels, in combination with the increased temperature of the testis).[127,128] Fetal and adult Leydig cells are the chief source of circulating, and the serum concentration of INSL3 can even serve as an index of the functional status of Leydig cell steroidogenic capacity.[132] The gubernaculum is the main site of LGR8 expression, but this protein is also localized to Leydig cells and germ cells. In germ cells the binding of INSL3 to LGR8 prevents apoptosis, but the function of the LGR8 pathway in Leydig cells awaits elucidation.

Oxytocin

Leydig cells produce and secrete oxytocin, as do (to a lesser extent) epididymis epithelial cells.[133] Oxytocin produced in Leydig cells is regulated by LH.[134] Oxytocin stimulates testosterone production.[135] It has been suggested that the function of testicular oxytocin is to stimulate contraction of the peritubular myoid cells that surround the seminiferous tubules, moving spermiated sperm to efferent ducts.[136] Oxytocin receptors are located in Leydig cells[137,138] and Sertoli cells[138] and peritubular myoid cells.[139]

Summary

Testosterone is the most well known of the products synthesized and secreted by Leydig cells and that have a defined involvement in the regulation of spermatogenesis. However, the Leydig cell is the main source of testicular estrogen and estrogen action has both positive and negative effects on spermatogenesis that can no longer be ignored. In addition, two protein

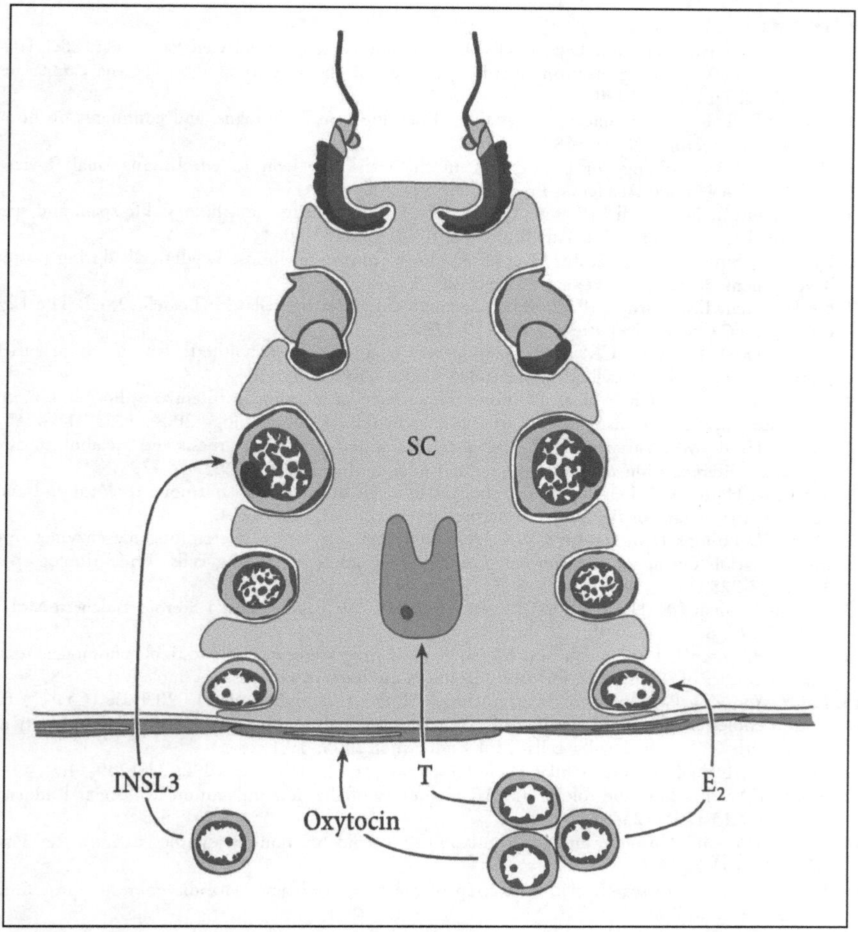

Figure 3. Leydig cell factors that play an important role in spermatogenic function. Leydig cells synthesize and secrete testosterone (T), which diffuses into Sertoli cells (SCs) and binds its receptor androgen receptors (ARs) and the T-AR complex then enters into the SC nucleus to induce transcription of AR targeted genes, promoting spermatogenesis. Leydig cells also produce E_2 via $P450_{arom}$, which binds ERβ to stimulate the proliferation of spermatogonia. Leydig cells have recently been shown to express several proteins, such as insulin-like protein 3 (INSL3) and oxytocin, the former binding to LGR8 to promote sperm meiosis and the latter may stimulate peritubular myoid cells to contract, moving sperm to the excurrent ducts.

products of the Leydig cell—INSL3 and oxytocin—influence spermatogenic function by stimulating, respectively, testis descent and movement of mature sperm to the excurrent ducts (Fig. 3).

Acknowledgements

We thank Dr. Dianne Hardy for comments on the manuscript, and Evan Read for the preparation of figures. This work was supported in part by NIH R01 grants HD33000, HD32588 and ES010233.

References

1. Schulze C. Sertoli cells and Leydig cells in man. Adv Anat Embryol Cell Biol 1984; 88:1-104.
2. Connell CJ. A scanning electron microscope study of the interstitial tissue of the canine testis. Anat Rec 1976; 185:389-401.
3. Prince FP. The triphasic nature of Leydig cell development in humans, and comments on nomenclature. J Endocrinol 2001; 168:213-6.
4. Haider SG. Cell biology of Leydig cells in the testis. In: Jeon K, ed. International Review of Cytology. New York: Academic Press, 2004:181-241.
5. Huhtaniemi I, Pelliniemi LJF et al. Leydig cells: Cellular origin, morphology, life span, and special functional features. Proc Soc Exp Biol Med 1992; 201:125-40.
6. Faria MJ, Simoes ZL, Lunardi LO et al. Apoptosis process in mouse Leydig cells during postnatal development. Microsc Microanal 2003; 9:68-73.
7. Ge RS, Shan LX, Hardy MP. Pubertal development of leydig cells. In: Lussell D, ed. The Leydig cell. Vienna: Cache River Press, 1996:159-173.
8. Ge RS, Dong Q, Sottas CM et al. Development of androgen biocynthetic capacity in an enriched fraction of stem Leydig cells. Bio Reprod (Quebec City) 2005; 104.
9. Lo KC, Lei Z, Rao Ch V et al. De novo testosterone production in luteinizing hormone receptor knockout mice after transplantation of leydig stem cells. Endocrinology 2004; 145:4011-4015.
10. Ge RS, Hardy MP. Variation in the end products of androgen biosynthesis and metabolism during postnatal differentiation of rat Leydig cells. Endocrinology 1998; 139:3787-3795.
11. Shan LX, Hardy MP. Developmental changes in levels of luteinizing hormone receptor and androgen receptor in rat Leydig cells. Endocrinology 1992; 131:1107-1114.
12. Shan LX, Phillips DM, Bardin CW et al. Differential regulation of steroidogenic enzymes during differentiation optimizes testosterone production by adult rat Leydig cells. Endocrinology 1993; 133:2277-2283.
13. Benton L, Shan LX, Hardy MP. Differentiation of adult Leydig cells. J Steroid Biochem Mol Biol 1995; 53:61-8.
14. Coffey JC, French FS, Nayfeh SN. Metabolism of progesterone by rat testicular homogenates. IV. Further studies of testosterone formation in immature testis in vitro. Endocrinology 1971; 89:865-72.
15. Liu Y, Yao ZX, Papadopoulos V. Cytochrome P450 17α hydroxylase/17,20 lyase (CYP17) function in cholesterol biosynthesis: Identification of squalene monooxygenase (epoxidase) activity associated with CYP17 in Leydig cells. Mol Endocrinol 2005; 19:1918-31.
16. Liscum L, Dahl NK. Intracellular cholesterol transport. J Lipid Res 1992; 33:1239-54.
17. Stocco DM. Tracking the role of a StAR in the sky of the new millenium. Molecular Endocrinology 2001; 15:1245-1254.
18. Stocco DM. StAR protein and the regulation of steroid hormone biosynthesis. Annu Rev Physiol 2001; 63:193-213.
19. Papadopoulos V. In search of the function of the peripheral-type benzodiazepine receptor. Endocr Res 2004; 30:677-84.
20. Porter TD, Coon MJ. Cytochrome P-450. Multiplicity of isoforms, substrates, and catalytic and regulatory mechanisms. J Biol Chem 1991; 266:13469-72.
21. Cherradi N, Defaye G, Chambaz EM. Characterization of the 3 β-hydroxysteroid dehydrogenase activity associated with bovine adrenocortical mitochondria. Endocrinology 1994; 134:1358-64.
22. Lachance Y, Luu-The V, Verreault H et al. Structure of the human type II 3 α-hydroxysteroid dehydrogenase/Δ 5-Δ 4 isomerase (3 β-HSD) gene: Adrenal and gonadal specificity. DNA Cell Biol 1991; 10:701-11.
23. Nakajin S, Shively JE, Yuan PM et al. Microsomal cytochrome P-450 from neonatal pig testis: Two enzymatic activities (17 α-hydroxylase and c17,20-lyase) associated with one protein. Biochemistry 1981; 20:4037-42.
24. Nakajin S, Hall PF. Microsomal cytochrome P-450 from neonatal pig testis. Purification and properties of A C21 steroid side-chain cleavage system (17 α-hydroxylase-C17,20 lyase). J Biol Chem 1981; 256:3871-6.
25. Matteson KJ, Picado-Leonard J, Chung BC et al. Assignment of the gene for adrenal P450c17 (steroid 17 α-hydroxylase/17,20 lyase) to human chromosome 10. J Clin Endocrinol Metab 1986; 63:789-91.
26. Geissler WM, Davis DL, Wu L et al. Male pseudohermaphroditism caused by mutations of testicular 17 β-hydroxysteroid dehydrogenase 3. Nat Genet 1994; 7:34-9.
27. Andersson AM, Jorgensen N, Frydelund-Larsen L et al. Impaired Leydig cell function in infertile men: A study of 357 idiopathic infertile men and 318 proven fertile controls. J Clin Endocrinol Metab 2004; 89:3161-7.

28. Rich KA, de Kretser DM. Effect of differing degrees of destruction of the rat seminiferous epithelium on levels of FSH and androgen binding protein. Endocrinology 1977; 101:959-974.
29. Rich KA, Kerr JB, de Kretser DM. Evidence for Leydig cell dysfunction in rats with seminiferous tubule damage. Mol Cell Endocrinol 1979; 13:123-135.
30. Singh J, O'Neill C, Handelsman DJ. Induction of spermatogenesis by androgens in gonadotropin-deficient (hpg) mice. Endocrinology 1995; 136:5311-21.
31. Cattanach BM, Iddon CA, Charlton HM et al. Gonadotrophin-releasing hormone deficiency in a mutant mouse with hypogonadism. Nature 1977; 269:338-40.
32. Singh J, Handelsman DJ. The effects of recombinant FSH on testosterone-induced spermatogenesis in gonadotrophin-deficient (hpg) mice. J Androl 1996; 17:382-93.
33. Haywood M, Spaliviero J, Jimemez M et al. Sertoli and germ cell development in hypogonadal (hpg) mice expressing transgenic follicle-stimulating hormone alone or in combination with testosterone. Endocrinology 2003; 144:509-17.
34. Lei ZM, Mishra S, Zou W et al. Targeted disruption of luteinizing hormone/human chorionic gonadotropin receptor gene. Molecular Endocrinology 2001; 15:184-200.
35. Russell LD, Clermont Y. Degeneration of germ cells in normal, hypophysectomized and hormone treated hypophysectomized rats. Anat Rec 1977; 187:347-66.
36. Kerr JB, Maddocks S, Sharpe RM. Testosterone and FSH have independent, synergistic and stage-dependent effects upon spermatogenesis in the rat testis. Cell Tissue Res 1992; 268:179-89.
37. Ghosh S, Sinha-Hikim AP, Russell LD. Further observations of stage-specific effects seen after short-term hypophysectomy in the rat. Tissue Cell 1991; 23:613-30.
38. Franca LR, Parreira GG, Gates RJ et al. Hormonal regulation of spermatogenesis in the hypophysectomized rat: Quantitation of germ-cell population and effect of elimination of residual testosterone after long-term hypophysectomy. J Androl 1998; 19:335-40.
39. Cunningham GR, Huckins C. Persistence of complete spermatogenesis in the presence of low intratesticular concentrations of testosterone. Endocrinology 1979; 105:177-86.
40. Awoniyi CA, Santulli R, Sprando RL et al. Restoration of advanced spermatogenic cells in the experimentally regressed rat testis: Quantitative relationship to testosterone concentration within the testis. Endocrinology 1989; 124:1217-1223.
41. Huang HF, Nieschlag E. Suppression of the intratesticular testosterone is associated with quantitative changes in spermatogonial populations in intact adult rats. Endocrinology 1986; 118:619-27.
42. Pakarainen T, Zhang FP, Makela S et al. Testosterone replacement therapy induces spermatogenesis and partially restores fertility in luteinizing hormone receptor knockout mice. Endocrinology 2005; 146:596-606.
43. Shetty G, Wilson G, Huhtaniemi I et al. Gonadotropin-releasing hormone analogs stimulate and testosterone inhibits the recovery of spermatogenesis in irradiated rats. Endocrinology 2000; 141:1735-45.
44. Shetty G, Wilson G, Hardy MP et al. Inhibition of recovery of spermatogenesis in irradiated rats by different androgens. Endocrinology 2002; 143:3385-96.
45. Shetty G, Wilson G, Huhtaniemi I et al. Testosterone inhibits spermatogonial differentiation in juvenile spermatogonial depletion mice. Endocrinology 2001; 142:2789-95.
46. Shetty G, Weng CC. Cryptorchidism rescues spermatogonial differentiation in juvenile spermatogonial depletion (jsd) mice. Endocrinology 2004; 145:126-33.
47. Lindzey J, Kumar MV, Grossman M et al. Molecular mechanisms of androgen action. Vitam Horm 1994; 49:383-432.
48. Lyon MF, Hawkes SG. X-linked gene for testicular feminization in the mouse. Nature 1970; 227:1217-9.
49. Vanha-Perttula T, Bardin CW, Allison JE et al. "Testicular feminization" in the rat: Morphology of the testis. Endocrinology 1970; 87:611-9.
50. Bremner WJ, Millar MR, Sharpe RM et al. Immunohistochemical localization of androgen receptors in the rat testis: Evidence for stage-dependent expression and regulation by androgens. Endocrinology 1994; 135:1227-34.
51. Vornberger W, Prins G, Musto NA et al. Androgen receptor distribution in rat testis: New implications for androgen regulation of spermatogenesis. Endocrinology 1994; 134:2307-16.
52. Kimura N, Mizokami A, Oonuma T et al. Immunocytochemical localization of androgen receptor with polyclonal antibody in paraffin-embedded human tissues. J Histochem Cytochem 1993; 41:671-8.
53. Zhou Q, Nie R, Prins GS et al. Localization of androgen and estrogen receptors in adult male mouse reproductive tract. J Androl 2002; 23:870-81.
54. Lyon MF, Glenister PH, Lamoreux ML. Normal spermatozoa from androgen-resistant germ cells of chimeric mice and the role of androgen in spermatogenesis. Nature 1975; 258:620.

55. Johnston DS, Russell LD, Friel PJ et al. Murine germ cells do not require functional androgen receptors to complete spermatogenesis following spermatogonial stem cell transplantation. Endocrinology 2001; 142:2405-8.
56. O'Shaughnessy PJ, Johnston H, Willerton L et al. Failure of normal adult Leydig cell development in androgen-receptor-deficient mice. J Cell Sci 2002; 115:3491-6.
57. Murphy L, Jeffcoate IA, O'Shaughnessy PJ. Abnormal Leydig cell development at puberty in the androgen-resistant Tfm mouse. Endocrinology 1994; 135:1372-7.
58. Kerr JB, Millar M, Maddocks S et al. Stage-dependent changes in spermatogenesis and Sertoli cells in relation to the onset of spermatogenic failure following withdrawal of testosterone. Anat Rec 1993; 235:547-59.
59. O'Donnell L, McLachlan RI, Wreford NG et al. Testosterone withdrawal promotes stage-specific detachment of round spermatids from the rat seminiferous epithelium. Biol Reprod 1996; 55:895-901.
60. Zhu LJ, Hardy MP, Inigo IV et al. Effects of androgen on androgen receptor expression in rat testicular and epididymal cells: A quantitative immunohistochemical study. Biol Reprod 2000; 63:368-76.
61. Grossmann ME, Lindzey J, Blok L et al. The mouse androgen receptor gene contains a second functional promoter which is regulated by dihydrotestosterone. Biochemistry 1994; 33:14594-600.
62. Chang C, Chen YT, Yeh SD et al. Infertility with defective spermatogenesis and hypotestosteronemia in male mice lacking the androgen receptor in Sertoli cells. Proc Natl Acad Sci USA 2004; 101:6876-81.
63. De Gendt K, Swinnen JV, Saunders PT et al. A Sertoli cell-selective knockout of the androgen receptor causes spermatogenic arrest in meiosis. Proc Natl Acad Sci USA 2004; 101:1327-32.
64. Holdcraft RW, Braun RE. Androgen receptor function is required in Sertoli cells for the terminal differentiation of haploid spermatids. Development 2004; 131:459-67.
65. O'Donnell L, Robertson KM, Jones ME et al. Estrogen and spermatogenesis. Endocr Rev 2001; 22:289-318.
66. Lubahn DB, Moyer JS, Golding TS et al. Alteration of reproductive function but not prenatal sexual development after insertional disruption of the mouse estrogen receptor gene. Proc Natl Acad Sci USA 1993; 90:11162-6.
67. Robertson KM, O'Donnell L, Jones ME et al. Impairment of spermatogenesis in mice lacking a functional aromatase (cyp 19) gene. Proc Natl Acad Sci USA 1999; 96:7986-91.
68. Pak TR, Chung WC, Lund TD et al. The androgen metabolite, 5α-androstane-3β, 17β-diol, is a potent modulator of estrogen receptor-β1-mediated gene transcription in neuronal cells. Endocrinology 2005; 146:147-55.
69. Thompson EA, Siiteri PK. Utilization of oxygen and reduced nicotinamide adenine dinucleotide phosphate by human placental microsomes during aromatisation of androstenedione. J Biol Chem 1974; 249:5364-5372.
70. Aquilano DR, Dufau ML. Cellular localization of rat testicular aromatase activity during development. Endocrinology 1985; 116:38-46.
71. Rommerts FF, de Jong FH, Brinkmann AO et al. Development and cellular localization of rat testicular aromatase activity. J Reprod Fertil 1982; 65:281-8.
72. Papadopoulos V, Carreau S, Szerman-Joly E et al. Rat testis 17 β-estradiol: Identification by gas chromatography-mass spectrometry and age related cellular distribution. J Steroid Biochem 1986; 24:1211-1216.
73. Levallet J, Bilinska B, Mittre H et al. Expression and immunolocalization of functional cytochrome P450 aromatase in mature rat testicular cells. Biol Reprod 1998; 58:919-26.
74. Nitta H, Bunick D, Hess RA et al. Germ cells of the mouse testis express P450 aromatase. Endocrinology 1993; 132:1396-401.
75. Janulis L, Bahr JM, Hess RA et al. P450 aromatase messenger ribonucleic acid expression in male rat germ cells: Detection by reverse transcription-polymerase chain reaction amplification. J Androl 1996; 17:651-8.
76. Carreau S, Bilinska B, Levallet J. Male germ cells: A new source of estrogens in the mammalian testis. Ann Endocrinol (Paris) 1998; 59:79-92.
77. Levallet J, Mittre H, Delarue B et al. Alternative splicing events in the coding region of the cytochrome P450 aromatase gene in male rat germ cells. J Mol Endocrinol 1998; 20:305-12.
78. Carreau S, Levallet J. Cytochrome P450 aromatase in male germ cells. Folia Histochem Cytobiol 1997; 35:195-202.
79. Eckstein B, Ravid R. On the mechanism of the onset of puberty: Identification and pattern of 5 α-androstane-3 β, 17 beta-diol and its 3 α epimer in peripheral blood of immature female rats. Endocrinology 1974; 94:224-9.

80. Luu-The V. Analysis and characteristics of multiple types of human 17β-hydroxysteroid dehydrogenase. J Steroid Biochem Mol Biol 2001; 76:143-51.
81. Cochran RC, Schuetz AW, Ewing LL. Age-related changes in conversion of 5α-androstan-17β- ol-3-one to 5α-androstane-3β,17β-diol and 5α-androstane- 3α,17β-diol by rat testicular cells in vitro. J Reprod Fertil 1979; 57:143-147.
82. Luboshitzky R, Kaplan-Zverling M et al. Seminal plasma androgen/oestrogen balance in infertile men. Int J Androl 2002; 25:345-51.
83. Korach KS, Couse JF, Curtis SW et al. Estrogen receptor gene disruption: Molecular characterization and experimental and clinical phenotypes. Recent Prog Hormone Res 1996; 51:159-86.
84. Eddy EM, Washburn TF, Bunch DO et al. Targeted disruption of the estrogen receptor gene in male mice causes alteration of spermatogenesis and infertility. Endocrinology 1996; 137:4796-805.
85. Hess RA, Bunick D, Lee KH et al. A role for oestrogens in the male reproductive system. Nature 1997; 390:509-512.
86. Toda K, Okada T, Takeda K et al. Oestrogen at the neonatal stage is critical for the reproductive ability of male mice as revealed by supplementation with 17β-oestradiol to aromatase gene (Cyp19) knockout mice. J Endocrinol 2001; 168:455-463.
87. Honda S, Harada N, Ito S et al. Disruption of sexual behaviour in male aromatase-deficient mice lacking exons 1 and 2 of the cyp19 gene. Biochem Biophys Res Commun 1998; 252:445-449.
88. Kuiper GG, Enmark E, Pelto-Huikko M et al. Cloning of a novel receptor expressed in rat prostate and ovary. Proc Natl Acad Sci USA 1996; 93:5925-30.
89. Tremblay GB, Tremblay A, Copeland NG et al. Cloning, chromosomal localization, and functional analysis of the murine estrogen receptor β. Mol Endocrinol 1997; 11:353-365.
90. Mosselman S, Polman J, Dijkema R. ER β: Identification and characterization of a novel human estrogen receptor. FEBS Lett 1996; 392:49-53.
91. Enmark E, Pelto-Huikko M, Grandien K et al. Human estrogen receptor β-gene structure, chromosomal localization, and expression pattern. J Clin Endocrinol Metab 1997; 82:4258-65.
92. Saunders PT, Fisher JS, Sharpe RM et al. Expression of oestrogen receptor β (ER β) occurs in multiple cell types, including some germ cells, in the rat testis. J Endocrinol 1998; 156:R13-7.
93. Minucci S, Di Matteo L, Chieffi P et al. 17 β-estradiol effects on mast cell number and spermatogonial mitotic index in the testis of the frog, Rana esculenta. J Exp Zool 1997; 278:93-100.
94. Colborn T, vom Saal FS, Soto AM. Developmental effects of endocrine-disrupting chemicals in wildlife and humans. Environ Health Perspect 1993; 101:378-384.
95. Witorsch RJ. Low-dose in utero effects of xenoestrogens in mice and their relevance to humans: An analytical review of the literature. Food Chem Toxicol 2002; 40:905-912.
96. Akingbemi BT, Hardy MP. Oestrogenic and antiandrogenic chemicals in the environment: Effects on male reproductive health. Ann Med 2001; 33:391-403.
97. Steinberger E, Duckett GE. Effect of estrogen or testosterone on initiation and maintenance of spermatogenesis in the rat. Endocrinology 1965; 76:1184-1189.
98. Meistrich ML, Hughes TH, Bruce WR. Alteration of epididymal sperm transport and maturation in mice by oestrogen and testosterone. Nature 1975; 258:145-7.
99. Nielsen M, Bjornsdottir S, Hoyer PE et al. Ontogeny of oestrogen receptor α in gonads and sex ducts of fetal and newborn mice. J Reprod Fertil 2000; 118:195-204.
100. Sar M, Welsch F. Oestrogen receptor α and β in rat prostate and epididymis. Andrologia 2000; 32.
101. Fisher JS, Millar MR, Majdic G et al. Immunolocalisation of oestrogen receptor-α within the testis and excurrent ducts of the rat and marmoset monkey from perinatal life to adulthood. J Endocrinol 1997; 153:485-95.
102. Pelletier G, Labrie C, Labrie F. Localization of oestrogen receptor α, oestrogen receptor β and androgen receptors in the rat reproductive organs. J Endocrinol 2000; 165:359-70.
103. van Pelt AM, de Rooij DG, van der Burg B et al. Ontogeny of estrogen receptor-β expression in rat testis. Endocrinology 1999; 140:478-483.
104. Jefferson WN, Couse JF, Banks EP et al. Expression of estrogen receptor β is developmentally regulated in reproductive tissues of male and female mice. Biol Reprod 2000; 62:310-317.
105. Atanassova N, McKinnell C, Williams K et al. Age-, cell- and region-specific immunoexpression of estrogen receptor α (but not estrogen receptor β) during postnatal development of the epididymis and vas deferens of the rat and disruption of this pattern by neonatal treatment with diethylstilbestrol. Endocrinology 2001; 142:874-876.
106. Couse JF, Lindzey J, Grandien K et al. Tissue distribution and quantitative analysis of estrogen receptor-alpha (ERα) and estrogen receptor-β (ERβ) messenger ribonucleic acid in the wild-type and ERα-knockout mouse. Endocrinology 1997; 138:4613-21.

107. Rosenfeld CS, Ganjam VK, Taylor JA et al. Transcription and translation of estrogen receptor-β in the male reproductive tract of estrogen receptor-α knock-out and wild-type mice. Endocrinology 1998; 139:2982-2987.
108. Saunders PT, Sharpe RM, Williams K et al. Differential expression of oestrogen receptor alpha and beta proteins in the testes and male reproductive system of human and nonhuman primates. Mol Hum Reprod 2001; 7:227-36.
109. Taylor AH, Al-Azzawi F. Immunolocalisation of oestrogen receptor β in human tissues. J Mol Endocrinol 2000; 24:145-55.
110. Pelletier G, Luu-The V, Charbonneau A et al. Cellular localization of estrogen receptor β messenger ribonucleic acid in cynomolgus monkey reproductive organs. Biol Reprod 1999; 61:1249-55.
111. Pentikainen V, Erkkila K, Suomalainen L et al. Estradiol acts as a germ cell survival factor in the human testis in vitro. J Clin Endocrinol Metab 2000; 85:2057-2067.
112. Shughrue PJ, Lane MV, Scrimo PJ et al. Comparative distribution of estrogen receptor-α (ER-α) and β (ER-β) mRNA in the rat pituitary, gonad, and reproductive tract. Steroids 1998; 63:498-504.
113. Taylor HC, Pillay I, Setrakian S. Diffuse stromal Leydig cell hyperplasia: A unique cause of postmenopausal hyperandrogenism and virilization. Mayo Clin Proc 2000; 75:288-92.
114. Weihua Z, Makela S, Andersson LC et al. A role for estrogen receptor β in the regulation of growth of the ventral prostate. Proc Natl Acad Sci USA 2001; 98:6330-5.
115. Weihua Z, Warner M, Gustafsson JA. Estrogen receptor beta in the prostate. Mol Cell Endocrinol 2002; 193:1-5.
116. fertility WHOTFomftrom. Contraceptive efficacy of testosterone-induced azoospermia in normal men. Lancet 1990; 336:955-9.
117. Remy JJ, Bozon V, Couture L et al. Suppression of fertility in male mice by immunization against LH receptor. J Reprod Immunol 1993; 25:63-79.
118. Madhwa Raj HG, Dym M. The effects of selective withdrawal of FSH or LH on spermatogenesis in the immature rat. Biol Reprod 1976; 14:489-94.
119. Matthiesson KL, McLachlan RI. Male hormonal contraception: Concept proven, product in sight? Hum Reprod Update 2006; 12:463-82.
120. Finkelstein JS, O'Dea LS, Whitcomb RW et al. Sex steroid control of gonadotropin secretion in the human male. II. Effects of estradiol administration in normal and gonadotropin-releasing hormone-deficient men. J Clin Endocrinol Metab 1991; 73:621-8.
121. Bagatell CJ, Dahl KD, Bremner WJ. The direct pituitary effect of testosterone to inhibit gonadotropin secretion in men is partially mediated by aromatization to estradiol. J Androl 1994; 15:15-21.
122. Hayes FJ, Seminara SB, De Cruz S et al. Aromatase inhibition in the human male reveals a hypothalamic site of estrogen feedback. New Orleans, LA: 80th Annual Meeting of the Endocrine Society, 1988.
123. Akingbemi BT, Ge R, Rosenfeld CS et al. Estrogen receptor-α gene deficiency enhances androgen biosynthesis in the mouse Leydig cell. Endocrinology 2003; 144:84-93.
124. Lee KH, Hess RA, Bahr JM et al. Estrogen receptor alpha has a functional role in the mouse rete testis and efferent ductules. Biol Reprod 2000; 63:1873-80.
125. Burkhardt E, Adham IM, Brosig B et al. Structural organization of the porcine and human genes coding for a Leydig cell-specific insulin-like peptide (LEY I-L) and chromosomal localization of the human gene (INSL3). Genomics 1994; 20:13-19.
126. Overbeek PA, Gorlov IP, Sutherland RW et al. A transgenic insertion causing cryptorchidism in mice. Genesis 2001; 30:26-35.
127. Nef S, Parada LF. Cryptorchidism in mice mutant for Insl3. Nat Genet 1999; 22:295-9.
128. Zimmermann S, Steding G, Emmen JM et al. Targeted disruption of the Insl3 gene causes bilateral cryptorchidism. Mol Endocrinol 1999; 13:681-91.
129. Adham IM, Steding G, Thamm T et al. The overexpression of the insl3 in female mice causes descent of the ovaries. Mol Endocrinol 2002; 16:244-52.
130. Kumagai J, Hsu SY, Matsumi H et al. INSL3/Leydig insulin-like peptide activates the LGR8 receptor important in testis descent. J Biol Chem 2002; 277:31283-6.
131. Ferlin A, Simonato M, Bartoloni L et al. The INSL3-LGR8/GREAT ligand-receptor pair in human cryptorchidism. J Clin Endocrinol Metab 2003; 88:4273-9.
132. Bay K, Hartung S, Ivell R et al. Insulin-like factor 3 serum levels in 135 normal men and 85 men with testicular disorders: Relationship to the luteinizing hormone-testosterone axis. J Clin Endocrinol Metab 2005; 90:3410-8.
133. Assinder SJ, Rezvani A, Nicholson HD. Oxytocin promotes spermiation and sperm transfer in the mouse. Int J Androl 2002; 25:19-27.
134. Nicholson HD, Hardy MP. Luteinizing hormone differentially regulates the secretion of testicular oxytocin and testosterone by purified adult rat Leydig cells in vitro. Endocrinology 1992; 130:671-7.

135. Frayne J, Nicholson HD. Effect of oxytocin on testosterone production by isolated rat Leydig cells is mediated via a specific oxytocin receptor. Biol Reprod 1995; 52:1268-73.
136. Maekawa M, Kamimura K, Nagano T. Peritubular myoid cells in the testis: Their structure and function. Arch Histol Cytol 1996; 59:1-13.
137. Bathgate RA, Sernia C. Characterization and localization of oxytocin receptors in the rat testis. J Endocrinol 1994; 141:343-52.
138. Frayne J, Nicholson HD. Localization of oxytocin receptors in the human and macaque monkey male reproductive tracts: Evidence for a physiological role of oxytocin in the male. Mol Hum Reprod 1998; 4:527-32.
139. Howl J, Rudge SA, Lavis RA et al. Rat testicular myoid cells express vasopressin receptors: Receptor structure, signal transduction, and developmental regulation. Endocrinology 1995; 136:2206-13.

Index

F

G

H

I

J

L

M

N

O

P

R

S

T

U

V

X

Z

FSC
www.fsc.org
MIX
Papier | Fördert gute Waldnutzung
FSC® C083411

Kolibri 360 GmbH
Ferdinand-Jühlke-Straße 7
99095 Erfurt, Deutschland
produktsicherheit@kolibri360.de